Taking Flight

Inspirational Stories
of
Lung Transplantation
~More Journeys~

Compiled by: Joanne Schum

Order this book online at www.trafford.com
or email orders@trafford.com

Most Trafford titles are also available at major online book retailers.

Printed in the United States of America.

ISBN: 978-1-4269-6731-3 (sc)
ISBN: 978-1-4269-6874-7 (e)

Trafford rev. 05/04/2011

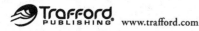 www.trafford.com

North America & international
toll-free: 1 888 232 4444 (USA & Canada)
phone: 250 383 6864 ♦ fax: 812 355 4082

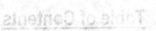

Table of Contents

Table of Contents

Author   Page Title

Author		Page	Title

Author		Page	Title

Author		Page	Title

Acknowledgements & Thank You…from Joanne

To my loving and giving family…George Schum (Daddy) & Katherine Schum (Mommy); Dolores & Stony Lohr, Bill & Melissa Lohr – their children, **Olivia** and **Madison; Keith & Gen Lohr** – their children, **Andrew, Ellie, Henry, Amelia** and **Randall; Stony & Janelle Lohr** – their children, **Raine, Mica** and **Corvus; Roseann Schum, Brent Malloy; Noella Schum, Safia Gravel** – her daughter, **Afraah Gravel; Mary Lou & Ed Allocco, Megan, Eric, Laura,** and **Lisa; Karl & Debbie Schum, Kari** and **Jessie; Trudy & Jim Pellman** and **Mitch Radcliff** for the care and love you provided over the years. To all my aunts, uncles, cousins, the many friends of my parents, siblings and a very special mention of my **"Aunty Sister"** – **Sister Mary Rose Schum** and **Sister Howard** – "Your prayers are so appreciated and they work miracles."

To my many friends…I am not going to attempt to name all of you, I have over 3,500 friends on Facebook, in addition to many friends from over the years. You're all amazing, kind and supportive, and I am very happy to have you all in my life. May we all be blessed with many additional years of happiness and good health.

To the many medical professionals…My entire life you have been great offering consultations, advice, listening and caring. With you, I live on with the "Gift of Life", when long ago, I never dreamed I would be alive this length of time. **Dr. Robert Schwartz, Ann McMullen, Judy McSweeney, Ken Davis, Dr. Linda Paradowski, Dr. Robert Aris, Bill Kanasky, Dr. Isabel Neuringer, Dr. Margaret Bergin, Dr. Rob Horowitz,** the entire **Lung Transplant Team at University of North Carolina Hospitals, Chapel Hill,** the many doctors and nurses, and **medical professionals at Strong Memorial Hospital, Rochester, New York** who were part of my care both pre and post lung transplant at the **Cystic Fibrosis Clinic at Strong Memorial Hospital** and **Culver Road Medical.** Special gratitude to my lung transplant surgeon, **Dr. Thomas Egan** and his team for performing one of their many miracles on me, which allows me to live a life of breathing, health and happiness.

To those professionals… In other parts of my life…**Cheryl DiFrancesco** – you continue to make this girl smile and glow, and you create the hair of my dreams. How convenient of you to move your salon "Full Circle Beauty Bar" to my street!!! **Wegmans** pharmacists, and pharmacy professionals… you keep me healthy and your guidance is appreciated.

To those who submitted stories for the 2nd Edition of Taking Flight...If it weren't for you, this book would not exist. By contributing your story, you have helped many others realize that lung transplantation does work. We are able to live, breathe, attain dreams, achieve our goals and our family and friends continue to be thankful that lung transplantation is an accomplishment for those gifted with the talent of their career in lung transplantation, and are able to give us that "Flight" of a new life.

To those who helped create this edition of Taking Flight...Shannon VanValkenburg, only 16-years-old, and the daughter of my "one and only friend" Eileen VanValkenburg, designed the front cover that was described by many as, "eye catching" and a book that would capture a person's curiosity. "Shannon you perfected the whole theme behind the idea of, "Butterfly wings are the shape of new, healthy lungs, and when that moment of connection in surgery is performed, the lungs expand like the new wings of a butterfly, preparing for their first flight." Jessie Schum, another young woman of 19 years, and also my niece, took an idea I had, and she presented me with the back cover that I could not even imagine...I gasped when I saw it. "Jessie, you simply created a cover of my dreams...how did you know?" Both of these young women hope to have a creative future with the careers they choose. All those that will be reading this book, will truly agree these two women are truly talented. To my editor, BreAnn McFarland, "Your thoughts, ideas, and skills with the English language are invaluable. You taught me a great deal with your editing, and your style was easy to follow. Thank you for making the stories "Shine" and your expert advice." Also a note, no one who submitted their story, or those who worked on the creation of this book are perfect...we are human so...if you find an error in spelling, punctuation, grammar, know this, "The error may be intentional, or may of not been seen, but imperfection is part of being human – for only God is perfect, and I never proclaim to be anywhere near to God's perfection."

To my donor and my donor family...you have given me the ability to "Take Flight" in many ways I never imagined. Thank you for your kindness at such a difficult time. You are in my prayers daily.

To God...you have created amazing, kind, and gifted people on this earth, allowing all of us to achieve dreams, and goals. My dreams are never ending, and my achievement is a lifelong joy.

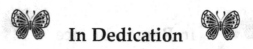

In Dedication

My dedication of, "Taking Flight: Inspirational Stories of Lung Transplantation – More Journeys" is for two of the most important women in my life! My sister **Mary Lou Schum Allocco**, and my mother, **Katherine Semler Schum.**

My Sister: Mary Lou Schum Allocco

Mary Lou passed away on April 19, 2005, due to ovarian cancer. For those of us left behind on this Earth, this was a time of great sadness. She was my big sister, though "twins" would be a more truthful description. We shared our Cystic Fibrosis trials, tribulations and joys with one another. Who else would know better what it felt like to, "Have an elephant sitting on your chest." Who else would know better than us the thrill of, "Shoveling snow, raking leaves, running, traveling, laughing, talking and breathing clearly for the first time in many, many years, and what receiving new lungs provided us." We were two peas in a pod.

Thank You - Barbara **Ann Earby-Davis** for the gift of lungs, March 3, 2001 to Mary Lou. Thank You - Barbara's daughter, **Temeka Earby-Turner** for making this decision. Temeka and I are now friends and having a friend who decided to donate life to a complete stranger – is truly the "Gift of Life".

Mary Lou's husband **Ed**, and their children **Megan, Eric, Laura** and **Lisa** and the entire **Schum** and **Allocco** families, and friends, miss our Mary Lou dearly. But she is in Heaven, healthy, happy and home.

My Mommy: Katherine Semler Schum

My Mother was my rock, my foundation from the day I was born on July 18, 1963, to the day she went home to be with Mary Lou in Heaven on July 18, 2007. To have such a gift of nurturing, love, kindness, optimism, gentleness and fairness for exactly 44 years of my life, no better gift can be given.

I now can say, "On my 44th birthday I received the best gift – Mommy went to Heaven – happy, healthy, quietly in her sleep – a gift I prayed for my entire adult life." God gave me that gift. Bless you Mommy. You are still here with me, every day.

In Remembrance

I would like to remember some very special people that have moved onto Heaven since the 1st Taking Flight book. They still continue to inspire me, with their spirit, creativeness and happiness. Thank you my dear friends. No particular order, not an entire list, these individuals played a role in my life these 13 years with my new lungs.

Susy Dirr – Designed the cover of the 1st book, From Georgia
Erin Masling – From Rochester
Shelley Whitney – From Rochester
Melissa Thompson Fleming – From California
Dave Messmer – From Rochester
Sandy McNitt – From Rochester
Piali Mukherjee – From India
Tamara Crafts – From Rochester
Tracy Fenyn Bussani – From Rochester

Note: This edition of Taking Flight took just a year in the making. During that time several of the story contributors passed away, but their story is included. My heart goes out to their families and friends, for the loss of their loved one.

INTRODUCTION

By Dr. Thomas M. Egan

It is an honor to be asked to write an Introduction to the second edition of Joanne Schum's anthology of inspirational stories about patients who have received lung transplants. I am delighted to know that Joanne continues to do well and has put her improved health to such good use, encouraging others who must embark on this journey. I have been privileged to serve the community of patients with end-stage lung disease by performing lung transplants. The surgeon gets a lot of credit for transforming the health of patients who get a lung transplant and do well, but a large team of dedicated health care professionals - nurses, respiratory and physical therapists, pulmonologists, intensivists and anesthesiologists, psychologists, social workers and transplant coordinators - play vital roles. Even before the transplant occurs, a team of emergency medicine technicians, physicians and nurses try in vain to save the life of a person who has an unexpected tragedy, and dedicated organ donor professionals and health care providers coordinate the task of approaching a grieving family and maintaining a donor until the teams can be put in place to orchestrate the removal of these precious gifts of life.

Lung transplant patients are an inspiration to all of us who participate in this Herculean effort to restore health. Many of you have inspired me as I struggled with my own health problems that ended my surgical career much earlier than I had planned. My own surgeries and recovery weren't easy, but I know my health problems pale in comparison to yours. You have been much braver; you had to be. And your recovery required much more hard work and determination. I learned a great deal from many of you and I thank you.

A lot has happened since Joanne put together the first edition of *Taking Flight*. Lung transplant outcomes have improved to some extent, but not as much as we all would like. There are still not nearly enough organs to meet the need for over 100,000 patients on the national organ transplant waiting list. For potential lung transplant recipients, the problem is further exaggerated because only one-fourth to one-third of lungs from organ donors work well enough in the donor to be used for transplant. How does one choose who gets access to such a scarce resource?

Earlier in this decade, I was pleased to chair the United Network of Organ Sharing (UNOS) Lung Allocation subcommittee to help make some major changes to the lung allocation system in the United States (U.S.). We still have a long way to go, but the Lung Allocation Score (LAS) that came into effect in May 2005 resulted in sweeping changes to the way lungs are offered to people on transplant waiting lists in the U.S.(1) Waiting time (the old way of allocating lungs) no longer matters. The new system offers lungs to waitlisted patients based on urgency (the likelihood of dying on the waiting list), and transplant benefit, calculated from expected waitlist survival and probability of dying after transplant. The lung allocation system is currently the only organ allocation system that takes post-transplant survival into account to try to reduce "wasting" organs by offering them to patients who are so sick that they are unlikely to survive.

The new U.S. lung allocation system immediately cut the number of wait list deaths by 50%. More importantly, the new system made allocation easier and more efficient for organ procurement organizations (OPOs). By offering lungs to patients who really needed them, lung transplant programs became more willing to use lungs that were considered "marginal" in the "old days". Fortunately, this change in practice did not result in higher death rates due to graft failure. So with the new system, we suddenly increased the number of lung transplants in the U.S. by 40 percent! Unfortunately, this is still not nearly enough to provide lungs for all potential victims of end stage lung diseases, currently the fourth leading cause of death. Because of its success, the U.S. lung allocation system, or variations of it, is now being considered for implementation in some European countries.

There are exciting developments on the horizon to help patients with end-stage lung disease who could benefit from transplant. At the University of North Carolina, we have been working on an idea for many years that has potential to dramatically increase the number of lungs for transplant. Currently, virtually all lungs, and most other organs for transplant, are obtained from individuals who sustain a massive brain injury and are intubated and ventilated before brain death occurs. After brain death is established, if consent for organ donation is obtained, organ procurement organizations (OPOs) orchestrate the removal of organs from brain-dead, but circulation intact conventional organ donors.

"All I need is the air that I breathe" are lyrics from a song popularized by Olivia Newton John when I was younger. Because our lung tissue gets oxygen from the air that we breathe, lung cells live for a long time after circulation stops when people die suddenly. Many years ago, we showed that lungs might be suitable for transplant, even if retrieved up to four hours *after* circulatory arrest and death(2-4). For years we have been working on this idea in our lab at University of North Carolina, Chapel Hill, North Carolina (UNC). If we can retrieve some lungs from the 750,000 Americans who die suddenly in the U.S. every year, we could solve the lung donor shortage. Initially our idea was met with a lot of skepticism; it remains a challenge to obtain grant funds from the National Institutes of Health (NIH) and other funding agencies to pursue these "non-heart-beating donors" as a solution to the lung donor shortage.

We have also been studying the injury that occurs when lung tissue has circulation interrupted (causing ischemia) and then started again (reperfusion). Ischemia followed by reperfusion occurs with all organ transplants, and causes injury to the organs when transplanted. Ischemia-reperfusion injury

(IRI) is the main reason why organs sometimes fail after transplant. We have been studying IRI because IRI occurs in organs transplanted from conventional brain dead organ donors, as well as organs retrieved from non-heart-beating donors. We and others have learned that IRI occurs because of activity of the innate immune system. This family of integrated cell receptors and molecular switches, or signaling molecules that suddenly change gene transcription, evolved over hundreds of millions of years to protect all animals from infection with bacteria, fungi, yeast and viruses. Activation of the innate immune system is a "call to arms" for our adaptive immune system, recruiting white blood cells to the newly reperfused organ, causing inflammation, tissue damage, and cell death. We discovered that TLR4, the innate immune receptor that recognizes gram negative bacteria, or endotoxin, also is responsible for development of edema, or fluid accumulation, in the lung due to IRI(5). This is puzzling, because there is no infection due to IRI, but the cells are responding as if there were an infection. We also showed an inhibitor of TLR4 significantly reduces lung edema due to IRI.(5) I incorporated a biotech startup company (X-In8 Biologicals Corporation) to try to commercialize some of my ideas about inhibiting the innate immune system to prevent and treat IRI.

The lung isn't the only tissue that lives after "death." The cornea, the clear tissue covering the front portion of the eye, also gets its oxygen from the outside air and can be retrieved for transplant hours after circulatory arrest and death - even from cadavers in a morgue. Over 50,000 corneal transplants are performed each year in the United States, with corneas retrieved and distributed by a national network of Eye Banks. I believe that there is potential to retrieve that many lungs for transplant -- far more than the 1500-1600 lung transplant procedures that are performed annually now. My wife, Lynn, and I founded Lung Banks of America, a 501(c)3 not-for-profit corporation (www.LBofA.org), whose mission is to educate individuals and health care professionals about the concept of lung retrieval from non-heart-beating donors, and become involved in assessing suitability for transplant of lungs retrieved after death. Eventually, we might have a national network of lung banks similar to the eye banks that retrieve and distribute corneas for transplant.

Now we come to what's on the horizon that is new and exciting. Because of the different circumstances and the variation in warm ischemic time that will occur when a potential lung donor dies suddenly, we need a reliable method to evaluate lung function to determine if lungs removed after death from a non-heart-beating donor are safe to transplant. Dr. Stig Steen, a lung transplant surgeon from Sweden, was the first to develop a system of perfusion and ventilation of lungs outside the body (ex-vivo), and used his ex-vivo lung perfusion system to document good function of a lung from a human non-heart-beating donor that was subsequently transplanted(6). Later, Steen used his perfusion circuit to evaluate lungs from conventional organ donors thought to be unsuitable for transplant(7, 8). He showed that some of these lungs seem to improve after removal from the brain-dead organ donor and a period of ex-vivo lung perfusion.

With Steen's help, and a research grant from the Cystic Fibrosis Foundation, we designed a modified cardiopulmonary bypass circuit to perform ex-vivo lung perfusion on human lungs. We used lungs from conventional brain-dead organ donors that were not suitable for transplant, and measured gas exchange capability and other measures of lung function, including performing CT scans of lungs ex-vivo(9). We then received a grant from the Division of Transplantation of the Health Resources and Services Administration to use our perfusion system to explore the possibility of assessing and transplanting lungs from non-heart-beating donors, victims of sudden death. We encountered several obstacles obtaining access to non-heart-beating donations (NHBDs) and arranging retrieval of lungs in a timely manner. Emergency Medical Services personnel, medical examiners, and law enforcement agencies aren't accustomed to the notion that deceased individuals might be organ donors. Obtaining consent to proceed with rapid cooling and retrieval for assessment, and getting appropriate medical history from a shocked family are other necessary and critically important steps in the logistical logjam. Clearly, Lung Banks of America has a lot of work to do.

Meanwhile, investigators at the University of Toronto, my alma mater, made refinements to ex-vivo lung perfusion. They learned how to safely perform lung perfusion for prolonged periods - up to 12 hours(10)! This is long enough to consider treatment strategies during perfusion. The Toronto group showed that gene therapy could be performed during ex-vivo lung perfusion(11), and hope to capitalize on this to reduce IRI when lungs are eventually transplanted after perfusion. The Toronto group also showed that many lungs thought to be unsuitable for transplant from conventional donors appeared to improve after a few hours of ex-vivo perfusion. At the April 2010 meeting of the International Society for Heart and Lung Transplantation, they reported 23 lung transplants after ex-vivo perfusion (12). This has piqued interest in ex-vivo perfusion on a global scale.

We have taken a slightly different approach to the utility of ex-vivo perfusion. The airway can be used not only to ventilate lungs in a non-heart-beating donor and during perfusion, but also to *treat* lungs. Recently, we showed that ventilation of lungs with nitric oxide (NO), begun an hour *after* death, and continued in the perfusion circuit and after transplant, resulted in dramatically improved lung function after transplant on our rat model of ex-vivo perfusion and lung transplant(13). Small amounts of carbon monoxide (CO) are also beneficial in this model(14). We are beginning to explore ways to inhibit activation of the innate immune system during ex-vivo perfusion, so that IRI might be prevented when lungs are transplanted.

Ex-vivo perfusion offers an opportunity to utilize some of the lungs that are currently being turned down because of poor function in the donor. We were recently awarded a NIH grant to

- optimize ex-vivo lung perfusion system with Vitrolife (the manufacturers of Perfadex™, the widely used pulmonary preservation solution), and Steen solution™, developed for ex-vivo perfusion)
- demonstrate safety of transplanting lungs after ex-vivo perfusion
- study EMS attitudes about organ donation, and lung donation after death, and
- plan a multicenter study of ex-vivo perfusion using lungs from non-heart-beating donors as a means to increase the lung donor pool.

If lungs can be retrieved from non-heart-beating donors and assessed with ex-vivo perfusion to establish safety of transplant, the shortage of lungs for transplant could potentially be eliminated. But there are even more enticing possibilities. As we understand more about IRI and the interplay between the innate and adaptive immune systems, a new paradigm about organ rejection after transplant is beginning to emerge. For decades, we were taught that the purpose of the immune system was to recognize "self" from "non-self". The discovery of the innate immune system led Polly Matzinger, a scientist at NIH, to propose another concept... that perhaps the purpose of the immune system is not so much to worry about self, but to detect and respond to danger(15). This Danger Hypothesis is consistent with another observation made by Dr. Land, who noted that if IRI could be reduced after kidney transplant using a free radical scavenger, that acute rejection episodes were reduced(16). This led to his "Injury Hypothesis" which proposes that it is the injury that occurs at the time of transplant due to IRI that primes the recipient's immune system to recognize foreign HLA antigens on the donor organ as Danger Signals(17).

But what if we could prevent IRI? Why is IRI the same as the response to infection? The innate immune system evolved to protect us from infection, but IRI is really something that man created - especially in the context of organ transplantation. Is it possible that the response to ischemia and reperfusion is a misread? .... a type of mistake?[1] This concept is the basis for the formation of X-In8 Biologicals Corp. While the innate immune system is vitally important to protect us from infection, temporarily inactivating it may be very helpful to reduce or eliminate IRI. And preventing IRI might have profound implications for recognition of the graft as "foreign" and episodes of acute rejection(18). There is already an established relationship between the degree of early primary graft dysfunction (PGD) - probably due to IRI - and the risk of developing chronic rejection, or bronchiolitis obliterans syndrome (BOS) after lung transplant(19). Brain death causes up-regulation of the innate immune system and a "pro-inflammatory state" in conventional organ donors(20). This raises the intriguing and exciting possibility that preventing IRI by temporarily turning off innate immunity, probably during EVLP, might provide lungs that work better immediately after transplant, and that might last longer than lungs we are currently using from conventional organ donors! Perhaps immunologic tolerance, eliminating the need for immunosuppression, is on the horizon for future lung transplant recipients with this strategy.

So for future lung transplant recipients, truly, the sky's the limit! Which means *Taking Flight* is such an appropriate title for these touching stories about the success of lung transplants over the adversity of end-stage lung disease. Thank you, Joanne Schum, for all your hard work!

Dr. Thomas M. Egan
Professor of Surgery
University of North Carolina at Chapel Hill, Chapel Hill, North Carolina

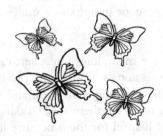 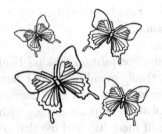

[1] IRI is a biologic mistake™ is a registered trademark of X-In8 Biologicals Corporation.

FOREWORD

By Dr. Marshall Hertz

"A human being is a part of the whole, called by us "Universe", a part limited in time and space. He experiences himself, his thoughts and feelings as something separated from the rest – a kind of optical illusion of his consciousness. This delusion is a kind of prison for us, restricting us to our personal desires and to affection for a few persons nearest us. Our task must be to free ourselves from this prison by widening our circle of compassion to embrace all living creatures and the whole of nature in its beauty." – Albert Einstein

I think that Einstein would have enjoyed Joanne Schum's books. Her stories are about a small part of the universe – the universe of lung transplantation – and the connectedness of everything within it. They provide vivid examples of the intimate relationships in organ transplantation between scientific progress and technology on the one hand; and human experience on the other. And they describe the entire range of human emotions – grief, joy, suffering, relief from suffering, guilt, compassion – in a way that only real stories about real people can accomplish.

I have been privileged to be part of the lung transplant universe for the past 25 years. I often reflect on how fortunate I am to be practicing medicine in one of the most profound and revolutionary fields in the history of science and medicine. Organ transplantation, which was only a dream 50 years ago, has now become a common therapy for thousands of individuals with organ failure. In my role as a non-surgical transplant physician, it has been extremely gratifying to contribute to the dramatic improvements in lung function, quality of life, and long-term survival of patients who literally would have and only months to live without transplantation. In fact, in my office I keep photos of hundreds of children who were born after their parent or grandparent underwent lung transplantation.

Joanne's first compilation, Taking Flight, has been a treasure for many lung transplant candidates, recipients, family members, donor families, and transplant professionals. When my pre-transplant patients are having a hard time deciding when or whether to have a lung transplant, and when my post transplant patients are dealing with "bumps in the road", I often tell them read "Taking Flight". Every one of them has told me that the book was enormously helpful for them because it tells the human side of the transplant experience – all the positives and negatives – in a way that doctors and nurses cannot.

I was pleased that five of my patients' stories were included in "Taking Flight", and have greatly enjoyed reliving their stories in anticipation of "More Journeys". One of my patients, Lee Starr (whom I often credited with being the worlds' second funniest man) wrote in order to pass the story of his life-changing experience along to others, which Joanne's books will enable him to do for many years to come. I think Lee summed it up best for everyone in the lung transplant universe when he wrote, "…being normal is something I will never take for granted again".

Thank you, Joanne. I can't wait to read more inspiring stories in "More Journeys"!

Dr. Marshall Hertz
Professor of Medicine
Director, Center for Lung and Health
Medical Director, Lung Transplantation Program
University of Minnesota Medical Center, Minneapolis, Minnesota

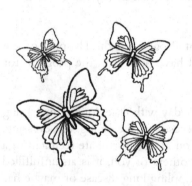

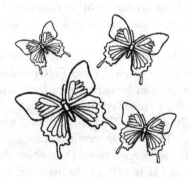

Lung Transplant Coordinator Contribution

A Walk in My Shoes
By J. Eric Hobson, MSN, CRNP

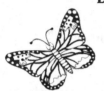

When the opportunity to write this story was presented, it was suggested that, "A Day in the Life of a Lung Transplant Coordinator" might be a good idea. My interest was piqued by the idea, but not captured by it. For me, discerning when the days begin and end has always been a challenge in the Transplant Coordinator role. I also feel that there is more to this experience than just one day and liken it to more of a journey. Therefore, I decided the theme of; "A Walk in My Shoes" is more appropriate.

I currently work as a Nurse Practitioner with the Lung Transplant Program at the Hospital of the University of Pennsylvania (HUP) in Philadelphia, Pennsylvania. I have been with the program for the last two years.

For some of you, walking is a dream you have of doing again someday with ease, long gone. Lung disease has limited your tolerance for the simplest of every day necessities like eating and dressing. For others of you, it is a fulfillment of a great dream come true. You are the fortunate recipient of a much-needed transplant, offering you a second chance. For still others of you, it is an unfulfilled prayer, as a family member or friend of someone who lives with crippling lung disease or maybe has already succumbed to its ravages. Or maybe, that second chance never materialized because of the degree of your lung disease or other concurrent diseases, which made transplant an impossibility due to medical risk, personal fear, or beliefs. So walk with me, if you will, for a spell.

I am awakened by clattering on my bedside table. The clock reads 2:15 a.m. Caller I.D. tells me it is the Transplant Information Center (TIC) at the Gift of Life. Calls that come at this hour are usually an organ offer and can be either from local centers or from centers out of our region as far away as 1,500 miles, which are called 'import offers'. The desk coordinator Matt states they have a patient presentation, "We have a 27-year-old, blood type B donor from Boston who was involved in a motor vehicle crash. The vehicle crashed into a tree". Matt proceeds to provide background donor information he has gleaned from DonorNet, the national donor database system for deceased donor organ allocation. It is part of the national transplant database system United Network of Organ Sharing (UNOS) developed to aid in the allocation of organs in the United States. The Computerized Tomography (CT) scan of the donor's chest has no concerning findings, while the bronchoscopy, a procedure to visualize the airways using a camera, done on the donor several hours ago, has identified some potential concerns. Despite these concerns the oxygenation status is reasonable. I inform Matt that I want to review all the data myself and will call back shortly.

Lung organ offers are sent to the recipient centers for review. The offer consists of two parts. The first part of the offer is comprised of donor specific clinical information including age, height, weight, cause of brain death, social and medical history, testing and procedure results, and the supportive requirements necessary to maintain their organ function since their brain is no longer working effectively to meet those needs. The second part of the donor offer is the list of patients for whom this offer is being made. That list includes all those patients eligible to accept those organs being offered based on body size, blood type, and disease process as they were entered by the Transplant Center staff who listed them as a candidate. Compatible patients are listed according to priority based on lung allocation score (LAS) and proximity to the donor location. Those patients listed in the local transplant centers appear first and are arranged based on LAS scores from highest to lowest. While patients listed at centers outside the local region appear lower on the list based on distance ranges from the donor hospital with the patients again arranged based on LAS scores from highest to lowest.

I log into DonorNet on my home computer. I further research the possible donor and all medical treatments he is receiving. This includes ventilator setting, an updated blood gas and a chest x-ray. I will have to make a decision. Either I need to get the pulmonologist on call involved and potentially the lung transplant surgeon or alternatively, or decide that I have enough information to make this call on my own. While in the DonorNet system, I noted that the first two HUP patients are acceptable, while the third patient has blood antigens that should be avoided if possible which takes that recipient out of the running. 4:30 a.m., Matt is calling back. He reports that they agreed to the changes with the ventilator and the repeat blood gas results show oxygen status that has fallen. I agree to contact the pulmonologist and upon review we decide to pursue this offer and notify the surgeon. In review with the surgeon, I presented the donor offer and the potential recipients for whom the offer is made. The surgeon voices concern that this is a borderline donor given the donor history and current testing results, though close enough that and we should go take a look. The surgeon agrees we should send our team to evaluate on site. I then call the patient we have selected to receive this set of lungs and make sure they have not experienced any changes in their health status and are healthy enough to accept a donor offer. The identified recipient and his wife are startled, but scurry to make the 100-mile trip that typically takes them one hour and 45 minutes to complete. I then call our in-house coordinator to notify them of this transplant. They will call the many other departments who will be involved in this potential transplant. In all, approximately 10 calls are made from the operating room (OR) staff to the security office. I then send an email to the lung transplant team notifying them of this potential transplant and specific orders for this recipients care during the operative event.

I awaken again at 5:30 a.m. in response to my alarm clock, to begin my morning routine. I make two children's lunches, shower and dress myself, wake and dress two of my children. At 6:00 am. Our procurement team is mobilized and departs on their trip to the donor site as the recipient arrives at HUP admissions. By 7:05 a.m., I am racing to the train station to catch my 7:26 a.m. train. I was scheduled to work in the office during the morning and see patients in the afternoon. I will arrive to work just after 8:00a.m., see the patients until my colleague arrives. When I arrive in the clinic, I am called by a pulmonary rehab program staff member who is concerned about the heart rate and oxygen saturation on a recent recipient who is in their area. The rehab team applied oxygen, so I instruct that the patient should be sent to get a chest x-ray and then come to the office for assessment. It is now 9:15 a.m. and I have seen the first two patients on my colleague's schedule and then have the patient from rehab placed in a room for their visit. I review the chest x-ray and note a new small to moderate-sized pneumothorax. At rest the oxygenation saturation is 94% with two liters of nasal cannula oxygen support. I inform the patient of the findings of the chest x-ray and my exam and tell the patient and his wife that an admission is necessary.

At the donor hospital, the procurement team reviews the actual imaging studies and the donor surgeon determines that there is suggestion of significant bruising to the chest wall and the oxygen status has fallen even further. The procurement team performs a bronchoscopy to determine if they can locate and remove any secretions to allow for improved oxygenation. The team finds no significant secretions and upon review with the recipient surgeon they determine that the radiology studies and assessments reveal too many problems to accept the lungs as it approaches 9:15 a.m. The surgeon calls to update me on the findings at the donor hospital and then goes to inform the recipient in the OR who is on the table waiting for the okay to be put under anesthesia. Then the surgeon goes to the family in the waiting room to inform them that the donor was deemed unacceptable upon visual inspection and that the offer was declined.

I send a quick email notifying the team that the transplant has been canceled and then call the admissions office to arrange for my sick patient to be admitted. It is now 10:30 a.m., and the recipient and his family are reunited. While accepting of the team's decision, the transplant candidate and family begin their return trip home disappointed, having been up since 4:30 a.m.

I return to the office to begin review of the voice messages while my other three colleagues see patients in office hours. There are several calls to address. The first is from a patient's wife who is concerned about the increasing oxygen requirements for her husband. The patient is now six months out from his bilateral lung transplant. He has struggled with complications at the connection site where the donor airway tissue and recipient tissue are sewn together. This is known as anastomotic site. I ask the patient to make arrangements to come to clinic the next day, to obtain pulmonary function testing, labs, a sputum specimen, and chest x-ray (CXR) prior to the office visit and prepare them that admission may be necessary. I review the lab results that have come in via fax and distribute those that are not my patients, and not with significant abnormalities, to the other coordinators. Among my patient results, I find a confirmatory blood type that I have been waiting for to place a patient on the list. I notify the patient that I have received the required results to clear the patient to be listed for transplant. She tells me that, she is not ready to be listed yet due to anxiety. She is having second thoughts and wants to talk with another female recipient who has been in similar circumstances. She asks me, "Do you think you can find a patient who would be willing to talk with me?" At lunchtime, I talk with my colleagues and we identify a patient that fits this criteria and I give her a call. This patient has been through a very challenging post-operative course but now, five years later, this patient is living her life again. Since her transplant she has attended the birth of her first grandchild, walked two of her three daughters down the aisle at their weddings. She is now the proud grandmother to four grandchildren (and counting), and has just returned from a family vacation at an island resort. The patient and her husband arranged this trip in celebration of her five-year anniversary since transplant and treated all of the family to a week in Bermuda! I am wondering why her Nurse Practitioner was not invited along to monitor her immunosuppression while traveling?? This recipient readily agreed to talk to the hesitant patient and I provide her with contact information for the patient having second thoughts.

At 3:00 p.m. my E-mail inbox alert signals that my colleague assigned to the inpatient service has a question about a patient currently admitted to the hospital. This patient was transplanted about six months ago and has been struggling with significant medical and social issues. His support system deteriorated while waiting for transplant. This has left the patient homeless since transplant and without family or social support. His family has been essentially absent in his care since the early post-transplant days dealing with their own issues. It is difficult to watch this patient's emotional status falter as he accepts his current life situation.

By 4:30 p.m. a few more voice messages are received and addressed. The coordinator on call tonight has been called about a local donor offer and moments later there is another call from the TIC about another import offer. I take the call regarding the import offer, which is unfortunately a 35-year-old donor with an asthma history that has required active treatment his whole life. I decline this donor offer and inform my colleague of this outcome. He has provisionally accepted an offer for two single lung recipients and is preparing to make the calls to those patients to have them come to HUP. At 5:15 p.m., I am walking to the train station to return home. I wonder if we will see an email notifying us that they will both move forward to transplant. The day is not really over. Instead it is carried onward by passing the torch to others until it is your turn to carry it again.

This journey, one we partake in together with our patients, is never ending. Lung Transplant is evolving with better outcomes, new technologies, and longer life expectancy. Often our relationships with patient families continue well beyond the life of the patient. As patients and families, you develop similar bonds with each other that reach outside the usual boundaries of time and space. Hopefully, these relationships propel us forward and extend the legacy of the meaningful and invaluable gift or organ donation. Over the course of my career in transplant, I have benefited from what colleagues and patients have taught and shared with me during routine and extraordinary moments. It is a privilege to walk on this journey beside you.

J. Eric Hobson, MSN, CRNP
Nurse Practitioner with the Lung Transplant Program
Hospital of the University of Pennsylvania in Philadelphia, Pennsylvania

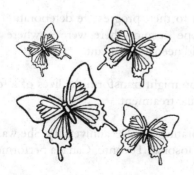
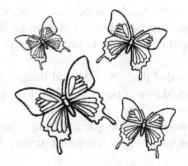

OPENING REMARKS

By Dr. Joel Cooper

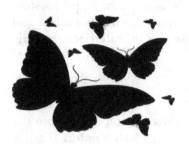 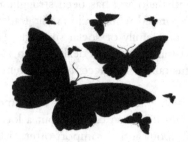

The patients waiting for a transplant and a member of their family often have to move to the city where there is a lung transplant center and live in an apartment for months or longer in the hope that a suitable donor organ will become available. At times we had 10 to 20 such potential recipients living in the same nearby apartment building hoping that the phone would ring in time announcing that we had a donor and they should come to the hospital immediately for their transplant. For many the phone did not ring in time.

I witnessed the marvelous effect that hope had upon these suffering patients and their families.

I attended the weekly get-togethers these patients and their families had to encourage and support each other.

I saw the genuine delight they showed when one of their group received a successful transplant even as they clearly must have been disappointed that their turn had not yet come.

The mutual love, respect, and support they showed for each other was a lesson for all of us and was inspirational for me. When we first successfully treated a person with cystic fibrosis – a genetic disorder that causes repeated lung infections and usually leads to a premature death – I wondered whether we had accomplished a good thing or not.

On the one hand – hope that there was a potential solution to their progressive deterioration and ultimate demise - but on the other hand perhaps false hope – since there were nowhere near sufficient donor lungs to provide for all the patients who would need a transplant.

I concluded that it was a good thing – that lung transplantation might transform the lives of a few – but would give hope to all – that there was, if needed, a potential treatment.

The longest surviving double lung transplant recipient is celebrating her 24th anniversary. She was the second, double lung transplant patient that Toronto General Hospital, Toronto, Canada performed.

For those who have received a transplant, each anniversary is considered a birthday and is celebrated as such, even more so than their true birthday. They have a new appreciation of life and treat each day as special.

One recipient told me, "I have no more rainy days. Every day is sunshine".

Another one said to me, "Dr. Cooper, I know you want me to live forever, and I hope you don't mind, but I am living for Thanksgiving – and after that I will live for Christmas – and after Christmas I will live for Easter".

Many recipients have expressed sentiments similar to the one who told me; "I have been given back my life and I want to spend whatever time I have giving back to help others".

I recently was the surprise guest at a special celebration held in Montreal, Canada, to mark the 20th anniversary of the lung transplant which I performed on the honoree – a young lady of great courage – who has established a charitable foundation to help those in need of a transplant and to promote awareness of the need for organ donation and the miracles it can accomplish. Many transplant recipients were at this event. I went over to a teenager who I had been told had received a lung transplant a few years earlier for cystic fibrosis. She did not know who I was or the role I had been privileged to play in developing the procedure, which had transformed her from a chronically ill child into a healthy, energetic teenager.

Speaking of miracles, I once heard a miracle defined as an event, which leaves you with an abiding sense of astonishment no matter how often you think of it – it always leaves you with a sense of wonderment. For me a lung transplant which transforms the life of a recipient and their family fits this definition.

So I would like to close by sharing with you some of the lessons I have learned –

- Live each day to the fullest.
- Cherish your health, your family, your friends, your teachers, and those who have encouraged and supported you.
- When a little something goes wrong, remember and appreciate all that is going well.
- Use your skills and your talents to better mankind.
- Be of service to others. There is no greater privilege or reward.
- Don't accept the status quo. Persistence and hard work pay off, and are the instruments of change.
- Never give up hope and do all you can to give hope to others.
- Miracles do happen. You can help make them occur, and many of you undoubtedly will.

I would like to close with a verse written by Ralph Waldo Emerson and sent to me by a transplant recipient:

"….To appreciate beauty, to find the best in others; To leave the world a bit better, whether by a healthy child, a garden patch, or a redeemed social condition; To know even one life has breathed easier because you have lived. This is to have succeeded."

Dr. Joel Cooper, Thoracic Surgery
Chief of the Division of Thoracic Surgery at the University of Pennsylvania Health System,
Philadelphia, Pennsylvania

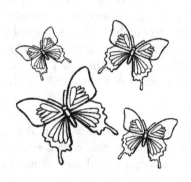

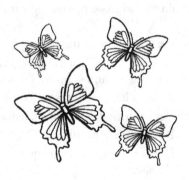

"REMEMBER ME"

I know you will remember me, I did not die in vain.

For God Chose special gifts of mine, to ease another's pain.

He gave these gifts to someone, who's time on Earth was near.

Cause I'll no longer use them, And Mom, I had no fear!

He called on me to help him, I said, "I don't know how".

He told me I could save the life of someone's loved one now.

He gave a baby sight, Mom. He healed a teen's weak heart.

And even though I'm gone now, we'll never be apart!

I live on now forever, I helped someone else live.

This precious gift of life, Mom, I'm so proud that I could give!

Don't remember me for my riches, my possessions or my grades.

(**Sarah** was 16, and killed by a drunk driver. She, too, knew she wanted to be an organ donor and her mom, **Sue Diotte,** gave me full permission to share this with the whole world. God Bless our Children! Thank you to **Deborah Blagojevic** for making this connection!)

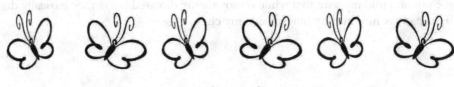

My Last Goodbye
By Mike Adams

"I sit here in the secret place to write my last goodbye.
I will be brave, I will be strong, I will not even cry.
The pills I take will make me sleep, for how long I do not know.
I hope that they will do the job and free my soul to go.
Some will say I was crazy, and some will say I was nuts.
Some will say it was amazing, and some will say it took guts.
I had my reasons for this act; it had to do with health.
It was not lack of money, because that is not true wealth.
I would have gladly given dollars if only I could stay.
But the lung disease I have, it will not go away.
Doctors say it could and family says it will,
"All you have to do Mike is take this little pill."
So this is it, now I must go, it is my time to fly.
So this is it, my time has come, to say my last goodbye."

I wrote this poem while lying in a hospital bed with a chest tube sticking out of the left side of my chest. I had just been told I needed to have a major surgery to repair my lung, which had collapsed.

I was feeling fed up with Cystic Fibrosis (CF), hospitals, doctors, and medications, and just not being able to live life like most of my friends. I would have never taken my life as expressed in my poem. I just needed to let people know I was hurting.

I have always been a fighter, and I did my best not to let CF take my life from me. On Thanksgiving of 2002, my disease tried its best to do just that. I was taken to our local emergency room (ER) gasping for air on eight liters of oxygen. The doctor told my wife and me there was nothing they could do for me. We were told to go home and wait for my transplant call, which I had been waiting for since 2000. I didn't want to go home and die. I asked my wife to drive me to Tarzana Medical Center, Tarzana, California where my lung doctor who had taken care of me for years would be. I told her that if I had to be placed on life support, he would know when to pull the plug.

As soon as we arrived at Tarzana, I was placed on a bi-pap machine, which finally gave me some relief from the hours of gasping for air. I spent the next two weeks in the intensive care unit struggling to hold on to every breath I could.

On December 5th, the pastor who married my wife and me was giving me my last rights before my pending death. On December 6th, the call came; it was time to get my life-saving pair of lungs. I was taken to Cedars-Sinai Medical Center in Los Angeles, California, where I had my transplant. The surgeon came out and told my wife that while removing my diseased lungs they basically dissolved in his hands; but I had my new healthy lungs inside my chest.

I spent fourteen days in the hospital before I got to go out into the world with my new lungs and new life. I soon found out that it was a young fifteen-year-old boy who saved my life. His name was Tory Howe, and to this day I am very close with his mother.

My young donor gave me life again and for that I felt the need to give back in some way. Soon after my transplant, I became an Ambassador with OneLegacy, a Donate Life organization. I volunteer my time, sharing my transplant story with high school and college medical students. I also wanted to give back to my transplant center, so I became a volunteer in the lung transplant department at Cedars Sinai.

My transplant not only saved my life but it also gave me the ability to enjoy my life! I have since played tennis at the United States Transplant Games, traveled to Europe, Canada and Mexico, gone whitewater rafting in the Grand Tetons, and in 2008, I was able to experience the joy of scuba diving in St. Thomas.

I have truly been blessed with my life-saving lung transplant. I give thanks everyday for these bonus years I have been given. My only wish is that many of my friends who lost their lives to CF could have been given a second chance at a better life, too.

Mike Adams, 47
Rancho Cucamonga, California
Cystic Fibrosis
Double Lung Transplant, December 6, 2002
Cedars-Sinai Medical Center, Los Angeles, California

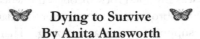

Dying to Survive
By Anita Ainsworth

I moved from my hometown of Tuam, County Galway, Ireland, in July 2003 to Bronx, New York where I worked as a chef in an Irish bar\restaurant. While in New York I met my partner Aidan Whelan. Life was going pretty good for us then I discovered I was pregnant. Although shocked we were very happy. At first things were okay, but I kept getting chest infections and my breathing slowly started to get difficult. I wasn't alarmed; as I was told I had mild asthma back in 2001. I also smoked, although not a lot. Fortunately I had a problem free birth on March 17, 2006 to my daughter Ayla Mai.

In 2006 when I returned home for the wedding of my sister, I fell ill and had 45% of my lung function left. I was told it was Lymphangioleiomyomatosis (LAM).

I never really thought I wasn't going to get new lungs, but sitting in the hospital, looking at the same four walls was difficult, and so I started to knit to keep my mind off what was going on. My daughters first Christmas was in my hospital room with Aidan and me. My family was staying in Dublin and brought us our dinner, it was lovely considering. Planning for Ayla's future without me was very difficult; I spent time writing goodbye letters.

Then on January 23, 2007, I was told they found a match. I kissed and waved goodbye to all my family especially Ayla and Aidan. It was awful, as I really didn't know if I'd see them again. The surgery took four hours and I woke up a day and a half later. Once the respirator was taken off and I took my first new breath, it was amazing. I was discharged two weeks later with a lot of medications, no oxygen, feeling sore, and kind of scared, but alive.

Now just over three years later it is starting to settle in what happened and the medications being reduced and I'm feeling great. I have had no rejection thank God. I now enjoy my life with my daughter, family and friends.

This whole ordeal has obviously affected my life and those around me. The first year was quite difficult to accept what actually happened. I do not know where the lungs came from. I have sent a letter to the donor's family, which took me three years to do. I just didn't know how to word my appreciation for the gift I was given. How brave of this family to make such a tough discussion at a very upsetting time.

Since the surgery Aidan, Ayla and I have been on holidays overseas together and had a great time. I have spoken to some senior students, in local secondary schools about organ donation awareness and about my experience and asking them to speak to there families about there wishes on donation which makes the decision easier for their loved ones.

At the moment my sister, friends and I are doing a walk to raise money for the heart and lung transplant unit in Dublin, Ireland in July 2010, and so looking forward to completing the walk.

I would like to thank Aidan, who was my solid rock through the whole ordeal, and Ayla who gave me strength and her love. My parents, brother, my two sisters, Aidan's family, and our friends and strangers for all their prayers and support which was amazing. Thank you also to my medical team; Dr. J. Egan (who I have such faith in); the staff at the hospital and clinic who looked after me so well.

My reason for doing this is for others who find themselves in similar situation, may find comfort in the great outcome of my ordeal. They may be scared but don't give up.

R .I .P.
Sweet donor

Anita Ainsworth, 31
Galway, Ireland
Lymphangioleiomyomatosis
Double Lung Transplant, January 23, 2007
The Mater Misercordiae, Dublin, Ireland

My Second Chance
By Crystal Akins

Hi, my name is Crystal Akins. I am a 48-year-old mother with Cystic Fibrosis (CF), and I've had a double lung transplant.

Growing up I was pretty healthy only having bronchitis or pneumonia. I was 19 the first time I was hospitalized needing intravenous (IV) antibiotics. For the next few years I was in and out of the hospital often. Each stay was for at least two weeks. It was then discovered that I had pseudomonas, a bacteria that lives in the lungs.

In my mid 30's I met and married my husband. I had a very healthy pregnancy despite the risks. I am also a diabetic. As our son began to get older, I noticed a gradual decline of my lung functions.

In September 2006, my pulmonologist convinced me to go to Boston to learn about lung transplantation. At that point I was not on oxygen and wasn't convinced I wanted or needed a transplant. The statistics of success rate and survival rate did nothing to encourage me.

At the same time, my brother who also has Cystic Fibrosis started pursuing a lung transplant in Pennsylvania. He was on oxygen and was finding it limiting. He went back and forth for a couple of years before going to Florida to try another hospital. They referred him to Duke University Hospital, Durham, North Carolina, late in 2008. He was successfully transplanted in May 2009. My brother told me to contact Duke. He did not want me to allow myself to get as sick as he had become.

Duke felt I had potential to be a candidate and told me that I would need to gain weight and suggested a feeding tube. They also wanted me to enroll in their rehab program to build up my strength.

My husband and I flew back to New York. Unfortunately no one had told me that flying with diminished lung capacity is a bad idea. On the flight, while using portable oxygen, my oxygen level fell to 77%. That night I went to the emergency room because I was still having difficulty breathing. They gave me some fluids for dehydration along with oxygen, and then sent me home. I was flown back to Duke, on a medical flight, to be treated. At that point I weighed 89 pounds and had to walk with a walker because I had no muscle strength.

I started my rehab at The Center for Living, which consisted of one hour of floor exercises, 20-30 minutes of walking and 20 minutes of weights. In three weeks I gained 10 pounds. Officially listed, two days later I got my first call. This ended up to be my first 'dry run' and had four more 'dry runs'.

Then on January 7, 2010 I got the official "it's a go" call, and I got my lungs. The following day I was taken off the ventilator and gotten up to walk. I was moved out of intensive care unit the following evening and continued to walk.

Twelve days after my transplant I was released from the hospital to begin my outpatient rehabilitation at The Center for Living.

My last bronchoscopy in August I got a clean bill of health with no rejection!

Crystal Akins, 48
Queensbury, New York
Cystic Fibrosis
Double Lung Transplant, January 7, 2010
Duke University Hospital, Durham, North Carolina

🦋 The Gift that Changed Our Lives Forever 🦋
By Debra Aparicio

My name is Debra C. Aparicio; I was born in New York, but raised in Puerto Rico. I am a retired Army Nurse Corps officer, and served proudly for 21 years, taking care of soldiers and their families until I became ill. My husband Felix and I have four wonderful children and eleven grandchildren. After my retirement, I do volunteer work, and I continue to do so. This is my story.

In 2000, I requested a military assignment to Europe for my last duty station so that my husband and I could retire in Italy. We were so excited when my assignment came for Landstuhl Regional Medical Center (LRMC), Landstuhl/Kirchberg, Germany. Our dream to retire in Italy was coming closer and closer, not knowing that God had other plans for us. We arrived in Germany in December 2000 and immediately started looking for a place in Tuscany, Italy. By spring of 2001, I started experiencing problems while running the two-mile military fitness test. By the next spring, I noticed that I could not take a deep breath and it was getting harder for me to walk fast. I was referred to a Rheumatologist, and a computerized Tomography (CT) scan was done and I was given a possible diagnosis of an interstitial disease in the lungs, but a lung biopsy was needed to confirm the diagnosis.

My son's wedding was approaching and I did not want to have any surgery before my son's wedding, so I put the biopsy on hold until July 2002. Subsequently, a Video Assisted Thoracic (VAT) surgery was done in Germany, and I was diagnosed with Idiopathic Pulmonary Fibrosis (IPF), which causes hardening of the lungs. I was sent to Walter Reed Army Medical Center, Washington, D.C., where I started treatment with Interferon Gamma injections since the Prednisone and Cytoxan treatment had not worked. I was immediately referred to University Transplant Center, San Antonio, Texas for evaluation. Although I only waited two months, the wait seemed extremely long. Especially, when December came and I thought I was not going to be alive to celebrate my favorite holiday of the year, Christmas. It was very difficult to see my husband sad and to inform my son that I may die soon. The biggest pain I had in my heart was to leave my loved ones behind.

Early on the morning of December 23, 2004, I received a left lung from Kevin, giving me a second chance in life. We received the call the day before, and that call changed our lives forever! A grieving family, in the midst of losing their loved one, decided to donate their son Kevin's organs. I remember waking up and taking deep breaths…it was a miracle in the works. The doctor came to my room and told me that my lung was from a healthy 16-year-old male, and all I thought in that moment was about Kevin's parents. While I was celebrating my second chance in life, they were mourning the loss of their beloved son. Every year, on December 23, I celebrate life and at the same time I grieve for his parents and honor his memory. I pray and ask God to comfort them and give them peace.

I was discharged to go home on December 28 (five days post-op) and spent New Years with family. Like all transplant recipients, I went home with lots of medications, including anti-rejection and other pre-existing medical conditions medications. At first, I was taking up to 23 pills a day, but now only 16 pills a day. I do not complain because I can breathe!

Since my lung transplant I have been able to travel to Italy where I go every year and to Puerto Rico twice a year to see my family. I also travel in the United States to visit friends and other family members. When I'm not traveling, I volunteer at Brooke Army Medical Center (BAMC) at Fort Sam Houston, Texas as the Nurse Recruiter Assistant; at Texas Organ Sharing Alliance (TOSA) as guest speaker; and health fairs promoting organ, eye, and tissue donation; and continue to volunteer for Vital Alliance; and Chair for the Annual Tree Planting Ceremony honoring the memory of donors. I also mentor patients that are diagnosed with pulmonary diseases and require lung transplants.

Words cannot express how grateful my family and I are for my donor family's decision to donate life. Because of their decision to donate Kevin's organs, I was able to breathe again, see my granddaughter and grandson born, and tell my husband and my family how much I love them. I now see life in a different way, helping people, and Praise God for His miracles. Last year, I was able to meet my donor family and tell them how grateful my husband and I are for the "Gift of Life."

Debra Aparicio, 57
Schertz, Texas
Idiopathic Pulmonary Fibrosis
Single Lung Transplant, December 23, 2004
University Hospital, University of Texas Health Sciences, San Antonio, Texas

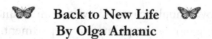

Back to New Life
By Olga Arhanic

Part One

My illness took time to develop throughout my life. It started in my youth with various pains in my back. I recall one day I went to the Celje hut (ski resort) and in the hut I had a total blockage of breathing. Very serious sensation, as I did not know what I did wrong. Also during this period of time I had severe headaches and many times I lost consciousness. Several times I went to the doctor, but no cause was found for my malaise.

I was married in 1983 and my husband and I wanted a child. We adopted in 1991, and we received a beautiful baby girl, one-month-old. Months later I went into the Military Service, which was a big surprise.

Part Two
In 1996 I experienced the first of six spontaneous lung collapes. The first doctor who took me was Dr. Zorko Anton of the University Medical Centre Maribor, Slovenia, Europe.

Part Three
I felt good and carried on. I rode my bike, went for walks. My health was slowly deteriorating, and I sought to answer why. I went from doctor to doctor.

Part Four
My pulmonologist, Dr. Meznar Brane, suggested that I retire, and I did in 2003. Before retirement, I was twice at sea, and in 2002 when my daughter desired to swim with me, and when I came from the water, I coughed pure blood. I needed two days to gain my state of repair. This is when I learned about lung transplant. My first reaction was not to go, as my culture, they prefer to die. I chose to look further into lung transplant but it meant leaving my home. My Mom was sad that I chose to do it alone.

Part Five
In late 2003, I went for another review by the pulmonologist, and that is when my saturation was measured for the first time. It was about 70%.

My friend Tekrat, who is also a doctor, said that I was panicking and I was not as bad as I imagined. I returned to the pulmonologist and looked at the pictures of my lungs and once again I was told I needed a lung transplant. Finally in 2004 I began to use oxygen.

I arrived in Topolsica, Slovenia, and wandered in the darkness and seeked answers to my situation and here in Topolsica, I at last had answers which I had been looking for all the years of my illness. At the hospital a friendly doctor told me the possible treatments. This was my first bright spot, as for almost eight years, I wandered in the dark.

From Topolsica I was taken by ambulance to Univerzitetni Klinicni Center Ljubljana, Slovenia (University Medical Centre Ljubljana) to the pulmonary department. For me it was all new. In the pulmonary section, I met with people who have had various problems with breathing. I met many new friends. I am most happy that I met and was able to meet friendly doctors and other medical staff. All the people are beautifully cared for, we were people, not numbers.

My doctor at the University Medical Centre Ljubljana, pulmonary section has been Mrs. Barbara Salobir. She prepared all the paperwork necessary for transplantation of my left lung. Ordinarily you would receive two lungs, but they were unable to perform a double lung transplant because of my plevrodeze lung (pneumothorax, or collapsed lung). Collapsed lung repair could not allow removal of both lungs as they sometimes "attach", "glue" the lung to the rib cage.

Before the transplant I had to present myself to the Vienna General Hospital, Vienna, Austria (AKH), where they examined me and took pictures. So I got on the list for organ transplants. My health situation had visibly worsened. All things which I needed for AKH Vienna, I packed in a suitcase.

Part Six

I was called 15th October 2005. I remember the words of my daughter, "Mom why do you have to go to Vienna today?" I replied to her, "I am getting new lungs". The ambulance arrived quickly at our house, I said goodbye to my husband and daughter, took the suitcase and we drove to Vienna. I remember that we were waiting for the Vienna police, so that we would be rapidly brought to AKH.

After the transplant surgery I was at AKH Vienna for four weeks. My parents, sister and daughter, came several times to visit. Also visiting me was Dr. Turel Matja. I remember his visit was very happy and that I hugged his neck and gave him a kiss on the cheek. I had some hallucinations, which were difficult. One of my hallucinations, I traveled in space. My biggest wish was to get back to University Medical Centre Ljubljana, and be with my doctor, Mrs. Barbara Salobir. She was my guardian angel for me.

Part Seven

From the hospital I returned home. What a great feeling it was when I returned home and again sleep in my own bed. My husband was with me all the time at home. He helped me. I could not even eat alone, because my hands were shaking from the medication.

In the spring when it was warmer, I went to have a short walk around the house. I watched how the flowers bloomed, and the very first butterflies were emerging. I live near the forest, so every morning I could hear birds singing. My health has slowly returned to normal. During this time I went to regular checkups. At home I am able to perform almost all the work. I walk the dog for long walks through the woods and enjoy myself. I am so glad with my life, as I returned to normal and not dependent on oxygen, or other people. Alone, I am able to go into town to shop and enjoy the small things.

Part Eight

In 2009 I went with my mother to New York, because they have a day with an association set up for organ transplants. There I met a lot of people who had transplanted hearts and lungs. It was interesting to see all these people and meet with them, as they too share the same concerns as I. Some were real athletes. I myself do not see transplants as a disease, but a transplant brings better quality of life.

Part Nine

I now have chronic rejection of my transplanted lungs. Vienna, suggested that I try taking new drugs. They treated me with the following medicines: Sandimmune Neoral, Medrol, and Certican - (Everolimus).

Thank God that medicine is always advancing and more opportunities for better quality of life after organ transplantation. Slovenia is small country but we have excellent doctors. Every night I pray and thank our Creator that I have such good doctors. I'm happy and grateful for each day. My thinking is that I live right now; everything else is the past or future.

In Slovenia there is another woman diagnosed with Lymphangioleiomyomatosis (LAM). She is much younger than me and post-transplant about ten years. I feel good. Her name is Nina and I wish her many happy and healthy days.

I pray every night for my sisters around the world who have LAM. I ask that God protect them and give them a long and quality filled life.

Sending beautiful greetings from Slovenia.

Olga Arhanic, 53
Skofja vas, Slovenia
Lymphangioleiomyomatosis
Single Lung Transplant, October 15, 2005
Vienna General Hospital (AKH), Vienna, Austria

🦋 My Life Changing Journey 🦋
By Jane Aula

I was born on June 19, 1967, and was diagnosed with Cystic Fibrosis (CF) two days later. In March 2007, I became dependent on oxygen. It was later that year that my doctor started to talk to me about the possibility of needing a double lung transplant; 2008 the wait began. I did receive a call that a pair of lungs were available and looked good. Unfortunately it did not work out for me. My doctor felt I was doing too good at that point to compromise with the lungs presented to me so I was sent home, very sad and disappointed. In 2009, I was admitted to the hospital because both of my lungs collapsed. I was admitted to our local hospital, William Beaumont Hospital, in Royal Oak, Michigan and subsequently I was then transferred to the University of Michigan Medical Center, Ann Arbor, Michigan by Life Flight. My doctor, Dr. Tammy Clark Ojo, told me I could not go home until I received a lung transplant.

On April 28, 2009, I was sitting in my hospital bed when my phone rang. It was Jenni, my pre-transplant coordinator. We were waiting to hear if United Network of Organ Sharing (UNOS) had granted my appeal to change my status on the list and thought it was about that. Instead it turned out to be "the call". My husband was working so I called him and he immediately left for the hospital. He had a 45-minute drive.

I was taken into surgery that night and to recovery the next morning. There were some complications with my right lung and they placed me on the heart/lung by-pass machine for a period of time. They woke me about five hours after the surgery to be sure there were no deficits from that procedure. I left the hospital three weeks after my transplant.

I knew that my life would change but I really had no idea exactly how much it would change. I had been treating myself for CF for so long that I had performed my daily routine without blinking an eye. I had all new medicines and had to create a new daily routine. I didn't know where to start...I was completely overwhelmed and suffered from severe anxiety the first weeks I was home. It was a struggle but I worked myself out of it with the support and love of my husband Steve, my amazing parents and three sisters, in-laws and countless others. I took it one day at a time and eventually I created a new routine.

I have not returned to work and have no plans to return at this time. I am fortunate to have full disability benefits through Social Security. I am currently concentrating on advancing my quilting skills and hope to turn it into more than a hobby some day. I have joined a gym and do my best to go three to four days a week.

At my last appointment back on February 10, 2011, my Pulmonary Function Test (PFT) that day showed my lung capacity up to 105%. That day Dr. Ojo was looking through my test results and said she was trying to find something to fix and wasn't able. I did have an episode of minor rejection back in July 2009, which was treated with steroids. I was hospitalized because of complications from Cytomegalovirus (CMV). I have been doing very well since.

I no longer need oxygen, nebulizer treatments or vest treatments. I have several pills I take in a day but I'm used to taking pills, which doesn't require me to be home to do. I was also diagnosed with, Cystic Fibrosis Related Diabetes (CFRD), and am now insulin dependent. I am now comfortable with that part of my daily routine and again, this is something I can monitor when away from home.

The past year and a half has been challenging, but a lot of fun. My husband and I are back to one of our favorite things to do and that is travel. Our travels have included a nine-day tour of the coast of California along with a few days in Yosemite. It was amazing. We traveled to Las Vegas and Phoenix this past month and had a great time. We can't wait to plan our next adventure.

My youngest sister issued a challenge and I have decided to take her up on it. I will be running in a 5K on March 20, 2011. There will be a 5K and ½ marathon on Grosse Ile, Michigan, to raise awareness and money for the Cystic Fibrosis Foundation. I have started training for a half marathon that I will run with some of my family members on April 2, 2011, in Wisconsin. I look forward to challenging myself for many years to come.

I am quickly approaching the two year anniversary of my transplant and hard to believe it has gone so fast. I had the privilege of meeting my donor's mom and stepfather and was able to thank them in person. I know I wouldn't be here if it weren't for my donor, Jessica Varney, and her family. I am forever grateful to them for a second chance at life. Always in my thoughts....thank you to Jessica and her family, Carol Varney, Bill Coffman, Rodney Varney and Melissa Varney, as well as her grandparents and many friends that lost an amazing person.

Jane Aula, 43
Royal Oak, Michigan
Double Lung Transplant, April 28, 2009
University of Michigan Medical Center, Ann Arbor, Michigan

Just Breathe
By Heather Beadle

"Just breathe. Steady. Okay, get ready…blow! Blow! Blow! Blow harder! A little bit more! Blow! Okay, that's great Heather." Matthew knew I had done a good job on my pulmonary function test (PFT), but he thought I could do a little better. My lung functions had been doing great, so we only had to do one more. That was my second annual evaluation, so there was a lot more testing after that. There was my bone densitometry test to see if the steroids had caused any osteoporosis, and then it was off to the x-ray department.

When I got down to the x-ray reception area there was a line of waiting patients, and they all had on little blue surgical masks. Great – that meant there were at least six transplant patients in front of me waiting for their own x-rays. I knew it was going to be a long morning. As I moved to the front of the line, I had to fill out the pregnancy forms. Let's see, Name: Heather Beadle; Age: 28; Could you be pregnant: No; Last menstrual cycle: uhm…last month? Have you had a hysterectomy: No; Tubal Ligation: Yes. You would think they would have gotten this in their system by now so I didn't have to fill it out every time. I sat down in the waiting area wearing my own little blue mask and realized it almost felt like a second home there. I spent so much time there that I recognized half of the staff walking through the halls. There was Luis, the crazy transport guy, and Marian, the lady that later did my sonogram. It was always the same around there.

1 – Mother Cow
"Heather! Come here!" My mom was calling for me. "Sit in my lap for a second." My esteemed mother then licked the length of my forehead. That confirmed it in her heart. She had just seen a commercial asking if she had licked her child today. What a strange commercial, and yet it wasn't. My pediatrician, Dr. Donaldson was called, "Doctor, this is LaGaytha; I think I know what's wrong with Heather. I just saw a commercial and she has almost all of the symptoms they described." At four years old, all I remember is going into his office and him sitting me on his lap. That is when this wise old doctor lifted up my bangs with one hand and licked my salty forehead like a mother cow. How could I keep from laughing?

I was sent to the hospital, there, the technician put a sensor on my arm, and then told my parents to put the coat on me. I cried - it didn't hurt, but it was strange and I was getting hot. But the sweat test was working and the salt in my sweat moved the indicator completely to the other side of the sensor. That's when my parents knew for sure that I had Cystic Fibrosis (CF).

My parents were taught to give me nebulizer breathing treatments and to clap my back to break up any mucus I might have building in my lungs.

2 – Caged Animal
"Mom! How many more minutes?" I couldn't stand sitting in the living room doing a breathing treatment when there was something exciting to do outside!

When it was time for me to go to pre-school, there was only one in town that would take me. They were all afraid of the liability if something happened to me while in their care. I loved playing duck-

duck-goose and singing on the merry-go-round with the other children. During kindergarten my mom enrolled me in ballet and tap. I loved dancing so much that I would keep my black tap shoes on when we went into the grocery store and I would dance for my mom down the aisles - tap, tap, tapping away.

3 – Needle Hater
When I was in the second grade I was in Mrs. Graham's class. I loved her fiery red hair. That was the first year that I was diagnosed with pneumonia and had to have intravenous antibiotics (I.V.'s). I had to do the I.V.'s three times a day, so Mom got no rest. The routine started at 7a.m., then again at 3p.m. and finally at 11p.m. I hated the I.V.'s because the needle in my hand hurt. Once, my nurse told me that if she missed the placement of the needle in my vein, then I could start an I.V. on her. Well, she missed (or my vein rolled), and I got to stick one of those nurses with a needle for a change. I was very excited! I got all of my supplies ready, placed the tourniquet on her arm, and then very gently placed the needle in that big vein on her hand. I had started my first-and only–I.V.

I remained pretty healthy during most of elementary school. I had to go into the hospital for a "tune-up" every August before school started in September.

4 – Growing up
At the end of sixth grade I decided to try out for cheerleading. After many hard hours of practicing with my friends, I made the squad!

I was a cheerleader and an honor roll student for the rest of my Junior High, and High School years. I was also fairly healthy, and I finally hit 100 pounds my junior year. My dad had told me almost daily that he would give me $100 the day I hit 100 pounds. I was ecstatic!

5 - Brandon
In November of 1993 (my junior year in high school), I met my now husband, Brandon. We started dating that fall and have been together ever since.

6 – Diabetes Calls My Name
My senior year I felt terrible. I had lost a lot of weight, and my vision was getting so bad that my dad decided to take me to the emergency room. When they checked my blood sugar, it was over 850. They freaked out! After that, I had to start checking my blood sugar at least three times a day.

7 – College Years
The main health problems I had in college started my sophomore year. The Ear, Nose, and Throat (ENT) doctor determined that I had a sinus infection and required surgery immediately. I had a few hospital stays during those four years, but they were mainly uneventful. The summer between my junior and senior year, Brandon and I were married. It was a big, beautiful wedding, and we had the time of our lives when we went to Cancun for our honeymoon.

8 – Getting Sick
In 2002, I had pneumonia once again. I developed Respiratory Syncytial Virus (RSV), and my PFT's went from the low 80's to the mid-30's. I also developed the Mumps. That was the first time any

physician had ever mentioned transplant to me. January of 2003, I was ready to be listed for lung transplantation. I had all of the tests, and, thankfully, passed.

On Sunday, December 21st, I received 'the call'. I was living with my sister and her boyfriend. As we sped towards the hospital, I called Brandon and told him to hit the road.

All I remember about the rest of that day is being wheeled on a gurney into the operating room. I really didn't want to see what was about to happen. They put me to sleep, and the next thing I knew I was waking up in the intensive care unit (ICU) with a breathing tube down my throat. They finally took out the breathing tube, and I immediately started hyperventilating. Those were the biggest breaths I had taken in a long time – and it scared me at first.

We were truly blessed to have received this great Christmas gift from God, but at the same time we knew that another family was grieving the loss of a loved one.

My new lungs were doing great – my new lung functions were approximately 110%, a lot higher than the 18% they were before my transplant. I had to do the typical Pulmonary Rehabilitation after I was released, even though I was very weak.

9 - Aftermath

The first year after my transplant, I was the Matron-of-Honor for my sister when she got married. I was so excited to be able to be there for her. When we tried on the dresses in April, I was a size 00. When we picked up the dresses in July, I had finally put on a little weight, though I was still tiny. We talked the ladies at the store into exchanging my dress for one that fit - I needed a size 0. If I had not received that precious Christmas gift, I never would have had the joy of seeing my sister get married.

The most important things to me are my nieces and nephew. I have an eleven-year-old niece Cailean that spends every summer with Brandon and me. Cailean is now a big sister to JC, who are the children of my brother Colin and his wife Candace. My sister, Jenelle and her husband Carl have had two daughters, Kamryn and Kaylor that I love as if they are my own. I was able to be in the room when Jenelle gave birth to Kamryn, who is now three and a half. I spend as much time with my nieces and nephew as possible. Kamryn actually spends the night with Brandon and me on occasion; she stayed with us last Tuesday night. We had a great time coloring and watching music videos on Country Music Television (CMT).

We have two Jack Russell Terriers that keep us busy. When I'm feeling well and the wind is not blowing, we like to take them for a walk. We love to travel; we've taken many trips around Texas into the hill country. Brandon and I went on a skiing trip to New Mexico with some friends. At the time my PFT's were approximately 95%. I loved being able to breathe in the mountains and I skied for the first time in my life. We had a great extended weekend. Afterwards I developed the flu and I went into rejection. I had to go through Photopheresis for three months until my lung function finally stopped dropping. They tried changing my Prograf to Rapamune, but my blood sugars kept dropping very fast. I had a few closes calls while driving, so I was put back on Prograf and they increased my Prednisone.

Brandon bought me an embroidery machine for Christmas last year, and I've gone crazy with it!

My seventh transplant anniversary is this December. If I had it to do again, would I choose to have a transplant? Absolutely!

Midland, Texas
Cystic Fibrosis
Double Lung Transplant, December 21, 2003
UT Southwestern University Hospital – St. Paul, Dallas, Texas

 Two Lungs, One Heart, 26.2 Miles
By Mark Black

When I was born, it didn't take long for doctors to realize that something was seriously wrong. Within hours of birth I began to turn blue. My 23-year-old, first-time parents were told that there was something wrong with my heart and if I was going to survive, I would need open-heart surgery—and quickly.

Hours later, I was put on a medical helicopter and flown to the Isaac Walton Killam (IWK) Children's Health Centre in Halifax, Nova Scotia, Canada (three hours from our home) for emergency open-heart surgery. The surgery was incredibly risky, especially for a newborn infant, but there were no other options.

It wasn't until I graduated from the Mount Allison University, Sackville, New Brunswick, Canada in May 2000 that things took a turn for the worse. That is when I began the journey that would change my life forever.

In October 2000, I began to notice that I was increasingly short of breath, and often fatigued and tired, much more than I should be. Chalking it up to stress and lack of sleep, I ignored the worsening condition for months until I went home at the end of the year and saw my doctor. The look on the doctor's face told me that I was much sicker than I realized.

After a undergoing a series of tests, my cardiologist came back with news that no one was prepared for. "You need a heart and lung transplant, and you need it NOW."

In September 2001, I was sent more than a 1000km from home, to be evaluated at the Toronto General Hospital for a rare and dangerous heart and double-lung transplant. The surgery is performed less than a handful of times in Canada each year; in fact, in 2001 there hadn't been a single one done in the whole country. There wasn't much hope that I would be accepted on the list because of my precarious health and the fact that I was so small, a donor would be difficult to find, but we had no other options; so we put all of our eggs in the transplant basket and hoped for the best.
October 2001, my father and I left the rest of our family at home, and moved to Toronto to start the wait. The first month of waiting was one of the hardest of that year. Every time the phone rang, I jumped wondering if it was "The Call." My heart had developed a life-threatening rhythm

abnormality causing me to remain in hospital under 24-hour surveillance until suitable organs could be found.

On September 6th, a nurse appeared at my door. "Okay, it's time to go!" I looked at my mom and my mom looked at me, both of us searching for the right words to say, knowing that this might be the last time we would speak to each other. I looked at my mom and said, "Mom, I'll see you soon." I wasn't going to mention the possibility of a negative outcome.

The surgery lasted seven hours. Despite a few hiccups, the surgery went well; after a few days in the intensive care unit, and a week in a step-down unit, I was discharged 16 days post-surgery. I've been blessed that things have gone very, very well.

Since those days, I've been fortunate to be healthy enough to run three marathons and five half-marathons. I've competed twice for Team Canada at the World Transplant Games, and became a 15-time medalist at the Canadian Transplant Games. Most recently, I was also a part of the first ever all-heart-transplant relay team to complete in an Ironman Triathlon in November 2010.

In 2003, I founded my own speaking and consulting firm, 'Mark Black Speaks'. In the seven years since then, I have given 200 presentations to more than 55,000 people across North America.

To anyone waiting for a transplant, as you read this you are probably feeling fearful and anxious, wondering if a donor will be found in time for you. I remember that feeling. When things get hard, please remember this: When I was listed, I was told I might wait two to three years for a suitable donor, and by four months into the wait I was admitted to the hospital because I was deteriorating so quickly. I wasn't supposed to survive, but I did. It's been eight years now, and things couldn't be better. So don't give up—ever. No matter how dire or hopeless things may seem, refuse to quit. If you can do this, amazing things can happen!

Also, I have written a book, <u>Live Life from the Heart: 52 Weeks to a Life of Passion and Purpose.</u>

Mark Black, 33
Dieppe, New Brunswick, Canada
Pulmonary Hypertension
Heart/Double Lung Transplant, September 7, 2002
Toronto General Hospital, Toronto, Canada

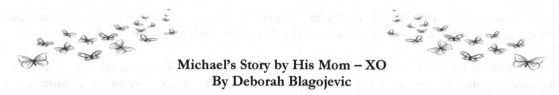

Michael's Story by His Mom – XO
By Deborah Blagojevic

My name is Debbie, and I am so proud to share Michael's story!

Mike was a proud father of a precious little girl who was only six-years-old when he passed away. He loved his daughter so much, and wanted so much to be a Dad that she would be proud of; but Mike, at the age of 26, had a terrible drinking problem. It was his drunken state that caused his death! In my heart, I feel as if Mike just passed away yesterday…actually it was June 20th, 2000.

On Father's Day weekend, Mike was at the bar with some friends watching a boxing match on the big screen, having the time of his life! He called our house and left a telephone message at 1 a.m. His message said he was changing his plans to go out for Father's Day lunch with his daughter, whom lived with us at the time, to dinner because he was going golfing with his friends. He said he couldn't wait to see what Gabrielle had made at school for him for Father's Day, and that he was treating for dinner! We know he went to the automatic teller machine at 2 a.m. to withdraw money for his golf game and for his Father/Daughter dinner plans. By 5 a.m. the police were knocking on our door! They informed us that our son was in the emergency room at the local hospital, and it did not look good. He'd had a tragic fall, which had caused brain damage! We called Gabrielle's Mom to come to the house to be with Gabrielle, and the police took us to the hospital. When we arrived, we went to see Mike; he looked like he was just having a peaceful sleep while all the nurses and doctors hovered over him. It was the strangest thing—he didn't look injured at all!

The doctor asked if he could talk to us, and he informed us that he believed Michael was brain dead. He asked if we would consider organ donation; my husband, Butch, and I both said, "YES" at the exact same time! We both knew how strongly Michael felt about donating his organs.

Mike had called us one day to tell us to look at our local newspaper; there had been a story in it about an old friend of his that he had played hockey with. Mike's friend had donated bone marrow through a bone marrow drive at his University, and he was so proud to know that he had saved a young mom with leukemia whom would have passed away if not for the donation. "ISN"T THAT COOL MOM?" Mike had said. Mike told us at dinner the next day how strongly he felt about donating, and how proud he was of his friend. He'd said, "If anything ever happens to me, I want all my organs to be donated. What good are they in the ground?"

I never, in a million years, thought we would ever see that day come. In the hospital, Michael was moved to the intensive care unit, and the doctors and nurses took such good care of him. We were informed that because of the alcohol in Mike's system and the heroic efforts the paramedics made to revive him, there was a possibility he would not qualify to be an organ donor. Butch and I were devastated-we knew it would have devastated Mike as well! After 2 ½ days of total numbness and shock from what was going on in our lives, the doctor informed us, with the hospital chaplain by our side, that Michael was gone. He had been tested twice, and it was confirmed that he was brain dead.

Since it had taken 2 ½ days, they were able to replenish his organs, and Mike was able to be an organ donor. As SAD as we were, we were also very HAPPY-if that makes any sense at all!

We met with the coordinator, who took all of Mike's history. Mike had been a heavy smoker, and he had damage cause by the paddles from the paramedics, so his lungs were never considered for donation. His heart valves were viable, but his heart wasn't, due to a heart disease problem in my husband's family! We knew immediately that a liver recipient was waiting at another hospital. Butch and I giggled when the doctor told us a liver recipient was a perfect match, and that Mike's liver was in excellent condition—after all his drinking problems, we couldn't imagine that his liver was healthy. Thank God it was! Michael also donated both of his kidneys, and to this day, we know that all three organ recipients.

In letters from the Trillium Gift of Life Program, we came to find out that Michael's gifts helped 29 people in total through bone, tissue, cornea, and organ donation! Knowing that Mike helped so many others in his passing has helped our family survive our grief. We know that many other families out there were saved from experiencing the pain we feel at losing a loved one, and we couldn't be more proud of Our Hero, Michael!

I'd like to thank Joanne for being such an inspiration to so many others, and for inviting me to share my story about Michael—even though this book is mostly about lung transplantation. The world now knows that Michael would have donated his lungs if he could have, and because of him, our whole community has now signed their donor cards!

Deborah Blagojevic, Donor Mother
Son, Michael Blagojevic – An Organ, Tissue Donor
Brighton, Ontario, Canada
Michael Passed Away, June 20, 2002
"Forever 26"

Scleroderma, Pulmonary Hypertension, Bilateral Lung Transplant – Oh My!
By Keith Bloomer

In 1997, my journey began. At the age of 26, I was recently married to my wife, Lynn, and diagnosed with Scleroderma, an autoimmune disease. Although diagnosed quickly, the disease was aggressive. In the short time between the first symptoms and the diagnosis, my lungs had been damaged with fibrosis, most pulmonary function test (PFT) values were around 50%, and the progression was showing no signs of stopping. The doctors responded quickly and began a course of Cytoxan (chemotherapy) treatments, which would last over two years. We also tried a number of medications including Cellcept, Imuran, and Rituxan. I also took the following medications to help with the symptoms of Scleroderma: Prilosec, Nexium, Protonix, Procardia xl90, and Pentoxifylline.

Whether it was the Cytoxan or just the disease slowing down, my lungs remained stable until 2006. During this time, our daughter Katie was born, our first gift. Life was good. Although over the years I had to give up some of the activities I enjoyed such as mountain biking, skiing and golfing, I was still enjoying life tremendously. I was very content and had forgotten the dangers of Scleroderma. In 2006 my lung function declined enough that I needed oxygen. I was able to continue working and help take care of Katie, but my quality of life began to decline. My need for oxygen continued to increase. In 2007, I was diagnosed with Pulmonary Hypertension (PH). I went on short-term disability with the hope of getting the PH under control, and then returning to work.

Tracleer, Revatio, Ventavis, and Remodulin were all tried as treatments for my PH. I never had a significant improvement from any of these medications. It was likely that the Pulmonary Fibrosis from the Scleroderma was controlling my breathing issues rather than the PH.

When I went on oxygen in 2006, my wife and I began to research, discuss, and pray about lung transplantation. We were led to this decision by the impact the damage to my lungs was having on my quality of life. For the first time fighting these diseases, my spirit was broken.

The evaluation process, at Brigham and Women's Hospital in Boston, Massachusetts, took six months. We had been warned that the average wait time is two years.

The day after I was listed, we had a routine clinic visit scheduled. The policy at Brigham and Women's Hospital is to not disclose the patient's Lung Allocation Score (LAS) or their place on the list. I was determined at this visit to ask "trick" questions designed to help us figure out where I was on the list. As the doctor entered the room, she noticed my list of questions and began answering them with a slight smile on her face. The last question was "Where do we go when we get the call?" She smiled and said, "You are going there now since we think we have lungs for you." Lynn and I looked at each other with surprised expressions on our faces. All we could say was, "We haven't completed our list of things to do before transplant." We were warned repeatedly throughout the day that this could be a false alarm and at any time we could be told to head home.

I received our second gift, the gift of new lungs as hoped, that day. I had complications, which meant a longer stay.

I was discharged on Christmas Eve. It was so great to be home with Katie. Lynn spent almost every day in the hospital with me but I didn't get to see Katie. It was a little scary to be home at first, away from the 24-hour medical care. It took me about two weeks to call my oxygen company and ask them to pick up the equipment I no longer needed.

I spent these two years doing whatever the doctors told me. I regained my strength, began exercising, and began enjoying life. I have gone bike riding, hiking, kayaking, and fishing. I have been to amusement parks and on a few vacations. It is so exciting to get to run, play, and swim with Katie. I couldn't have made it this far without Lynn and Katie.

I am thankful for my new chance at life and spend much of my time doing volunteer work. I am a volunteer with the Rhode Island Organ Donor Awareness Coalition, the New England Organ Bank, and the Rhode Island Blood Center. I have made presentations to various organizations encouraging and supporting organ and blood donation.

I am thankful to my donor, Brent, and his family. In their time of loss, they made the decision to donate Brent's organs to help others. I have been in touch with them and hope to meet them eventually. Since Brent cannot be brought back, I have made the choice to do volunteer work to honor his life.

Keith Bloomer, 39
Exeter, Rhode Island
Scleroderma, Pulmonary Hypertension
Double Lung Transplant, November 12, 2008
Brigham and Women's Hospital, Boston, Massachusetts

 The Beginning of a New Life, Where we "Appreciate Everything"
By Jerry Bluff

My name is Jerry Bluff. I am 67-years-old, and I live in Upstate New York with my wife Diane, who has shown me the real meaning of caregiver. She has been there for me every step of the way during my transplant experience. Without her, I don't know where I would be. I refer to this as 'our transplant' because she was as much a part of it as I was.

In 1998, I was diagnosed with chronic obstructive pulmonary disease (COPD) as a result of smoking and unhealthy working conditions (chemicals that I worked with and years of woodworking and breathing the dust without a mask).

At the time of my diagnosis I had 31% of my lung volume left; I had gone to my doctor for what I thought was bronchitis. I was put in the hospital and diagnosed with double bacterial pneumonia. A few days later I was told that I had COPD, and that I would be on oxygen the rest of my life.

Diane and I were devastated, to say the least. At first I looked at the diagnosis as a death sentence because COPD is a progressive disease, but it can be slowed with medicines and a good exercise program.

Shortly after this, my lung function dropped to 18%. My pulmonologist, along with The Cleveland Clinic Foundation, Cleveland, Ohio, felt that I would benefit by undergoing Lung Volume Reduction Surgery (LVRS). In February 2002, I had the LVRS at the Cleveland Clinic; they removed 33% of the upper lobe of each lung. This increased my lung volume capacity from 18% to 36%. In June 2003, the Cleveland Clinic told us that my lung volume had dropped to 18% again, and that without a lung transplant, I would have less than two years to live. We were stunned.

Our faith was undergoing the hardest test of our lives, but through that faith, my wife and I were brought closer together. We knew that we were in God's favor and never gave up. After evaluation, a phone call told us that I was on the transplant list. The anxiety was overwhelming, but we never gave up. We kept a suitcase packed so we would be ready at a moment's notice. I had one 'dry run'; we got a call that it was time, but when we got to the hospital, the surgery was canceled. After the 'dry run', our hearts sank, but we had to realize that lung just wasn't the perfect lung for me.

Then on February 22, 2004, we got 'the call.' They sent a Lear Jet to pick us up, and a police van was waiting to take us directly to the clinic when we landed in Cleveland. Diane and I said a prayer, praying to God for a successful surgery, and a healthy lung.

After the surgery it was only two hours when they removed the breathing tube out, and I took my first breath. I knew that everything was wonderful. Yes, we are in God's favor, and we are thankful. I was discharged from the hospital after eleven days.

This transplant has given me a new life, a life which I will never take for granted. The freedom is wonderful. I can now walk up to six miles, and I have been blessed with the chance to watch our grandchildren grow up. It has given me the opportunity to enjoy life with my wife, family and friends. In the six plus years since transplant, I have been doing volunteer work helping others through the transplant process. We also volunteer for the Finger Lakes Eye and Tissue Bank to bring awareness to organ and tissue donation through health fairs, blood drives, and speaking in schools. When we went through transplant, we had nobody to talk to about the process, so now we try to talk to people going through the same thing.

The biggest event since my transplant was attending the 2010 Transplant Games in Madison, Wisconsin. The experience far surpassed any expectations that I could have had. The thrill of each and every event was wonderful, but more importantly, it was the spirit of the games and all of the people involved that made everything so special. Also, there was a Lung Gathering where most of the lung recipients gathered together for a general meeting and discussion.

At the games, I was able to participate in the ballroom dancing competition with Diane as my partner. Even though we didn't win a metal, I won because I had the most beautiful partner. Then it was on to the 1500-meter race/walk. All I can say is that I finished the race—well actually, I did come in third (FROM THE LAST!). However, the games are not about winning, but about being able to finish. My wife was as proud of me as if I had been in first place. Then there was the long jump, or in my case, the short jump—that's enough said about that. I am looking forward to the 2012 Transplant Games, but I will definitely skip the long jump.

A dear friend told me, "You have to experience the games at least once in your life time." She was wrong. One time is not enough!! We will be going back.

To sum it up, I am living my life as if I have thirty years to live. When either Diane or I pass, we want the remaining partner to be able to say, "We had a good life together."

We all have our 'pity parties', but life is too short to waste it. Embrace it. Enjoy it.

Jerry Bluff, 67
Hilton, New York
Chronic Obstructive Pulmonary Disease
Single Lung, February 22, 2004
The Cleveland Clinic Foundation, Cleveland, Ohio

 Journey of Encouragement
By Sherri Bradley

Our son's name is Eric Bradley, and he was diagnosed with Cystic Fibrosis (CF) at birth, as was his older brother James.

Eric was diagnosed at nine months with hydrocephalus. A Ventricular-Peritoneal Shunt (VP shunt) was placed in his head to help his body release the extra fluid on his brain (this was a birth defect and had no relation to his CF history).

Eric was in and out of hospitals several times during his young life. For the most part it was CF related, pneumonia, bronchitis, chronic coughing, fevers, or regular tune up visits. Eric's doctor always kept a very close eye on him, and even at such a young age, his doctors knew that Eric would need surgery someday. As parents we were in disbelief, but we tried not to dwell on it. Instead, we focused on all the positive things, and encouraged Eric to be the best he could possibly be in school, sports, and activities. I never wanted him to feel like he couldn't do something because he had CF.

Eric was happiest when he was with his family and friends. He enjoyed school, basketball, Legos, and playing pool. Even though every day was a constant battle to breathe, eat and exercise, he always had a smile on his face, no matter what. Eric was nine-years-old when his lung transplant journey started.

In November 2006, during our stay in the hospital, our doctors advised us that it would be in Eric's best interest if we moved to have him close to the University of North Carolina Children's Hospital, Chapel Hill, North Carolina (UNC). Eric was showing signs of decreased lung function and air movement. Eric and I were at UNC for nine months waiting for the news of a donor.

On March 26th, Eric's nurse wakened me; she was so excited that Eric might get his new lungs that day. I quickly made airline reservations for his Dad and brothers to fly up and be with us. They arrived and were able to spend time with Eric before his surgery began. It was an all day and all night process. Eric was wheeled into surgery that night, and he has a 'NEW' birthday of March 27, 2007 that we celebrate every year, in addition to his June birthday.

Over the next couple of days, they had him up and walking twice a day and doing some light chest therapy. Many wonderful nurses and doctors have blessed Eric during every step of his journey. During his time in recovery, the nurses never saw a patient more loved and cared for than Eric, from all the visitors and phone calls to the doctors who came to check on him—even though Eric wasn't their patient. His determination to get better and overcome any obstacles in his path showed his doctors that, 'Eric was a true trooper.' The third day after his surgery he was having a pizza party in his room, and on another day he was having Kentucky Fried Chicken.

Eric will still have CF in other organs, but his new lungs give him a better quality of life. He is able to play basketball, run, skate, swim, and ride a bike. He likes to go paintballing, play sports, and he is learning to play the tuba in the school band. He calls it, 'The Beast', and puts 100% effort into his practice sessions. There's no getting winded, tired, or having to stop because he needs to cough. He is able to do anything and everything like other nine-year-old boys.

Eric has triumphed over many obstacles in his young life. He has a wonderful outlook on life and a giving, loving spirit, and he is grateful to God. He is also grateful to his family and friends at Foundation Academy for supporting him and loving him unconditionally during his many times of need. Eric puts himself fully into whatever the task before him, and has given hope and encouragement to everyone he meets. Eric never lost faith that God would bless him while in the hospital, and he even did question and answer interviews with many teams of doctors and nurses so they could learn more about him and his Cystic Fibrosis, his emotions, strength, attitude, and courage, his outlook on life, and so much more. God has a plan for Eric, and we thank God for our blessings and using Eric in such a mighty way.

Sherri Bradley, Mother of Eric Bradley
Eric Bradley, 13
Groveland, Florida
Eric, Cystic Fibrosis
Eric, Double Lung Transplant, March 27, 2007
University of North Carolina Hospitals, Chapel Hill, North Carolina

 Ten Years Post Double Lung Transplant 🦋
By Susan Burroughs

Hi. I have cystic fibrosis. I was born in 1960 and I am proud to say that I just celebrated my 50th birthday. I had a double lung transplant in May 2000, just one month before my 40th birthday. I have been married for 22 years and have a 16-year-old adopted daughter. I am a Certified Public Accountant (CPA) and I am the founder of the Cystic Fibrosis-Reaching Out Foundation Inc. Eight years post transplant I was diagnosed as being in chronic rejection.

OMG! Using the lingo of my 16-year-old is the best way to describe what the last 10 years have been like post transplant. I honestly thought I would be trading one set of problems for another but that is just not how I view it. Yes, I have had a few bumps in the road but my quality of life has improved 1000%. Since my transplant I have taken up the tennis. I had never even dreamed of choosing that activity as something I would grow to love. I have traveled.... We recently celebrated my 50th birthday and 10th anniversary of my new lungs by visiting Greece and Italy. This was a lifelong dream come true. I have watched my daughter grow into a little lady. I have been there when she lost her first tooth, when she went to her first homecoming and when she bought her first car.

Eight years after my transplant my pulmonary functions had dropped to the low 70%. That didn't seem like such a big deal to me because prior to transplant they were in the mid-teens. But the transplant team was concerned because they had dropped over 20%. They suggested it was chronic rejection and wanted to treat me with photopheresis. Of course… "What in the world is photopheresis"? My research revealed that:

"In medicine, photopheresis or extracorporeal photopheresis is a form of apheresis in which blood is treated with photoactivable drugs which are then activated with ultraviolet light."

Luckily for me, the University of Alabama Hospital in Birmingham where I received my transplant was one of the few centers that used photopheresis as a treatment for chronic rejection. Photopheresis consists of 30 treatments over a course of 18 months. With only two treatments left someone asked me…. "Does Photopheresis work?" I am not a scientist but with an all time HIGH of pulmonary function test showing 97%... I would say YES!!! Praise the Lord. It was well worth it.

If you would like to see a video of my transplant surgery, look for "Susan Burroughs" in a CNN video on YouTube.

Susan Burroughs, 50
Lilburn, Georgia
Cystic Fibrosis
Double Lung Transplant, May 23, 2000
University of Alabama Hospital, Birmingham, Alabama
Read Susan's Lung Transplant Story in the 1st Edition of Taking Flight

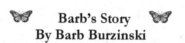

Barb's Story
By Barb Burzinski

The second time it occurred, January 2003, John (my husband) and I were in Monterey, California, on vacation. I was scared. I thought I had some serious heart problem. I was having difficulty breathing during a morning walk. That was not typical for me. I was active. At home, my girlfriends would tell me to slow down when we were shopping because I walked too fast for them. I never had a problem doing all of the house and yard work, and besides that, I was only 62.

After several visits to doctors and numerous tests, I learned that I did not have a heart problem. Our family doctor, Dr. Bruce Hyman, sent me to see Dr. Philip Sheridan, a pulmonologist. I had two conditions, chronic obstructive pulmonary disease (COPD) and emphysema. WOW! Why? I had quit my minimal smoking five years prior, and that was, only three or four cigarettes a day—and never when I was with my husband.

It was time for the exposure of one of the best-kept secrets of the past half-century. My husband had seen me with a cigarette only once, and that was before we were married over fifty years ago. Neither my son nor my grandchildren knew that I had this terrible habit. None of our friends knew, and only two or three of my very close girlfriends knew. Most were shocked when they learned that I had smoked.

Dr. Sheridan told me to use the oxygen about 16 hours a day, and throughout the night. I started with the small capacity portable liquid oxygen, and a year later I was using the Hercules Helios. To ensure we could travel, John ordered an extra tank of liquid oxygen and tied it down in the van; and travel we did, one trip to the West Coast, two to the East coast, two trips to Florida, two cruises and then the 'trip to hell.'

The 'trip to hell' was a vacation to the Big Island of Hawaii in March 2006. I got very sick. We arrived home March 15th, and the next day I did something that was never done at the Burzinski household. I felt poorly and I had John cancel our annual St. Patrick's Day get together. Twenty pounds of corned beef were put in the freezer.

It was back to the doctors, and it was then that I was told I had Pulmonary Fibrosis. That was five years after being diagnosed with emphysema and COPD. I was now living with three lung diseases. The only cure for pulmonary fibrosis is lung transplant. The next step was going to Loyola University Medical Center, Maywood, Illinois. Loyola rejected my case mainly because of my serious osteoporosis condition. They also mentioned my diabetes and my atrial fibrillation condition. When speaking to them, they also mentioned that I was too old for a transplant. I certainly did not think so! I then went to the University of Chicago Medical Center, Chicago, Illinois, and they rejected me for the same reasons.

John began researching the topic on the Internet—not only about the disease, but also about hospitals that had lung transplant programs. He discovered that Duke University Hospital in Durham, North Carolina gave the most information, and stated at their site that they evaluated high-risk cases. I contacted Dr. Mark Steele at Duke.

One of the requirements before being listed for transplant at Duke was entering a 23-session rehab program; each daily session was about four hours that included floor exercises, workout machines, weights, walking track and the bike.

My first call came on August 18th, but it was a dry run. The next call was August 25th, and this one was a 'go.' When the operating room personnel came to get me, they didn't give John much time to say good-bye, but he did deliver a letter from our granddaughter Alyssa. What a beautiful letter! The MAZE procedure (a fix for the atrial fibrillation) was also completed during my transplant.

Before I could leave the hospital, I had to walk a mile in one day—I was out of the hospital on the 11th day. I was 68-years-old, and one of the oldest patients to have a bi-lateral lung transplant. I was also told that my osteoporosis condition was the most serious of a patient that had been considered for transplant. Dr. Duane Davis, the transplant surgeon, had also had success with another transplant patient about my age. Our surgeries led to Dr. Davis stating that he was no longer considering age as a factor for transplant, but rather he is evaluating the individual. The last time I went for my check up at Duke, there was a gentleman who was 77-years-old and he had just had a single-lung transplant—and was doing quite well.

I did have a stent placed in the right airway where the new lung was attached. The stent was in place for three months, and now the airway has opened to about 60%. However, I can walk two miles and do five miles on the bike.

Prior to transplant, I was asked about my goals of living with a successful lung transplant. Other than the obvious, I said that I wanted to dance at our 50th wedding anniversary, and I did that. I wanted to see my grandson graduate from college, and he graduated from the University of Illinois last May. I'm not stopping there. I have two granddaughters who are continuing their education, and I want to see them graduate from college. I am now 70-years-old, two plus years out of transplant, and I love my life.

I thank you for reading my story, one that is probably not much different than most—except if it hadn't been for Duke taking high risk cases, I wouldn't have a story to tell.

Before signing off, I have to say that my husband John is 'God Sent.' Without his care, I would not be writing this story. My son nicknamed my husband 'Trapper John'—remember M.A.S.H? Anyway, he did it all. His care giving would be a whole other story. John, "thank you"; you are my love! I also send out a heart filled "thank you" to my wonderful family and friends, who kept me going with prayers and love, love, love.

Barb Burzinski, 70
Prospect Heights, Illinois
Pulmonary Fibrosis
Double Lung Transplant, August 26, 2008
Duke University Hospital, Durham, North Carolina

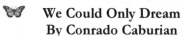 **We Could Only Dream**
By Conrado Caburian

I met Maribeth on 4th August 1994 on the Internet. I know a lot of couples tend to meet online these days, but back in 1994 it was different. The Internet wasn't as common as it is now. We met in our first semester at University. I was at one campus and Maribeth at another (about 40km apart). We had a friendly chat, and it started from there. I met her in person on August 8, 1994 (show's how eager I was). At that stage I had no idea on her medical circumstances. It was that afternoon that Maribeth explained her medical history. I was intrigued and interested to know more about what she had gone through and what she was going through at this time with her bronchiectasis.

From there our relationship took off. While Maribeth was able to walk to places, I was mindful that she couldn't walk long distances. I visited her often at her campus, to the point where I decided to transfer to her campus two years later.

During those years her health deteriorated. It wasn't an easy sight; she was getting worse. She had been hospitalized as least every year with pneumonia or infections. I visited her every day and would drive to the city to make sure I had transport to visit her in the hospital, and that I had a way to get home late in the evening after visiting hours (I lived about 1 ½ hours away).

It hit hard when she was told to start using a supplementary oxygen concentrator at home. We called it R2D2 (from Star Wars). We also had an oxygen tank in the back of the car in case she needed it urgently.

While Maribeth was on the waiting list, at her work, we would meet at the underground car park for lunch where she would put on the oxygen (as she didn't want to do it at work in front of colleagues).

On the evening of her transplant, I was at a golf driving range when the hospital called her to come to emergency ward as a lung was available. She called me and I felt weak. I was silent when I walked home and we readied her clothes.

That night was one of the worst nights of my life. The most difficult thing was see her get wheeled into theatre all bubbly and smiling, and the thought of not seeing her again, hit my family and I hard. We all started crying. We waited outside intensive care unit (ICU) for over seven hours until her surgeon told us she was okay and the transplant went well.

On the road to recovery, Maribeth recovered well. We were able to do things like travel around the world - something we could only dream about since I've known her. She also ran from one side of the football park to another. I caught it on video and it is a great moment in my life seeing her run for the first time in decades. She did have setbacks with hip replacements, but that didn't stop us doing things we've missed out for years.

Our life has been on the up since her transplant.

Conrado Caburian, Husband of Recipient, Maribeth Caburian
Maribeth Caburian, 34
Currans Hill, New South Wales, Australia
Maribeth, Bronchiectasis
Maribeth, Double Lung Transplant, March 19, 2004
St. Vincent's Hospital, Sydney, Australia
Read Maribeth Caburain's Lung Transplant Story in this Edition of Taking Flight

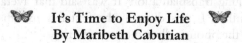

It's Time to Enjoy Life
By Maribeth Caburian

I would say my childhood started off quite normal. I was born in Manila, Philippines on October 6, 1975. By age of four, my parents and I migrated to Sydney, Australia, gained a younger brother soon afterwards. I went to school like all the other children, loved to climb swings and fences, sports, riding adventures with my bicycle. I was such a tomboy, always getting into mischief. I was a healthy and happy kid. I even remember being somewhat envious of my younger brother, Brian, getting so much attention because of his asthma. I too wanted to use the nebulizer! At the age of 10, my life totally back-flipped. From that moment on, my life was like being on a roller coaster. There were times when I went to hell and back. Somehow, through faith, determination, and the love and support from my family and friends, all the pain, heartache, and sacrifice is now a part of my history and has made me the person I am today. With a deep breath, I can finally say I am now living a life I once could have only dreamed of. I was given life three times. I was third time lucky.

At the age of 10, I was diagnosed with Chronic Myeloid Leukemia (CML). I went to hematology/oncology specialist at the Prince of Wales Hospital in Sydney, Dr. Marcus Vowels. I began taking medication that put me into remission for about a year. It then was time to have a bone marrow transplant. I was fortunate that my mother was a close match and became my donor. All I can say is this was the worst experience I ever had to face. I endured heavy radiation therapy and chemotherapy. After six weeks in an isolation room, I left the hospital.

My battle to breathe starts here. I was soon diagnosed with bronchiectasis due to; Graft-Versus-Host disease post Bone Marrow Transplant. The new antibodies from my new bone marrow started to attack my own lungs, thinking it was foreign tissue. I guess you could say it was reverse rejection. Anything that required breathing became difficult. Like others who have lung disease, it gradually got worse through the years when more and more lung infections further damaged my lungs. Stubborn like I am, I refused for any disability to hinder me from accomplishing my goals. I kept up with school and even graduated from the University with a Bachelor of Business degree. I scored a successful job and career with a leading financial institution. Got married to the best man in the entire world – Conrad, and built our dream home all before the age of 25. I was all set – except for the fact that I was now on oxygen 16 hours a day and slowly dying from lung disease.

My respiratory specialist, Dr. Frank Maccioni believed it was time for me to consider a double lung transplant and sent me off to St. Vincent's Hospital, Sydney to get assessed. At first, I was very hesitant about the idea of having a lung transplant. I had gone through so much in my life until that point. I didn't know how I could cope through another major operation. I was in denial of the whole thing. I went back to see Dr. Maccioni and confronted him with the most frightening question I've ever had to ask my entire life, "How long have I got to live if I don't have this transplant?" The answer I got was even more frightening, "two to three years". I thought okay, it's time.

I went through a lot of soul searching at this time. I read a lot of self-help books and inspirational ones such as the first edition of "Taking Flight". This helped me get some comfort that I was doing the right thing by choosing lung transplantation. It was said that average waiting time for lungs in Sydney was about eight months. It was difficult the first few months for Con and me; we were always on "edge" waiting for the phone call or the pager to ring.

March 18, 2004. We got home from work. I was struggling but still managing to work four days a week at this time. Con went off to the golf driving range. I'd just finished making pasta for dinner. While eating and watching television, the phone rang. It was the nurse from the lung clinic saying they had lungs for me. I called Con, who was on his way home, and at first he thought it was a joke.

My parents, in-laws and my husband were there to send me off, all looking very worried and trying hard to hold back their emotions until I was wheeled into the operating theatre. The last thing I could remember before they knocked me off to sleep was the most gorgeous blue eyes I've ever seen. I'm guessing it was the anesthetist behind that surgical mask. According to my family, I was in surgery for about seven hours. It didn't seem like that at all when I woke up in intensive care. The first people I saw were my brother and my husband. I had to ask if the surgery actually happened. I spent four-days in intensive care with the first two connected to a breathing machine. I had absolutely no sensation that I was breathing. The breathing machine did it all while I recovered from surgery. Still quite groggy, I tried to pull the breathing tube from my mouth by myself!

Recovery from the surgery went so well. I walked out of the hospital 11 days later, chest still sore from the surgery. I do regular exercise like Zumba! Travel, travel, travel!

Life is so precious. So much time to make up for. It's time to enjoy life and make the most of what my organ donor has given me. A life to live to the fullest.

Maribeth Caburian, 34
North South Wales, Australia
Bronchiectasis Due to Graft-Versus-Host Disease
Double Lung Transplant, March 19, 2004
St. Vincent's Hospital, Sydney, Australia
Read Conrado Caburian's Story in this Edition of Taking Flight

 Sharing My Story is Easy
By Charles Carpenter

I was transplanted on July 25, 2009. The first three months were rough. Besides my wife Linda, many others were very thoughtful and caring.

My wife Linda passed away a month ago. I am continuing to heal emotionally, and my health has never been better, according to all my doctors. I am back to my regular exercise program at the local Pulmonary Rehabilitation facility, and set new goals each week, 95% of which are reached! How does 30 repetitions at 220 pounds on a leg press sound? This week my target is 240 but we'll see. I use two other leg machines and two arm machines. I do 15 minutes on a bike/arm and a Nustep, which is also for arms and legs. Usually I walk a mile each time as well. I did the 5K walk, DAL – (Dead Ass Last) but I finished in 48 minutes, clock said 50, but I had to make a pit stop. I can actually see an improved upper body now and even losing some of my potbelly. Some of my jeans now need a belt to hold them up. But my weight remains pretty consistent so that is a good thing.

All in all, I feel great. Being able to do things that were impossible a year ago is magical. Being able to be Linda's caregiver was another blessing. Please do not take the above as "bragging", it is not meant to be that way. But I owe a lot to the team at New Lung Associates, and the Tampa General Hospital staff, especially those in intensive care unit (ICU), and Dr. Sheffield's team. Without all of these people, I doubt I'd be here today.

I must also thank the good Lord above us all, for his daily blessings, and my church family for providing spiritual help, meals for us, and other help. Through this period of time, not only has my health and spirits improved, I have also become a better person. I must mention my helping out here at OBC (One Breath Chat – Helping Lung Patients Connect) because not only do they think I'm a special person (really I don't know why), but they consider me a spiritual leader of this family. How amazing is that?

Many others have thanked me for my efforts at helping them and this community, but I'm no "hero", it's what I do now and costs me nothing while providing much satisfaction.

I will say one more important thing – I have zero time for any negativity anywhere, and if I can't turn it around, I'm gone. But best of all, I have no anger in me anymore.

For those still waiting for your transplant; believe that it will happen; we just do not know when God's plan for you will reveal itself. Just watch for the path He puts in front of you, as invisible as it may seem. Please be patient, and try to maintain a positive outlook.

Charles Carpenter, 66
Clearwater, Florida
Chronic Obstructive Pulmonary Disease/Emphysema
Single Lung Transplant, July 25, 2009
Tampa General Hospital, Tampa, Florida

A Light at the End of the Tunnel
By Chanin Carr

As a child, I was never considered sickly. Although I suffered from irritating allergies and often experienced upper respiratory infections, I was strong and managed to lead a normal childhood. I was a competitive gymnast for ten years, and then a cheerleader in high school, before showing any symptoms of lung disease.

At the age of fourteen, my health took a turn for the worse. I was first hospitalized in early 1994 with full-blown double pneumonia, which led to months of further hospitalizations with similar symptoms. By the end of the year, I finally underwent an emergency, open-lung biopsy. The results came back that I had a very progressive form of a rare, obliterative and inflammatory, small airway lung disease known as Bronchiolitis Obliterans Organizing Pneumonia (B.O.O.P.). This was further complicated by the diagnosis of Bronchiectasis, which results in repeated lower respiratory infections and eventually the loss of ability to move air in and out of the lungs.

Unfortunately, by the time my lung condition was given a name, my lungs were already irreversibly damaged. Additionally, the major surgery required to make my diagnosis, had also taken its toll on my weakened body. It took me months to recover, and at times it did not appear I would ever recover. But, with the help of my doctors, and many prayers from family and friends, I became confident that there would be a light at the end of the tunnel.

Because of side effects from treatment, and my lack of oxygen, I lost my hair and became too weak to walk. While most fifteen-year-olds were making the tough decision of how to style their hair, for their next high school dance, I was dealing with sacrificing my hair in hopes that I might be able to walk and be healthy again.

My decline was rapid, and soon my doctor was informing my family and me that I needed a double lung transplant. The idea of a transplant was very frightening to us, but we knew it was my only hope for survival. We placed our faith in God and decided to go for it. I was evaluated at the University of California San Diego Medical Center, San Diego, California (UCSD), and was listed in 1995.

On September 30, 1996, at the age of seventeen, I received my life-saving, double lung transplant. After the nearly eight-hour surgery, I was rolled on my bed into the intensive care unit (ICU). My many family members, waiting to see me, told me that I gave them the thumbs-up. Three days later, I was taken off the ventilator. And just one week after my transplant, I was placed in a regular hospital room, where I quickly was up and learning to walk again. My hospital stay lasted fourteen days, during which I experienced one bout of mild rejection. My mom and I then temporarily relocated to San Diego for the next three months, to be close to the hospital for my clinic appointments and physical rehabilitation.

During my time in San Diego, I completed the second quarter of my senior year of high school. After returning home, I graduated with honors alongside the friends I had started my freshman year with, before becoming sick.

Because of my transplant, I have been able to accomplish many things. I graduated high school, received my Bachelor's degree in Psychology, worked full-time, became an aunt, got married to my husband, James, bought a house, traveled overseas, and became a mommy to my son, Gavin. To honor and remember my donor, my husband and I even named our son's middle name after my donor.

I have led a very happy, rewarding life during my fourteen years post-transplant. I have had some complications, but nothing that remotely compares to what I went through prior to my transplant. Eight years post- lung transplant, I went into kidney failure, due to medication toxicity, and on November 17, 2004 I received a living, related, kidney transplant from my loving and supportive dad. I have since recovered from that transplant extremely well.

I will be forever grateful to my donor and his family, for their generosity and kindness, for making such a tough decision during an extremely sad time. I have now had my donated lungs longer than my donor had them during his much too short life. I hope someday I will have the opportunity to tell my donor's family how truly appreciative I am of them.

Chanin Leanne Carr, 31
Maricopa, Arizona
Bronchiolitis Obliterans Organizing Pneumonia/Bronchiectasis
Double Lung Transplant, September 30, 1996
Living Related Kidney Transplant, November 17, 2004
Living-Related Kidney Donor: Father, Ruben James Rodriguez
University of California San Diego Medical Center, San Diego, California
Son by Surrogate Pregnancy: Gavin Timothy, November 22, 2008

Amanda is Growing Up!
By Janice Caruso

Amanda was only four-months-old in April 1997 when I knew something wasn't right. Her subtle cough and poor appetite led me to the pediatrician. After an x-ray "just to be sure", we were immediately sent to emergency, and from there she was admitted for two weeks of testing, eventually leading to an open lung biopsy. A generic diagnosis of Interstitial Pneumonitis was given initially, which was just recently determined to actually be ABCA3 transmitter gene mutation. Oxygen therapy, steroids, and other medications were tried, with no success. It was a matter of only a few months until transplant was recommended. In November 1997, on her first birthday, we moved to St. Louis to await transplantation, which would be performed at St. Louis Children's Hospital at Washington University Medical Center, St. Louis, Missouri.

When Amanda was sick I worried constantly about her survival. When we decided on transplant, my fears changed. Initially, I remember being afraid that she wouldn't recover from the transplant, that she would reject the new lungs entirely. If she did survive the operation and her body accepted the lungs, I feared her life would never be normal - that her health would dictate and control her life due to medications, immunosuppression, and constant doctor visits. Boy was I wrong….

Since her transplant, at 17 months of age in April 1998, Amanda has enjoyed a childhood much like any perfectly healthy child. Amanda is almost 14, in ninth grade, and is growing more beautiful by the day. She is a high-achieving student in the public school system. She's an awesome dancer and gymnast, and was a member of the school's teams for both sports over the past two seasons. Drama is another love of hers, and she is performing in her third school production this year.

Yes, she is more breathless and tires more easily than other dancers, actors, and gymnasts, and yes, it is more difficult for her, but not so much that her determination and desire can't conquer these demons. True, there is the constant, ingrained awareness of hygiene and germ avoidance. It's all in a day's work, and all SO worth it!

Yes, there have been bumps in the road, including hospitalizations and illnesses. But we have been blessed with recovery and transcendence beyond these times. The experiences have given us the ability to realize that Amanda *can* get through illnesses, with God's blessing, and have thereby allowed us to relax our fears to a healthy level, from initial "post-transplant paranoia", which may have prevented her from illnesses, but would have limited her life experiences drastically.

I'm amazed by Amanda, and will always be awed by the gifts transplant has given her and us. The journey thus far has been entirely more positive than negative, and so much more than I had hoped for. I thank God, the doctors, and especially the donor family for our incredible blessings thus far and look forward to many more blessing's, I'm sure are to come.

Janice Caruso, Mother of Amanda Caruso
Amanda Caruso, 14
Webster, New York
Amanda, ABCA3 Transmitter Gene Mutation
Amanda, Double Lung Transplant, April 25, 1998
St. Louis Children's Hospital at Washington University Medical Center, St. Louis, Missouri
Read Amanda's Lung Transplant Story in the 1st Edition of Taking Flight

🦋 I Have Much Too Still Live 🦋
By Sandra Gallego Chiquillo

I have cystic fibrosis, and I was transplanted with my new lungs on September 1, 1997. I imagine that my donor was a victim of a car accident.

I still remember the operating room was so dark. I was in the middle of the room with a great light over, waiting for my new life, or maybe death. I've never been so scared—I wanted to run and leave, but I knew what I had to do if we wanted to get ahead—it was my last chance.

Suddenly, people started coming out everywhere—there were many. They were my guardian angels, protecting the people I was in the hands of—God, my donor, his family, doctors, nurses, and many people that made possible the miracle of life. I watched and felt like I was in another world.

The tears came out of my eyes. I told a nurse before I sleep, "Cogiera hand, your hand," without knowing anything, without knowing a name. The tears were for me a sedative, and I felt love, much love, and love of people who knew me, love of God. I felt fear, love…and home. (Cogiera is verb for 'take unconditionally')

In twenty-one days I was in my house, getting back to my life, doing aerobics, and for once did not have to worry about breathing. So for twelve precious years, in which I divorced and remarried; I learned much, and because after all, we are people with problems around the world, with the same failures and victories, and with the same dreams.

Now I have chronic rejection. I'm at 27% FEV1, but I will live because I am strong, and something inside of me needs to keep viviendo, living.

La conclusion, I feel inside me that I love people who I do not know. My life was saved, and there that day I learned that death and life are plucked by hand, and is a wonderful experience. What I like about my new life is how easy it is to do anything; going by public transportation, up hills, unwittingly walking down the street and nobody is walking ahead of me, or is faster than me—because before transplant, older women were faster than me. It is fun to do. I also meditate and talk to my lungs and tell them I love them, how grateful l am.

Since my transplant, I had the urgent desire to know where my lungs came from, who was my donor, what happened. I have asked, but I have not been told anything. Here in Spain, they do not tell you or share any information about the donor and their family. I feel it is unfair because for me, it is as if I fell into a well, and the well begins to fill with water, and I was going to die, but suddenly someone takes your hand and pulls you out of there, and saves your life. I do want to know whose hand pulled me out to live. My lungs are a miracle, a miracle with thanks to people who donate their loved ones organs so that we may live longer and be with our families, watching sunrises and sunsets, and enjoying things more—that means 'to live'.

I have two American friends, twin sisters with cystic fibrosis who have taught me much. Both are lung transplant recipients and are an example for all. I have to thank my American friends, the Stenzels, Modlin, Evans, and of course, my friend Joanne Schum who is writing this testimony for her wonderful book. Thank you all for coming into my life.

In my time since I have been transplanted, I have traveled, do aerobics and I remarried. Three years ago, I met the man of my life. We are very much in love, and want to live together for years. My experience with transplantation has not yet completed, there are many pages in my life yet because we have to face everyday life around the world, the problems at home, work, and also our poor health.

When I was little, my parents told me I would not live to adolescence. I have 36 years, and I have much still to live.

I would like to dedicate this testimony of mine especially to my husband Austin. He gives meaning to my life, and I love it.

Sandra Gallego Chiquillo, 36
Gvengirola, Malago, Spain
Cystic Fibrosis
Double Lung Transplant, September 1, 1997
Vall d'Hebron Hospital, Barcelona, Spain

Good Things Come in Two
By Kathi Novelli-Clapham

"I am Kathi person; not Kathi Cystic." My Mother had that printed on a pin for me some 39 years ago. Moreover, that was pretty much how my parents raised me. Cystic Fibrosis (CF), a genetic illness, did not run our lives; yet it was always hovering in the background now and then popping its ugly head out less we forget about it. Sadly, my family could never forget how bad CF could get. My siblings; John born in 1950 and Cecilia born in 1963 also had CF. they were robbed of their short lives and neither one made it to their 5th birthday.

Then in 1971 I was born, my Mother's sixth baby but only third one living. In addition, all the tell tale signs of CF were there. I was sweat tested shortly after birth; and the diagnosis was confirmed. Not much stopped me according to relatives. I was feisty and had a zest for life... especially laughing. I learned to take my pancreatic enzymes at the age of five. As I grew, I became more aware of what having CF could ultimately mean. Once after viewing a TV ad I saw, I ran to my Mom and said, "Mommy they said children with CF die! Am I gonna die?" She simply replied, "Do you want to die?" "No" "Well then you are not going to!" And that was pretty much how I lived my life.

My first CF exacerbation came at age 15. I went in the hospital for a two- week clean out or 'tune up' as they are commonly known in the CF community. When I came out, I was healthy as ever except for a cough that was ever increasing. Then I went away to college in Miami, Florida and claimed more responsibility over my health needs as I was now 'on my own'. I fell in love with the Theatre Arts and began acting on stage. At times, my disease would make itself known, but I was always able to triumph over it and pursue my dreams.

After college, I came home to Philadelphia and managed a family business during the day, while burning the night candle on stage at various local theatres. I had a wonderful system of doing my treatments backstage right before curtain and they would keep my health reasonable during my performance.

In 1999, I met my future husband Drew; we fell in love and were married September 2001. It was an awesome time, fulfilling my dream of finding a soul mate. Even my CF doctor was there to celebrate with us.

In July of 2003, another dream became a reality. I was pregnant and we soon found out there was not one heartbeat but two! It became clear it was no ordinary pregnancy, but we were determined to have our family. It was at this time that my Mother became seriously ill. My heart was breaking watching her suffer and ultimately she passed away in October 2003.

My son Paul Anthony was born at one pound, twelve ounces and Sarah Dorothy was one pound, nine ounces. Meanwhile, two weeks after their birth I went into a respiratory failure.

While waiting for my transplant I was blessed to have my little ones home and their curious spirits kept me happy and focused on the future. Yet, I felt like I was slowly dying while waiting for a life once more.

Then on May 29, 2006, after only 1 ½ months of waiting my call came. My husband said, "We should pray for the donor family." It was at this moment we were aware of how deeply another family was suffering while we were rejoicing in the chance of a second life.

I kissed my sleeping angels heads and we headed for the hospital. When my surgeon came out to inform my family that the surgery was finished, he told them they were "beautiful lungs, just beautiful!" He could not have been more right. I was out of bed in a day, and two weeks to the day, I went home. I completed pulmonary rehabilitation and I continue to exercise in a daily routine.

Life could not be better. I swim with the kids, chase them as they ride their bikes. I can read bedtime stories without even a throat clearing. We traveled to Disney World, and I walked morning, noon to night without a problem. One of my favorite things to do is speak on behalf of Organ Donation. I have told my story over and over to various groups and organizations so they can understand and make the decision to be organ donors. It is also a way of honoring my donor and his family. The love and courage shown by the family of my donor is unlike anything I have ever known. They agreed to save a complete stranger's life. They gave my family the greatest gift of all, the gift of me back.

Kathi Novelli-Clapham, 39
West Chester, Pennsylvania
Cystic Fibrosis
Double Lung Transplant, May 29, 2006
Hospital of The University of Pennsylvania, Philadelphia, Pennsylvania

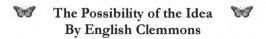

The Possibility of the Idea
By English Clemmons

Being born with Cystic Fibrosis means always having the thought of a double-lung transplant in the back of your mind. The idea is to push it back as far as possible. The idea is to do everything you can to not let it happen. The idea is always there, lingering in the words 'Cystic Fibrosis'. That means, when it does happen, you feel defeated. For 19 years that idea haunted me…and motivated me. I tried every hour of every day (not always happily) to push my double-lung transplant back as far as possible. Then March 2009 came. Hospitalized on the 5th floor, at Children's University of North Carolina Hospitals, Chapel Hill, sitting up tall with a smile on my face and an oxygen cannula in my nose, I was evaluated for a double-lung transplant. I was listed at spot number three for about three months. I stopped going to school. I stopped hanging out with my friends. I stopped living my life. I tried to teach myself to paint, and quickly realized I wasn't an artist. I watched a lot of TV and basically lived through the characters that were in the shows I watched. Three months is nothing as far as time to wait for lungs in the transplant world—I was incredibly lucky. However, you never know how long you are going to wait until the day comes, so every day feels longer than the last.

I have a 1909 Olivetti Typewriter that was given to me by a dear friend. When I get frustrated about life, about the hand I've been dealt, the only thing soothing to me is the sound of those keys when I press down on them. Those keys were even loud enough to drown out the consistent humming of my oxygen compressor. I love to type on that typewriter. Even when I couldn't make my legs take me from my car to my apartment, I could make my fingers type whatever was on my mind. I wrote the first six drafts of my donor letter on my typewriter. If ever there was an "out of the box" security blanket, that typewriter is it—my security blanket. Some people like to eat when they feel out of control, some like to run, some like to sleep. I like to type.

My birthday is May 14th. Last year, on May 14th, 2009, I typed a lot—random poetry, lists, stories…really anything that could be put into words. I know I wouldn't have typed as much if I had known that exactly two weeks later I would be wheeled into the operating room for a 7 ½ hours surgery, getting new lungs put inside me. It was the best birthday present I have ever gotten (my boyfriend has some big shoes to fill as far as gifts go). 7.5 hours, four pints of blood, and two lungs later, I was awake, attached to more tubes than I can imagine, and writing wearily on a white board trying to tell the people around me what it's like to breathe.

This is a frequently asked question when you're a lung transplant recipient, "What's it like to breathe?" After trying many different approaches, I have finally found the best way to answer this question. The feeling is like when you dive down deep in the water holding your breath, and then you attempt to shoot back up to the surface, making it just in time, and you inhale so vigorously and deeply that you can feel the air hit the bottom of your lungs; it's one of the most invigorating feelings in the world.

Lungs are pinkish-white, firm, like other internal organs, but not something most people look at and think "awe-inspiring." I do, and so do the people that love me. Sometimes it is hard to be the only one that observes the beauty in situations. It's not something you can ever explain to someone who hasn't climbed stairs with bad lungs. I have to remember that I see things a certain way, and that I have enriched vision because of it.

I am in college now, almost a junior. I am majoring in English and Economics. I am on the Model United Nations Team; taking dance classes, rock climbing, and doing all the things I never thought I would be able to do. I can sing along to the radio while I'm driving in the car now (one of my new favorite things to do). It's been almost two years now, and I have been so lucky in every endeavor I have put my mind to.

I love my new lungs; I even have a t-shirt that says so. Not only do I have a second chance at life (I am at a loss of words to describe that feeling), but I also feel like I am part of a special, selective club. Like after 19 years of being inducted, I finally have my letterman jacket. This club is full of stress, hurdles, pain, emotions, guilt, love, support, kindness, meaning, inspiration, and one experience that encompasses all of that. Would I ever choose to be part of this club? No. Would I ever give it up now? Not a chance.

My dream is to show the rest of the world how amazing this club is. These people, the ones I am lucky to call my peers, would inspire the coldest of hearts. This book is an amazing stride for us as individuals, but an even more amazing bound for us as a group. Our wisdom and experience came at a price, but I know I am better for it.

English Clemmons, 20
Cary, North Carolina
Cystic Fibrosis
Double Lung Transplant, May 27, 2009
University of North Carolina Hospitals, Chapel Hill, North Carolina

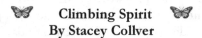

Climbing Spirit
By Stacey Collver

Unknowingly, I was about to reach the crux of my life. But I remember shedding only a few tears in the doctor's office on that fateful August afternoon.

"I have some good news, and some bad news," the doctor had begun. "The good news is that we have answers for you. We know why you're short of breath. You don't have asthma; you have a rare lung disease called Lymphangioleiomyomatosis, or LAM for short." He paused for a second, getting ready for his next announcement. "The bad news is that there is no cure for this disease, except to get a lung transplant. The average survival rate is five years past the transplant. I know that doesn't sound great, but without the transplant we expect you to live less than two more years."

"Two years?" I whispered in a feeble voice. I became numb, and shivered in my tank top, both from the diagnosis and the cold air of the air conditioning. Confusion set in. At 35, I prided myself on being in the best shape of my life, competing in rock-climbing competitions and coaching a beloved youth climbing team. I was also the president of a national women's climbing organization called SheClimbs, Inc. and managed a climbing gym for a living. Life was about rock-climbing and the pure joy of being physically strong and part of a community of friends. Terminal illness was a nearly incomprehensible concept for me.

By October 2003, I started using oxygen 24 hours a day (24/7). Daily chores were more difficult, and my mother, Laura Jeanchild, moved in with me to help me cook and clean. On my 36th birthday, I had a big fundraiser at the gym where I worked, Twisters Climbing Gym. About 80 people attended.

My friend Carolyn McHale started an international campaign called "Summits for Stacey" in which climbers obtained sponsors and climbed mountains in my honor. Members of SheClimbs, who climbed Mt. Washington, on Sept. 11, 2003, kicked it off. At the age of 20 months, my niece Sophia climbed the highest point in the country of Latvia, and soon after attained the highest peak in Estonia. Other peaks done by climbers included Stone Mountain, Georgia; Mt. Quandary, Colorado; Mt. Williamson, California; and Mt. Orizaba, Mexico.

I officially joined the waiting list at Stanford hospital for a single or a double-lung transplant. I also exercised as much as I could, to stay strong for the transplant. I climbed with friends at the gym, though my ability level started to decline. After attending a climbing seminar by Hans Florine, I started a game called, "Race to 10,000" in which the goal was to do 10,000 each of the following five exercises: push-ups, pull-ups, ab rollers, leg lifts and flights of stairs. I was very motivated, and practiced and recorded my exercises on a daily basis. While I was living on oxygen, I logged over 5,000 push-ups and over 1,000 pull-ups, but had a lot of trouble with flights of stairs.

By October of 2004 I could not stand up while I cooked, and used a stool to sit as I chopped vegetables. I invited my friend, Dave Allen, over for dinner most nights. Dave helped me in the evenings, and promised to take care of me for three months after the transplant, when the real call came.

I was starting to get depressed, because I didn't have the energy to do fun things and it was hard to be alone most of the day. Then the physical fear set in…at night. I was short of breath and could not sleep, even with the oxygen turned up full blast. I had trouble talking and laughing. I was dying. My lungs were failing, and I was at the end-stage of lung disease. Would I live to the transplant? One third of patients die waiting for their transplants. It was beginning to look grim.

On November 21st, the "call" came! My friends and family came to the hospital, and I was wheeled into the operating room at midnight. The surgery went very well, and I was making a strong recovery. In the intensive care unit (ICU), I could not talk because of the tube in my mouth, and I feverishly wrote notes to my friends, and waved at the doctors and nurses. On the third day, I could stand up out of bed, even with the myriad of tubes connected to my body. I was released from the hospital and lived with my mother and Dave at the home apartments.

Due to the excellent food provided by my mother, and exercise sessions with Dave, I continued to grow stronger over the next couple months. Each week, I could breathe easier, and go further and faster than before. In between medical appointments, Dave and I became obsessed with climbing flights of stairs. By two and a half months out, I was able to complete 100 flights in a couple hours.

Six years after the transplant, I again sit down to write about my experience. By now, tiny Netbook computers are popular, and I write my story in the comfort of a café. I am recovering from a transplant-related stomach surgery, and using these few weeks to write, plan and recuperate.

The extremes of emotion that I felt during the waiting period and the first year after transplant have settled. Back then, I swung from feelings of hope and despair, and back to hope again as my health and strength leveled off. In the first two years, I concentrated on my health only, and dedicated my time to efforts at the climbing gym. Much to my surprise, I eventually gained back most of my strength and was able to climb almost as well as before the transplant!

Some of the highlights of my life were attending the United States Transplant Games, as I dreamed of before the transplant. In 2006, I was thrilled to compete in badminton, and win a gold medal in my age group. In 2008, there was tougher competition, and I played harder, and happily took home the silver, losing to a ten-year champion. By 2010, I had trained hard, and was able to win the national title back! The Transplant Games were not only a fun sporting event, but also a chance to celebrate life after transplant, and honor our organ donors.

Today, I relax in this café all day, writing and getting ready to start work as the head coach of the Varsity Badminton team at Carlmont High School, Belmont, California. I am excited to lead the team this year, and I am carefully planning fitness tests and skill drills for the season. Life after the transplant is more relaxed. I have time for family and friends, and I have a budding new career. I move at a slower pace, but I feel more balanced.

The waiting game and the transplant experience turned my world inside out. It gave me a new respect for life, and for the people who showed compassion for me throughout my crisis. It taught me about humility, some broken dreams, and my own mortality. It was the worst of times, but in some ways, the best of times--at certain points I had never felt more loved. My recovery was a team effort of my mother, Dave and all my family and friends. The support from the climbing community was a warm surprise, and continues to this day. And through it all, I strive to keep up the climbing spirit and stay strong.

I appreciate the lessons I learned, and hope others can look forward to this second chance at life.

To check out the journal for the latest recovery news, Google: Stacey Li Collver and you will see, the Windsong Foundation site.

Stacey Li Collver, 43
Sunnyvale, California
Lymphangioleiomyomatosis
Double Lung Transplant, November 22, 2004
Stanford University Medical Center, Stanford, California

 "Ringing Phone?…Pick It Up!"
By Leon Cooper

I was diagnosed with Idiopathic Pulmonary Fibrosis in 2003. When diagnosed, the doctor figured I had already had it for about three years. I was the type to not go to the doctor for things, but I noticed a shortness of breath doing the smallest of tasks. My wife and I thought it was because I had gained a little weight (as we all do as we get older).

I was referred to Dr. Wynne, a pulmonologist in Gainesville, Florida; we tried different medications, but none worked. I was also put on oxygen and Continuous Positive Airway Pressure (CPAP) twenty-four hours a day (24/7). I worked in construction, and I really did not want to quit my job; so at first, I would take the portable oxygen tanks and 'drag' those behind me trying to do my job as much as I was able to. Finally, I was sent to Dr. Maher Baz at Shands Hospital at The University of Florida, Gainesville, Florida to get my name on the waiting list for a lung transplant.

One night our phone kept ringing. We had been getting prank phone calls, so at first we did not answer it, but the person kept calling back. My wife finally answered it, and it was Shands Hospital calling to ask us if I wanted a lung. We said yes and hopped in the vehicle to get to Shands. On January 12, 2004, I had my lung transplant. I was connected to the ventilator for about the first 24 hours, and then it was removed. Only two days in intensive care unit (ICU), and I was out of the hospital six days after transplant!

Before I got my new lung, I was denied time and time again for Social Security Disability. My wife wrote a letter to both the Governor of Florida, who at that time was Jeb Bush, and the President of the United States, President George Bush. Within two to three weeks we got a call at home from Washington, D.C.—it was the head of Social Security. He said the President had told him to call us, and we would have a check within a couple of weeks…and we did indeed receive that check!

About the second week home after I was discharged, the nurse coordinator, Melissa Kuhlmann, called and asked my wife what I was doing and how was I acting. My wife told her I was acting fine, what was wrong? Melissa told her that my labs had come back showing my glucose was 799, and I needed insulin in me right away.

I've had some problems with rejection; instead of doing the entire treatment in the hospital, they would put in a peripherally inserted central catheter (PICC) line and let us do some of the intravenous therapy's (IV's) at home each time. I was removed from Imuran, as Dr. Baz said that Rapamune might work better for me.

My lung transplant gave me a new lease on life. I can now enjoy times with my child and my family that I thought I would never have. It felt so good to no longer be attached to 'the leash,' my oxygen tubing, 24 hours a day. That feeling alone is worth a lot more than people can realize. I can now climb a flight of stairs without being out of air; I can walk to the mailbox without having to drag an oxygen tank behind me.

My passion is gardening, and I know I am not supposed to do that, but I take extra care so I can continue with my labor of love. I have been planting my flowers and bushes, and basically enjoying life to the fullest each and every day. I can get outside and mow my yard and plant some of my roses or lilies or fruit trees. I was never allowed to go back to work since the environment in construction may be harmful to my new lung. One thing I know is that if I had not had my lung transplant, I would be dead! My lung transplant has given me a chance to get closer to our Lord and to be saved; so once that day does come, I know where I will be going.

In 2009, I went into chronic rejection, and I hope to be placed on the re-transplant list. Re-transplant might be a sticky issue for me as I also have Stage 3 Chronic Kidney Disease (CKD), but I have learned that hope and faith in the Lord can make anything possible!

Leon Cooper, 54
Starke, Florida
Idiopathic Pulmonary Fibrosis
Single Lung Transplant, January 12, 2004
Shands Hospital at The University of Florida, Gainesville, Florida

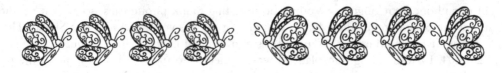

If Ever
By Bree Cordick

If ever I saw your grave
I would reach down and touch it
Oh no, you are not gone
You are right here
With me...

The words came to me as I lay in bed, as I knew they would, as I expected them to. On a dark, damp, cold, rainy fall night, as I lay silently, I thought of you, as I often did. Thoughts fluttered through my mind of the things I longed to say to you, to your family for what they have given me, and the things that I cannot say, that words simply fail to express.

I take a deep breath in. A deep clear breath. I hold it. I let it out. I do it again and again, over and over, the way one plays their new favourite song that they just cannot get enough of. It never gets old, the feeling, the rush of fresh oxygen spilling into my lungs and into my heart, racing through my veins to feed me the life that I once so longed for. Each deep breath my system craves. Each exhalation my body rejoices. My heart and lungs, my body and soul, feel like new lovers that just cannot get enough of one another.

It has been 13 months since my double lung transplant on August 7, 2009. How can I possibly begin to put into words about how my life has changed in just under a year?

After waiting for a painstaking 15 months on the transplant list, I finally got 'the call'. Ironically enough, that night I had gone to bed and realized that I would not be getting my new lungs before my 24th birthday, which was two weeks away. What were the chances that I would be well in that short amount of time? I sighed, closed my eyes, and drifted off into what I hoped would be another 13-hour sleep to squelch away the relentless exhaustion that chronically plagued me. And then...

The phone rang. It rang maybe four times before my dad answered. I listened for his footsteps, and soon enough, my bedroom door opened. "The phone is for you..." he said calmly.

I took the phone and was informed a pair of lungs had been found for me. I was asked how long it would take to get to Toronto General Hospital, Toronto, Canada, and my dad said we could be there by 2:00 a.m. I hung up, informed my mum and sister, and thus my new life began.

On August 7th, 2009, one call changed my life. One moment, one word, one shining time that had been anticipated for the last 15 months had finally come true. And I was on my way...

I was off the vent in two days. I spent two weeks in the hospital and went home on Friday, August 21 – two days before my 24th birthday. I actually did it. What seemed impossible wasn't, and it was my first birthday since I was 16 where I was 100% healthy.

So what was wrong with me? What could possibly ail a 23-year-old girl to the point of needing a double lung transplant at such a young age? Well, I had a condition called Bronchiectasis, a disease that is symptomatically a lot like Cystic Fibrosis (CF), but whereas Cystic Fibrosis is genetic, Bronchiectasis is not. Rather, it is caused by chronic and prolonged infections, which over time, scar and damage the lungs and airways beyond repair. It attacks the cilia – the tiny hair cells – that flush out and clear away debris that may invade the lungs. Instead, that debris stays in the lungs and mucus collects as a result of the irritation, and in return, that mucus is what causes the damage because it clogs the airways and harbours infections. Once infections begin, they do not go away, but rather, they spawn and become super bugs that are hard to treat. It is a vicious cycle. It depletes your lung capacity and in severe cases such as mine, the only option is lung transplant. Because Bronchiectasis is a progressive disease, it just gets worse over time, and because it is an infectious disease, both lungs need to be replaced. A week before my transplant, my total lung capacity was 21% out of a predicted value of 100%. I couldn't even brush my teeth and breathe at the same time. I was using five litres of oxygen 24 hours of the day (24/7). I had to lean over the counter and take breaks just to finish. Rolling over in bed at night left me gasping, as did putting on seatbelts and sandals. It was robbing me of any and all independence I had. Any scrap of energy I could muster had to be preserved. My body was dying in front of my eyes, but my mind remained as sharp as ever. I don't know which is worse: physically dying, the life slowly draining from your body, or mentally knowing you're dying, and knowing that although your body is on its way out, your mind is not ready to go.

But I was lucky...

I left that life behind me. My journey since transplant has been spectacular, and I have been fortunate enough to have no complications. I am more physically active than I have ever been, and nothing slows me down. Nothing leaves me out of breath, and I relish every moment that I have because of this beautiful gift I have been given. To know that in the event of my donor's death, their family cared enough to give a complete stranger the gift of life is something that I am so grateful for, and I cannot even begin to express how I feel with words.

Organ donation – to put it simply – is a miracle. To be restored surpasses any gift that one can be given. It is not just tangible, but it is also livable. It is a gift that you live, day in, day out, hour after hour, minute after minute…because without that gift, those days, hours, and minutes would not be possible. You live for yourself, and for your friends who were not lucky enough to receive their gift, or for those who simply did not survive; you pick up and carry on the journey where your donor left off.

So to my donor, and the friends that I have lost along the way of this transplant journey...

If ever I saw your grave
I would reach down and touch it
Oh no, you are not gone
You are right here
With me…

Bree, Cordick, 25
Guelph, Ontario, Canada
Bronchiectasis
Double Lung Transplant, August 7, 2009
Toronto General Hospital, Toronto, Canada

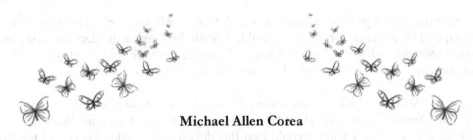

Michael Allen Corea

Organ Recipient 1997
Organ and Tissue Donor 2006
By Lynda Corea

As Mike's mom, I know the joy of receiving and the bittersweet joy of giving. I thank God everyday for loaning Mike to us for 22 wonderful years. He has made us all better people for having him in our lives. Now I will share his journey and my family's journey through organ and tissue transplantation and donation.

Mike was born full term on December 17, 1983. When he was four weeks old, his skin and eyes began turning yellow. He was diagnosed at five weeks with a rare liver disease, called Biliary Atresia, the lack of bile ducts in the liver. He had surgery to construct a common bile duct and an ostomy bag to collect the bile, which he had to drink in his special formula. Despite the success of the surgery, we were told to" take him home and love him", because he would die in six months. We cried and we prayed. Shortly we came to the realization, that instead of asking, "why us?" We should be asking, "why not us?" We realized we were not special and that God gave us Mike for a reason. He entrusted his life to us and we were going to do our best to help Mike live. Despite all the other times we were told he might die, he survived and actually, with the help of another surgery and medications, Mike had a fairly typical childhood. We decided early on that we would not treat him "special" and we would not overprotect him. He participated in many typical childhood activities: swimming, playing basketball, baseball, riding his bike, and going to camp. His low to no fat diet presented some challenges, but overall Mike accepted his life. We never used Mike's illness as an excuse and neither did he.

At age 11, his body outgrew his cirrhotic liver and he was placed on the transplant list. His health deteriorated during the waiting years. We actually prepared for him to die, because he was so sick and in and out of the hospital frequently. He wrestled with his own mortality and the concept of death and dying. He made out his will twice; because he was convinced he was going to die on the operating table. It was during this time that he formulated his philosophies of life and how to live each day to the fullest and to have no regrets.

Two years and two months after being listed, Mike received his life saving liver transplant. The hours before his transplant changed his whole life. When we received the call, Mike's first response was, "Tell them, no thank you, I'll take the next one". He went in his room and cried. He then informed us that he was going in his closet and would come out when he was ready. Two hours later, he came downstairs a different child. He announced to us that he was no longer afraid to die. He had come to terms with death and was at peace. He kept this peacefulness the rest of his life.

He was home from the hospital in one week and back to school in six weeks. Not a day went by that he did not express his gratitude for his donor and her family for making the decision to donate. Mike didn't waste a moment of his new life. He knew well how to make priorities and goals and he knew what was important and what to "let go". He wanted to live and make a difference.

Two years after Mike received his transplant, I was diagnosed with breast cancer. Mike was devastated, but I wasn't. I lived through Mike's challenging years and I watched him fight so hard to live and never, ever give up. I knew I could beat this disease and I did. Two years later, his sister, Jessica, was diagnosed with a brain tumor. She, too, witnessed her brother take medication everyday without complaints. She lived through his daily struggles with death and dying. It was Mike's inspiration that carried her through her challenges. She also is fine today.

Mike graduated from high school with honors and attended the only college he would even apply to: The Ohio State University where he Majored in Finance and was on his way to law school. He wanted to be a corporate lawyer and clean up the world. On the last day of finals, six days before attending his college graduation, Mike was hit while riding his motorcycle. It was not his fault and he was wearing a helmet.

I spoke with him after he finished his last final. He was, "On top of the world" and he was free. He was going to celebrate by eating his favorite meal, my meatballs, and then he was going to do his two passions in life: lift weights and ride his motorcycle. We got the midnight call that no parent wants to receive. We were told that Mike was in an accident and we needed to come to the Ohio State University Medical Center, Columbus, Ohio. His dad, sister, and I drove those two and a half hours to Columbus, but it felt like eighteen hours. When we got there, Mike was on a ventilator and they could not stop the swelling in his brain. We knew he was dying. The hospital staff was wonderful and constantly asked what they could do for us. Jessica had the presence of mind to request Ohio State University to deliver Mike's diploma to the hospital. Jess read the diploma to Mike so he could die a graduate.

We knew Mike was passionate about being an organ donor. The last thing he told us before he had his liver transplant was, "If I die, let them take anything they want so others can live". After he was declared brain dead, we mentioned Mike's wishes. We were gently reminded that organ recipients were rarely organ donors, due to medications, steroids, etc. However, Mike was almost on no anti-rejection medications and had not been on steroids for nine years. He was healthy and strong. In the end, Mike beat the odds and became one of a handful of people in the United States to be an organ recipient and an organ donor. He donated his heart, lungs, corneas, skin, ligaments, tendons, and long bones. In the midst of our sorrow and grief, we found peace in knowing we had fulfilled Mike's wish and had given life to others, just as life was given to Mike.

As we walked along our grief path, we decided that instead of being angry and bitter, we could best honor Mike by celebrating his life. We continue to do this whenever we can. My daughter and I share Mike's story when we speak for Lifebanc, the Northeast Ohio organ procurement organization. Mike's dad, Chuck, worked hard to establish an endowment fund at Ohio State for the Michael Allen Corea Scholarship for organ recipients and immediate donor family members. In the fall of 2009, we awarded the first scholarship to a woman who is a heart recipient. We have also established a scholarship program through Transplant Recipients International Organization (TRIO) in Cleveland and awarded several $1000.00 scholarships to organ recipients. Our mission is to give back for all the miracles that have been given to us.

A few months after Mike passed away, we received a letter from Barbara Roupe, the woman who received Mike's lungs. (You will find Barbara Roupe's story in this edition of Taking Flight also.) It was a beautiful letter full of love and gratitude for a gift that saved her life. We continued to write to each other (via the Organ Procurement Organization) for three years; always mentioning that we would like to speak to each other on the phone. Finally, the paperwork was all completed, and we were given each other's phone numbers and addresses. I will never forget the first phone call; we both cried. All I could think was, "Every word Barbara says is empowered by Mike's gift to her". We talked often and finally decided to meet.

I will always remember November 8, 2009; the bright, sunny afternoon when we met Barbara and her family. It was a wonderful reunion. We laughed, cried, and shared pictures and stories for hours. Barbara wrote us a poem, titled, "Michael's Gift", which resides in a prominent place in our family room. My daughter and I placed our heads on Barbara's chest and felt her breaths powered by Mike's lungs. It was one of the most amazing experiences in my life. It was then that I knew Mike's lungs had a wonderful home and they were no longer his lungs; they were Barbara's new lungs. We are all blessed!!

Lynda Corea, Mother of, Michael Allen Corea
South Euclid, Ohio
"Proud to be Mike's Mom"
Michael Corea: Liver Recipient
Michael Corea: Organ and Tissue Donor
Michael Allen Corea Passed Away, June 8, 2006
"Forever 22"
Barbara Roupe, Double Lung Transplant Recipient,
Read Barbara Roupe's Lung Transplant Story in this Edition of Taking Flight

Anya's Story
By Anya Crum

Anya, a young Virginia lady in her early 30's, has recently undergone a double lung transplant. She is the daughter of Larry Crum and Marion and Roger Pickenpaugh of Caldwell, Ohio. Anya grew up in rural Noble County and attended school at Bethel Elementary and Skyvue High School in Monroe County. After receiving a degree in Elementary Education from Marietta College, Marietta, Ohio, Anya taught in both private and public schools in the Washington, D.C. area for several years.

When Anya was just a few months old she was diagnosed with Cystic Fibrosis (CF). Anya has needed close medical supervision throughout her life. During her childhood she went through a 30-minute respiratory therapy twice a day. The treatment consisted of a mist form of medication that was inhaled into her lungs to help her breathe easier and prevent infections. Then her parents would cup their hand and pound (clap) her on the back and chest, to help loosen and clear the mucus from her lungs. Anya's CF also affected the ability of her body to break down and absorb food. It has been necessary for her to take medication her entire life before she eats a meal or snack.

Even with the excellent care her parents gave her when she was young, as Anya grew older, the infections grew worse and more difficult to treat. She was in and out of the hospital several times with infections that have led to serious lung damage. When Anya was in high school she was able to participate in cheerleading and track, but with the onset of the serious lung damage, just walking across a room left her struggling for her breath. With her deteriorating health, Anya was placed on the lung transplant waiting list where she remained for nearly three years.

On June 24, 2008, a pair of lungs became available, and Anya was transplanted from the generosity of an anonymous donor. After a month's stay in the hospital, Anya began her arduous recuperation that involved pulmonary rehabilitation and clinic visits twice weekly.

During her recovery, Anya decided to devote her free time to furthering her education. Though most of her income was devoted to paying her numerous and mounting medical bills, a determined Anya found the Boomer Esiason Foundation that accepted her application and provided her with a full scholarship to attend the University of Phoenix. Anya was the first recipient of the award given to a student at the University and graduated in April of 2010 with a Master's in Education.

As far as future plans are concerned, Anya is currently focusing her energies on training for the 2010 Transplant Games in Madison, Wisconsin. Running on August 2, Anya will return to her roots and participate in short distance sprinting events. Following the Transplant Games, she will resume her search for a career in the field of curriculum development.

Anya Crum, 35
Chantelly, Virginia
Cystic Fibrosis
Double Lung Transplant, June 24, 2008
Inova Fairfax Hospital, Falls Church, Virginia

Waiting to Breathe
By Barb Davern

For many years I struggled to breathe, but then one day I was given the "Gift of Life." My name is Barb and since I was a child I suffered with asthma and many episodes of pneumonia. Bronchiectasis was then a part of my life. At the age of 50 my doctors started telling me that I should consider a lung transplant. Of course this was way too much for me to think of at the time. Two years later my health took a turn for the worst. I was put on oxygen (O2) and sent home to survive as best as I could.

I was sent to University Medical Center, Tucson, Arizona for evaluation for possible lung transplant. I was still not sure that this was for me. I guess I just felt I was going to get better like I always did. My husband and I spent our 35th Wedding Anniversary going through all the testing needed to be listed. My son Brian's wedding was to be on March 16, 2006. I tried not to think of that call coming any time soon. March 12, 2006, a call comes in from University Medical Center. It is my coordinator Nancy, she says, "We have lungs for you. Can you be to the hospital in about four hours?" I am so overwhelmed I told her "My son Brian is getting married on Thursday". She tells me that I could go off the list until Friday after the wedding. I try to think, this may be my only chance again for a long time. I tell her "okay" we are on our way.

When I arrived I remember telling the wonderful nurse that I was scared. She said, "No problem that is normal. We will give you something to help." After that I don't remember anything until I woke up in intensive care unit trying to tell the nurse that the thing in my throat hurt. She comforted me with great love. The care I received in the next few days was wonderful. I gave all I could, to do all they told me. I walked as much as I could. The first week I had a slight rejection. Don't remember much of that either. As time went on I got stronger everyday. After about three weeks I was released from the hospital.

After transplant my sons and their families came to visit us as much as they could. It was great to have them around and see my wonderful grandchildren. That was the best medicine ever!!! Four months later, I returned home to Glendale, Arizona.

Life slowly returned to normal. Well I should not say that because before transplant, life was far from normal. The first thing I did was call the oxygen company to come pick up the three large O2 canisters from my home and threw away all that 50-foot tubing. I was free now. No longer tethered to that oxygen tank. Trips out with no more worry about getting home before my tanks ran out. Life was good. As time went by I felt stronger and better. I was in awe on how wonderful it was to be able to breathe.

My world is brand new to me now. I now am free to live in a world where every breath is precious to me. I sing in my Church choir, I have walked in a parade holding onto a hot air balloon, While traveling all over the country enjoying my family and friends it also meant visiting; California, New Mexico, Delaware, South Carolina, Ohio and Florida. I've hiked a forest, desert mountain trails, walked beaches and visited high altitude cities. I remember walking our capitals mall, two years ago and telling my husband, "This is what it is all about."

I now spend as much time as I can with Donor Network of Arizona. Volunteer work gives me great satisfaction and helps me give back to our state for giving me this wonderful, "Gift of Life".

Life after transplant is so amazing that there is no single word, sentence or story to describe it!

"Make Everyday A Great Day!"

Barb Davern, 59
Glendale, Arizona
Bronchiectasis
Double Lung Transplant, March 13, 2006
University Medical Center, Tucson, Arizona

 The Beginning of My Newlif95
By Paula Davis

I was diagnosed with a rare heart and lung disease when I was 22-years-old, called Primary Pulmonary Hypertension. At the time heart and lung transplants were unheard of. This was back in 1982.

At the time of my diagnosis they had told me that the statistics for this disease was to only live maybe three to five years without a transplant. I was lucky enough to hold on for ten years and was sent to Stanford University Medical Center, Stanford, California for an evaluation with the transplant team. They do not accept just anyone for their program. I had to see the team; the social worker and their psychiatrists, plus I had to have my family with me to make sure that I had a good support system.

In 1992, Martha the social worker informed me, that I had been accepted on the transplant list. I was instructed to go in and get my beeper. At that time there were no cell phones.

I forgot to mention that I lived in San Mateo, California, which was also a plus. Stanford was only 20 to 30 minutes away so when and if that call came it wouldn't be far to get there.

My wait on the list was long. Three and a half years. In early 1995 I started to take a dive and get sicker. I was on oxygen 24/7 and could hardly walk and get out of bed. My energy level was very bad and I was purple everywhere from the lack of oxygen my body was getting. On June 24, 1995 my husband and a friend had gone fishing and got home kind of late that night. We stayed up and talked a bit. I remember drifting off and then the phone ringing. It was now, June 25, 1995.

I remember waking up in intensive care unit (ICU) with that darn breathing tube down my throat and didn't like it at all and kept trying to pull it out. This was only about four hours after my surgery. I woke up and they were surprised. They had told Derle my husband, to go home and get some rest because I would probably be out for a while. Nope not me, I wanted that tube out. So the doctors said it was okay to pull the ventilator. Whew what a relief! I also told the nurse I wanted to talk to my husband.

Six hours after the surgery I am on the phone talking to my husband. He was amazed that I was awake and talking, which was a great sign. I don't remember a lot after the surgery, but a few days after they had me up and out of bed sitting up, and walking just a little. This was to get the lungs working and expanded and keep them from collapsing. In four days I was moved to what was called a step down to a regular room since I was doing so well. I was only in the hospital for 13 days and then was able to go home.

Here is a list of the medicines I have been taking over the 15 years. Prednisone (helps prevent rejection), Imuran (helps prevent rejection), Neoral (helps prevent rejection), Clotrimazole (helps prevent thrush in my mouth from all the meds), Azithromycin (treats/prevents bacterial infections), Bactrim (treats/prevents bacterial infections), Lipitor (lowers cholesterol), Lopressor (lowers blood pressure), Norvasc (controls blood pressure), Glipizide (controls my blood sugar), Advair Diskus (it keeps my lungs clear and my airways open), Flonase (treats nasal symptoms), Fosamax (prevents and treats osteoporosis), Calcium with Vitamin D, Magnesium, plus protein. They have been changed many times over the years.

I have had three rejections. Six years ago I developed what is called chronic rejection. The chronic rejection is not reversible and I was told that once diagnosed with it the life span is usually only three years. HA! It's been almost seven years and I am still here. I believe it's mind over matter and positive thinking.

I am very fortunate that I have had these extra years of life to see my son grow up. Derle and I adopted him when I was sick. He keeps me going. I made a goal after I had my surgery to hopefully see him graduate high school. I have two more years to reach that goal!

Also want to share that I did meet my donor family a year after I had my surgery.

UPDATE: Paula's family would like me to share, that Paula died, November 17, 2010, after writing her story. "She has touched so many lives with her story. 15 years was a great ride and we appreciated every extra day. Thanks to our donor family and to all her friends, and family members, for all the support through all the years."

Paula Davis, 49
Oakley, California
Primary Pulmonary Hypertension
Heart/Double Lung Transplant, June 15, 1995
Stanford University Medical Center, Stanford, California
Paula Passed Away, November 7, 2010
"Forever 49"

A Brother Speaks...
By Dr. Raja Dhar

A colleague, a friend, a confidante, a darling sister and my most difficult patient....blend all into one and there is Piali. I have known her just for a year now but thankfully calendar days have little to do with a relation as sweet as ours.

In the last few years she has gone through numerous upheavals, hospital admissions, bouts of coughing with sleepless nights, waking up bleary eyed every morning, ready to fight another day...a day of hard work in a hospital, where, there is no latitude because she was a sick girl striving to do her work to perfection. She thus developed a defense mechanism, which prompted her to put up a brave front and denied the very existence of her illness.

It was an intriguing situation. Here I was, a doctor who had just returned from the United Kingdom after about 10 years, fresh from my experience in one of the largest transplant centres in the United Kingdom having dealt with umpteen patients with cystic fibrosis (CF) and bronchiectasis. I was confident that dealing with a similar situation in India was going to be a walk in the park. Lo behold, I found this lovely feisty girl, with a 'never say die spirit', who could not walk straight for more than five minutes, and needed a wall to lean on with every few steps to catch her breath, but still would not accept that she was any different to a Susan, Dot et al!! She would cough her nights away in bed, stay up into the wee hours of the morning, but come to my chamber and ask me why I was not reducing her medications to a minimum!

It was an ongoing fight between the steroids she had to keep her asthma under control and the consequent lack of immunity resulting in numerous courses of antibiotics she needed (and still needs) to battle with the tough bugs in her lungs.

Gradually, we developed a relation, a deep bond, and I found a sister that I never had. It is a fine line we now tread.... a line where the demarcation between a patient and a sister gets blurred to a wonderful canvas of love, concern and affection.

I was the first doctor to tell her about her probable CF. Definitely not a very pleasant thing to do, but necessary for the sake of her health.

I can never forget the intense emotional turmoil she went through as I tried my best to lighten up things, while fighting my own share of grief. Little can I share with anyone the hard time I face trying to win over my worries each time she gets sick and admitted to hospital.

It hurts to see the emotional and social issues that she has to deal with beside her daily physical strife. Our country is still prejudiced against people with chronic illness. We expect the people around us to look 'normal'. Instead of going up and asking them about it straightforward, we stare uncomfortably at someone in pain, someone who needs support to walk, and someone in a wheelchair or with an oxygen tank or a feeding tube. The most wide-spread misconception about chronic pain is that it results from a psychological disturbance and has little to do with a physical cause and people with chronic pain should be able to tolerate pain better as time goes on. Often they are perceived as addicts, using pain as an excuse to obtain narcotics or secondary gains like sympathy or financial gain. Chronic pain often presents sufferers with a real "catch 22" dilemma. If they talk about their pain, they risk being labeled as hypochondriacs or even worse malingerers. On the other hand, if they hide their pain, others don't believe the pain is significant. It is enough to tax the patience of the most stoic person. Piali has gone through all this. People have told me that she has become a junkie, an opiate addict when she was trying to deal with steroid-induced osteoporosis and painful rib fractures.

Being her doctor, I try to prescribe her the multitude of treatments she needs to carry on and as her elder brother, I help her cope with stressful situations as best as I can. It is difficult to keep the balance at times but worth it every moment!

The future is a concern always, as we direly need to come out of the vicious cycle of infections, bronchospasm and weight loss. The first step would be to confirm her CF through a sweat test. Her bronchiectasis needs continuous aggressive management through medicines and chest therapies. It is surprising but sad that though these ailments are not very uncommon in India, often they are missed out and many patients succumb early! With her enthusiasm and concern Piali is keen to do her bit in raising awareness about these diseases and I encourage, support and guide her at each step.

Unfortunately, it will not be possible to reverse the lung damages already done but with continuous intensive treatment, I hope to slow down the progress of my sweet sister's disease. With her peripheral veins going bad, I advised her to opt for a Port a Cath and now she manages her own home intravenous (IV) therapies. To combat the weight loss, she may need a feeding tube soon. These procedures are not very common here, especially for young people and naturally there are plenty of fear and doubts. I am trying my best to break her inhibitions about tube feeds. A healthier body is better able to deal with bacteria and chronic lung infections and thus she needs a high-calorie, high-fat diet, which is vital to maintain optimal health. Exercise is also important for her as is rest and pacing herself. Like all CF patients, she needs to avoid unnecessary contact with people with contagious illness.

Piali is an adorable little girl with a captivating smile and innocent eyes that are bursting with the passion, and the promise to do much for the world around her. She is also a young girl living with a chronic lung disease that complicates an otherwise promising career and the very life that she so passionately enjoys. I hope my patient will adhere to a strict regime and manage to avoid the trials and tribulations related to a lung transplant. Even if she does need one, like so many of her friends in this book, she should be physically and mentally equipped with facing this challenge. I wish to see my dearest sister as a winner at each step, enjoying a life filled with hope and happiness and of course easy breaths…

Post Script – 'I write this with a very heavy heart. The demise of my dearest patient and sister happened about 4 months ago. She came into hospital to have a feeding tube inserted into her stomach (a PEG tube). She had not been eating well at all and lost a lot of weight. As a result she was ravaged by repeated infections and multiple prolonged admissions. Even her indomitable spirit was affected, doubts as to whether she would ever recover enough to pursue a normal life befitting a young lady. On this fateful admission she developed a stomach infection, which spread to the rest of her body. She fought tooth and nail but ultimately succumbed to the ferocity of her underlying illness. In her death, she taught the millions around her, who suffer from chronic debilitating lung disease, how to lead life to its fullest, smile in the face of adversity and to never give up. It also gave us a wakeup call to organize the lung transplant service in our huge country. It is a very difficult task due to the lack of an organized donor programme and infrastructure in our country. However, it is patients like Piali who will motivate us in getting our act together. I salute her spirit...her memory will stay with me forever. I miss her every-day. I just wish she was still with us....'

Dr. Raja Dhar
Pulmonologist to Piali Mukherjee
Apollo Gleneagles Hospital, Kolkata, W. Bengal, India
Read Piali Mukherjee's Story in this Edition of Taking Flight

🦋   **The Call**   🦋
By Lori Elizabeth Dietz

It was on the 23rd of May 2008, when my husband, Chris and I were sitting together in my hospital bed, watching the last movie in the Die Hard series, *Live Free or Die Hard*. My nurse interrupted us as she came into my room in the intensive care unit (ICU) at St. Michael's Hospital in Toronto, to say, "We are arranging your transport to Toronto General Hospital" Chris and I both stared at her, a bit confused, hoping that it meant that my new lungs had arrived. However, we had been told a couple of days earlier that I might be transferred as soon as there was a bed at Toronto General Hospital, Toronto, Canada, because if there wasn't one available when the lungs did arrive they would have to forego the surgery. That was a huge shock to us that, if there wasn't a bed in the ICU, the lungs would basically go to waste. Anyway, the nurse saw the confusion on our faces and said, "Oh, didn't anyone tell you, we got the call while I was on my break, they found you a match and you are scheduled for surgery at 2a.m.!" Luckily this also meant there was a bed available. This was it; I was finally going to receive the much-needed double lung transplant that we had waited so long for.

Chris and I looked at each other, completely shocked and yet so excited and happy. We hugged and kissed and cried! You see I had been tethered to that bed in the ICU, with numerous lines and machines attached to me, for about 25 days with the doctors telling me, "only a couple more days" for over three weeks. The long May weekend, and my 35th birthday, had come and gone, both of which we were all hoping would bring me my chance at a new life, but had failed to do so. When the call hadn't come by my birthday (just two days before) I started to lose a bit of hope. As it turned out, my time *was* running out. I was slowly wasting away, now down to 102 pounds from my regular under-weight amount of 120 pounds. As my husband wrote in his blog on the day the call came in, "Even though this is a major and complicated surgery, we are so excited to get it done and get on with her life. She has rarely gotten down while waiting, but did question how long she could survive in the condition she was in".

About a year and a half earlier, I was put on the list for a double lung transplant in Vancouver, British Columbia, Canada. My cystic fibrosis (CF), for which I was diagnosed at three months of age, had deteriorated to the point of end-stage lung disease. I had already been on oxygen at home for five years by the time we started the workup process. While waiting to be listed, I managed to contract a couple of nasty bugs. The first was the Methicillin Resistant Staph Aureus (MRSA). Intravenous (IV) therapy was done and I've never tested positive again for MRSA. Just as we got the results that we had beaten that, we found out that I had contracted the Multivorans strain of B. cepacia. *Burkholderia cepacia* is a bacterial organism that really only threatens the lives of CF patients.

Once listed, I was told by the Vancouver transplant team to expect to wait for about 1½ years but that it may be up to three years. However, 3000 miles away, in Toronto, Ontario, Canada, the wait time is four to six months. I will forever be thankful to Cheryl Nilsson, who being a CF patient requiring a double lung transplant around the same time as me, had decided to go to Toronto for her transplant, and helped to convince me to do the same.

While waiting, I had my share of worries; that I would maybe die while waiting, or perhaps during the operation or even in the first couple of weeks of recovery. I was afraid of leaving my six-year-old son without a mother and my husband without his wife. But I never let myself verbalize my worries; like by somehow speaking it out loud would perhaps allow it to happen. Instead, I made lists of things I wanted to do once I could run again or even walk without dragging an oxygen tank behind me.

And finally when the wait came to an end, we were so excited and thrilled. It was all good news: the operation was a complete success; no complications whatsoever and the surgery was done in four hours.

And that is when, on May 24th, 2008, the first day of the rest of my life began. I will forever be thankful to my friends and family and all the medical professionals that helped keep me alive while I waited. And to the doctors and professionals that were part of the surgery and recovery. But most of all I will forever be appreciative of my donor's family for allowing my life to continue in the midst of losing their own loved one. They may never read this, or realize that I am speaking of them, but I hope they do know that my family and I are truly thankful.

My life is fantastic now, better than I could have ever imagined! My recovery in hospital was only 3½ weeks, after which I returned to the townhome we were renting in the greater Toronto area. I needed to continue rehabilitation at the hospital three days a week for the next two months. At about eight weeks post surgery I was able to take my first airline flight since the surgery and we traveled to the Canadian Atlantic Provinces for a short six-day holiday. On August 28th, after my rehabilitation was done, we were able to return home to Vancouver, to my family and friends. Jace, my son, was able to return to his school just in time for the start of Grade 2 and Chris was able to go back to work. In December our entire extended family took a trip to Puerto Vallarta, Mexico for my new life celebration.

Now, I am able to volunteer at my son's school, both on the Parent Advisory Council and in the library. I have also been able to start my own at home business with Mona Vie. I am thrilled to say that my exercise tolerance is better than it has ever been in my life and I am truly very blessed to be able to be here, raising my son and living an amazing life.

For a more in-depth and personal account of this journey, I am writing a full-length book to be published in the near future. Please keep an eye out for it, being penned under Lori E. Dietz.

Lori Elizabeth Dietz, 37
Maple Ridge, British Columbia, Canada
Cystic Fibrosis
Double Lung Transplant, May 24, 2008
Toronto General Hospital, Toronto, Canada

A Precious Gift...
By Jennifer Dorman-Kaltreider

I was diagnosed with Primary Pulmonary Hypertension (PPH) in June 2006. That day changed my life forever. I thought I would just take some medicine and get better and go on with my life. Boy was I wrong. PPH is a rare life threatening disease where the lungs have high blood pressure and it affects the right side of your heart.

My doctor took me out of work; I was a nursing assistant for eleven years. I received a drug called Flolan, continuously infused. Flolan is the best thing they have to help better the quality of life in PPH patients. I was on that for a little over two years and felt a lot better but then I started getting a lot of fluid retention. They wanted to switch me to Remodulin another PPH drug, which only lasted for about four months because my PH was getting worse and I was admitted to the hospital for about a week every month for fluid retention. They would pull about 25–30 pounds of fluid off each time I was in. My breathing was getting worse to where I couldn't take more then 10 steps and I had to stop and sit.

My Grandmother had just come home on hospice care; they said she had about two weeks left. Our family had just found out she had lung cancer and I wanted to spend as much time with her and help her as much as I could. So I was happy to be out of the hospital.

My Grandmother passed away. But, I was admitted for my kidneys failing and I missed her funeral. My Grandmother was buried on February 25th. I was sitting in my hospital bed waiting for my husband. My phone rang it was Dr. Park she said, "Jenn we have a match for you." I just started crying and she was crying. The next morning, I was getting all my kisses and good luck wishes from my husband Tommy, and friends Cathy, Angie, Dave and Vito before I was taken to the operating room. Dr. Bartley P. Griffith (my lung surgeon) came out to talk to my family after surgery and said that I was doing fine.

Some complications made me feel like I was taking two steps forward and three steps back, but I was finally on my way to recovering. I started working with the physical and occupational therapists and eventually started walking again. Never knew how hard it was to do that.

I am seven months out and doing great; except for a few admissions for rejection and infection. I couldn't ask for anything better than to wake up everyday being able to breathe, spend time with my family and friends and doing things on my own again. I wouldn't have made it through without my husband, family, friends and medical staff that I had supporting me through all of this. I want to thank all of you from the bottom of my heart.

All the prayers and blessings people had said for me, thank you. Thank you God for helping me through this and giving me more time to be here. My attitude towards life has changed in a big way. I am grateful everyday I wake up. I smile and say, "Today is going to be great." I am most thankful for my donor and their family, there is not a day that goes by I don't think of you, and you are part of my family now. You are my true hero. I wrote to my donor family but have not heard anything back. I hope to hear from them one day.

I want to mention my great team of doctors; if it wasn't for their passion and dedication I would not be here today. Thank-You: Dr. Myung Park, Dr. Gautam Ramani, Dr. Aldo Iacono and Dr. Bartley Griffith.

What does the road ahead of me hold?? I am not sure but whatever it is, I am not going to waste a minute of it.

Jennifer Dorman - Kaltreider, 31
Baltimore, Maryland
Primary Pulmonary Hypertension
Double Lung Transplant, February 26, 2010
University of Maryland Medical System, Baltimore, Maryland

🦋 Make Everyday a Celebration 🦋
By Gina Douglas

My name is Gina Douglas. I am 46-years-old. I have been married 25 years and have two children; Amber who is 20-years-old and Eli who is 10-years-old. I live in Thomasville, North Carolina. The following essay is written to give thanks to my God, friends, and family, as a celebration of life.

I was diagnosed in 2003 with Bronchiolitis Obliterans a lung disease which in my case was thought to be brought on by rheumatoid arthritis. I was referred to Duke University Medical Center, Durham, North Carolina. Meanwhile, my family, friends, and church family began to pray.

I was on a ventilator and weighed 83 pounds when I received my transplant on March 23, 2005, after being on the active waiting list for only eight hours. Once I had those new lungs things improved rapidly.

In 2009 my doctor told me that due to chronic rejection there was nothing else to do but list me again for a second lung transplant. That was quite a blow for our family. We all had enjoyed five wonderful years and felt like all of the major surgeries were behind us. Once again I will say that it is the power of prayer and the Lord blessing those doctors at Duke with their abilities that has brought me to where I am today.

My prayers were most definitely answered because I lived each day having a peace about what the future held for me. I often thought of the verse from Jeremiah 29:11. "For I know the plans I have for you declares the Lord, plans to prosper you and not harm you, plans to give you hope and a future".

Before receiving "the call" I had five dry runs. I was on the active waiting list for one month to the day when I had my second lung transplant, which was on February 23, 1010.

I would also like to bring out some the positive similarities of the two surgeries. All of these I consider huge blessings from God. In both situations I have had a fantastic support system of a wonderful family and a church family that prays for all of us, and I have three pastors that we know personally who have supported, loved and prayed for our family. In addition I have wonderful coworkers and two best friends.

At this point I am trying to live each day for everything that it is worth, taking care of myself and living as stress free as possible. There is not anyone who is guaranteed tomorrow, so make everyday a celebration and a time to count your blessings and give praise. That is what I intend to do.

Gina Douglas, 46
Thomasville, North Carolina
Bronchiolitis Obliterans
Double Lung Transplant, March 23, 2005
Re-Transplant, Double Lung Transplant, February 23, 2010
Duke University Hospital, Durham, North Carolina

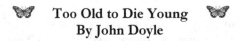

Too Old to Die Young
By John Doyle

It all started when I was a child. I was diagnosed as having a weak chest, which was later to be labeled 'asthmatic'!

My chest condition became much worse as the years progressed. I did however manage to work for a living as surveyor for a large national company and covered an area which took in the whole of Devon and Cornwall, Somerset, and Wiltshire, Avon and Gloucestershire, United Kingdom; right up until July 1992. This is when I experienced extreme difficulties with my breathing. My chest consultant told me that I had developed emphysema due to smoking, even though I hadn't smoked since 1984.

1998 I was diagnosed as having Alpha-1 Antitrypsin Deficiency, the next most common deficiency after cystic fibrosis. This put a whole new light on my prognosis. I was added to the waiting list for a lung transplant. It was Sunday 10th December 2000, Harefield Hospital in Middlesex, United Kingdom, when I received my lung transplant. Within days the ventilator was removed and my recovery was well on the way. I was released from the hospital to return home, the day before my birthday no less, what a birthday present!

In September 2001, I joined other transplant patients in the annual Harefield Jog. I managed to walk 10½ miles and won the cup that year for the furthest distance of any transplant patient, I had sore feet and lost two toenails but I managed to raise over £800 in sponsorship, it was a great sense of achievement for me as pre-transplant, I couldn't walk a hundred yards!

I am in my tenth year post transplant and doing quite well. I am still very positive in my attitude and hope to survive a good many years yet. I take regular exercise by way of walking and try to do three to four miles daily.

I also have a strict regimen for taking my medication which is documented daily along with my weight, temperature, and spirometry, and regularly attend my general practitioner (GP) to review my drugs: frequent blood tests are required to check the levels of my immune-suppressants to make sure that I stay at the therapeutic level; all part of a routine that I am used to living with.

Having a transplant has completely changed my life and given me the opportunity to pursue activities that prior to transplant would be impossible. I have traveled to Europe, and the United States of America. My whole life is busy and every day is filled; a couple of years ago I had a falconry day, something that I'd always wanted to do, it was amazing!

I also am a founder member of an Alpha-1 support group serving on the committee as Secretary /Treasurer. Both last year and this year I am organizing an annual get together for our members, this event will spread over two days and attracts about 35% of our total membership. (You can find the group online – Alpha 1- UK Support Group.)

There is so much more to tell, I have tried to keep it brief. Hopefully I can be an inspiration to those considering or awaiting transplants, I can highly recommend it!

In closing, I am forever grateful to my lung transplant surgeon, Professor Magdi H. Yacoub, Fellow of Royal Society (FRS).

Update: February 24, 2011, John E. Doyle, Jr. contacted me to let me know that his father passed away on January 24, 2011. "Dad worked relentlessly to make people aware, and wherever possible comfort and support them however he could. It was the motor neurons disease that got the better of him in the end. Here ends the life of a most beautiful giant of a man. John Edward Doyle, Sr."

John Doyle, 68
Plymouth, Devon, United Kingdom
Alpha-1 Antitrypsin Deficiency
Double Lung Transplant, December 11, 2000
Harefield Hospital, Middlesex, United Kingdom
Read John's Lung Transplant Story in the 1st Edition of Taking Flight

My Ship, You Finally Came In
By Sandra Johnson Driste – MacDonald

It was a beautiful June evening as I was preparing myself mentally and physically for another vest/respiratory lung treatment. This was my fifth treatment of the day, each treatment lasting slightly an hour. I swallowed the Demerol pain pills my body required to endure the pain from my chest vibrating, and all of the coughing that the regiment caused, in order to help me expel all of the mucus out of my lungs. It was very exhausting and so I prayed before each therapy session, for strength from God. He was always providing me with what I needed to get through a day in late stage Cystic Fibrosis.

I had just buttoned up the lifejacket-like device that I wore for each treatment, when suddenly my phone rang. I jumped, my heart started racing and a surge of panic and thrill cursed through me simultaneously, as had been the case for the last 12 months, every time the phone rang. Was this the call I had waiting and fighting for, in the past year? Or, maybe the call I had been praying for all 27 years of my life?

On the other end of the phone was a transplant nurse coordinator calling to tell me they believed they might have a pair of lungs for me. I started to shake and feel disbelief that this was indeed the call of anticipation. I had a false alarm just two weeks earlier; however, I was very confident and full of faith.

I notified family and friends and we traveled down to the University of Minnesota Medical Center Fairview, Minneapolis, Minnesota. It was June 20, 1994. Once put in a room, more family and friends arrived, more so than I had expected and the nurses began to refer to my guests as the "Sandy Johnson Entourage." It was such a warm feeling in that room and it felt so reassuring knowing all these people were there for me. I have never felt so loved in my entire life. The nurse told me they were ready for me. This was it. Each person in that room, all 20 of them, came to me to hug me, tell me they loved me, or to tell me that everything was going to be okay. I believed them.

Later, the surgeon came out and told the "entourage" that the surgery was complete, and there had been no complications and both lungs were working on their own. From what family and friends told me, everybody clapped, cried, hugged and thanked the surgeon. They were advised to head home and get some rest as I would likely sleep for about 12 hours. It turned out, however, that I was awake after six hours. I was in pain, but it was a "happy pain." I knew something incredible had happened despite the fact that I was still on a ventilator...my fingernail beds were pink; a gorgeous, rosy shade of pink. For several years, my finger and toenails had been blue to lavender from the oxygen-deprived blood that had been cursing through me for so very long. My sister Julie commented first on the fact that my lips were pink. They had been blue as well. It was so thrilling and so exciting and such a miracle from my dear Heavenly Father.

The evening progressed and more and more people came to visit and I was feeling giddy. Early the next day, they removed the ventilator and by noon, I was out of intensive care and in a regular room. On day three, a physical therapist came to get me up and exercising. What? Exercising? I was hooked up to so many tubes, wires, cords, and I wasn't planning on being tortured so soon after a bilateral lung transplant (two lungs). But the therapist was determined. We went for a walk and she asked me questions about family, pets, my job and I answered her and asked her questions in return when suddenly the most amazing reality hit me: I was able to walk and talk at the same time with no shortness of breath. Once I realized that, I just wanted to walk all day.

Physical therapy intensified quickly and soon I was riding the exercise bike, walking on the treadmill and for those who know me, talking...a lot. On day five, respiratory therapy came in my room and told me it was time to get off the oxygen I was still using. How could I? I needed it. It was my safety, and security, and I refused to give up my oxygen to a therapist who also had grown to become a very special friend. So, she backed off a bit. That evening as soon as my parents got arrived to visit, I asked them to go for a walk. We walked many hallways and covered a lot of area and I dragged the oxygen tank with me the whole time, because I was adamant that I still needed to use oxygen. When we got back to my room, I was going to shut off the oxygen tank and was startled to find that the oxygen had never been turned on in the first place. I felt fine, my lips and fingers were still pink. It was true: I no longer needed that oxygen. That was one of the biggest milestones in my recovery. I could not have been happier. As much as I depended on the oxygen, I hated it passionately.

After two weeks, I was released from the hospital and headed home. Who would have thought that you could have a lung transplant, and be home in two weeks? It actually felt strange to be able to breathe without having to concentrate on it or struggle to grasp a little oxygen. I could go up and down the steps in our split-entry house without assistance and without thinking twice. The huge liquid oxygen tanks were out of my bedroom and out of the house and I no longer had to spend several hours per day doing lung treatments. I was full of energy and really did not just feel like a new person, I was a very different person thanks to my Heavenly Father working through my donor family and my precious new lungs.

I started walking and cleaning. I would be up by seven in the morning ready to start the day, and I would go out for a power walk. Distance didn't matter anymore and I could walk at a good clip. I know my transplant was the reason for my ability to mosey around the neighborhood, a suburb of Minneapolis, but it was also an emotional feeling of excitement just because I could walk without fatigue or shortness of breath. It was so amazing. I could not believe that it was I, sick Sandy Johnson doing these things. I was so thrilled. It was almost surreal.

In addition to the walking, I was the cleaning. I lived with my parents at the time, and our house was already a clean house, but housekeeping became a hobby and I dusted the furniture, vacuumed, scrubbed bathrooms, did laundry every day and also cleaned out drawers, closets, and cupboards. I loved doing it and my mother did not mind coming home to a clean house everyday either. To most, cleaning like this probably does not sound like a lot of fun, but to me it was just a miracle that I was able to do all of that; and that I was able to use my new lungs any way possible. It was the most awesome feeling to be accomplishing something.

Additional activities I was able to participate in after my transplant included going to my boyfriend Brett's softball games, going shopping for hours at the Mall of America, traveling to places like San

Diego, Cozumel, and Jamaica, heading to the Metrodome to cheer on the Minnesota Vikings and Twins on many different occasions.

I am so happy and so very thankful for my transplant. I was unable to do any of the above prior to my surgery, which gave me my second chance at life. I enjoyed the things that I was doing, but I wanted to do more. I was not able to go to college previously, so I started looking at colleges I might attend, but my college plans got put on hold when I got the shocking news that I was going to have a baby. Yes, a baby! I always dreamed of having a child, but never thought it would actually happen. The news stunned Brett, my child's father, and even more so, my medical team. I was terrified that the anti-rejection medications I was on would harm the baby, but the Obstetrics/ Gynecologist (OB/GYN) I was referred to a high-risk pregnancy doctor who told me that I had as good a chance of having a healthy baby as anybody else. By the time I found out that I was pregnant, I was already 12 weeks along. I cannot describe my feelings, other than to say that I was completely in love with the tiny baby living and growing inside of me. Not only were my new lungs saving my life, they were making it possible for me to create new life. Thank you Jesus!

My pregnancy was pretty uneventful, and on March 31st, 1995, Jared Michael Driste was delivered by Cesarean section. He was a healthy baby boy. He brought so much joy and happiness to his father and me, and I just continued to thank God for what He had done in our lives through organ donation. Brett and I married soon after Jared's birth and I was more than thrilled about being a wife and mother. In the fall, I did go back to school, and received my Associates of Arts degree in June of 1998. I was four years post-transplant and sometimes I still could not fathom all the amazing things that I had been through. Life was so wonderful. Then things took a sudden and tragic turn. On October 15th, 1998, my husband died unexpectedly at the age of 32. He had a benign tumor in the stem of his brain.

Today, my life is good. I finally graduated with a Bachelor of Arts (BA) in Psychology in August 2002. I was surviving my loss as best I could, and in January 2009, I remarried. His name is Kent MacDonald, and he is a wonderful man. In June of 2010, I celebrated 16 years with my new lungs, my transplanted lungs. Overall, I am doing amazingly well as is my "baby" who will be 16 in March, and as I promised, I have been there for him.

I have not forgotten how fortunate that I have been. I thank God everyday for my lungs, my successful surgery and transplant, and my donor family. Written in loving memory of Berta, my donor, who continues to breathe through me.

Save a life. Please be an organ donor.

Sandra Johnson Driste-MacDonald, 43
Coon Rapids, Minnesota
Cystic Fibrosis
Double Lung Transplant, June 21, 1994
University of Minnesota Medical Center Fairview, Minneapolis, Minnesota
Sandra had son Jared, after her lung transplant – March 31, 1995

Nothing But Blue Skies
By Jeri Dubois

I opened my eyes and while trying to focus, looked around the room. I noticed family and friends surrounding me, and what seemed like the brightest sunlight I'd ever seen, streaming through the window. As I lay there and realized the magnitude of what I was waking up from, I sighed with relief that I was still alive.

Reflecting back on my life, I know that I am very lucky to be here today. Growing up I had a normal childhood. I climbed trees with my friends, played sports with my peers, learned how to drive and graduated high school. I was just a little different than the other kids. I would run out of breath easily, had curved shaped fingernails and toenails and was always sick to my stomach. My skin would get extremely salty when I would sweat and I was a constant cougher.

In the 5th grade my attendance started dropping due to frequent illness. At the age of 19, I had to have major surgery to have part of my intestines removed due to them being twisted. What I didn't know at the time was my surgeon had told my physician's assistant (PA), that I had a chronic lung disease and needed to be seen by a lung specialist. This is something my PA did not share with me, and a lung specialist didn't come into the picture until years later when I almost lost my life for the first time.

In 2000, due to many stomach issues and the loss of 42 pounds in just six months, my doctor tagged me as being a hypochondriac. A lung specialist in the hospital was 95% sure I had Cystic Fibrosis.

Never hearing of Cystic Fibrosis, I went home to do some research. I was shocked to see my entire life flashing in front of my eyes. One week later I was sent to Oakland Children's Hospital, Oakland, California, for a sweat chloride test and in January 2001, at the age of 24, received my diagnosis of Cystic Fibrosis. The emotions were running high that day, but I must say that relief was the biggest emotion of all.

I was sent to the University of California San Francisco Medical Center, San Francisco, California (UCSF) for treatment at the Cystic Fibrosis clinic. Immediately I was started on treatment and was told I would need to start evaluation for a double lung transplant. At that time under the old lung allocation system, it was a first come, first serve basis and approximately a two-year wait. My doctor was so amazed that I was even alive, he was certain I would not make the two-year wait. Not to mention the time it took to be evaluated. Only one week after enzymes, antibiotics, lots of medications and two liters of oxygen with sleep, I was packing on the pounds and feeling better already.

2003 I was deemed too healthy to need a transplant and was removed from the list. In 2005 my health started to decline again. I was placed on oxygen 24 hours a day and started having bile duct issues in the liver.

I checked into the hospital in 2008 due to very low FEV1, and by this time I was coughing up 1/2 cup of blood daily and on eight liters of oxygen. Luckily under the new allocations, transplant was based on a score. Kind of like whom needs the organs more type of thing.

My doctor started fighting for me to get a double lung and liver transplant. At that time there were only about 25 that had been done in the United States and it had never been attempted at UCSF.

Our youngest daughter was about to graduate high school and our oldest daughter, living clear across the country, had just given birth to our 1st grandchild. Knowing that the longer I waited or even if my transplant didn't take, there were so many parts of their lives I was going to miss out on and didn't even know if I would ever get to meet our grandson.

Three days after being listed, when my daughter and grandson were visiting, I got "the call". Shock was the only way I can describe the way I felt at that moment. When they wheeled me into surgery I was surrounded by my entire family and the fact that our daughter and grandson were here with us was priceless. I knew at that moment that even if I didn't come out of that surgery, I had lived a full and rich life surrounded by tons of love. After I woke up from my 15-hour surgery, I was walking 12 hours later and off oxygen the next day. I had minimal complications and was released from the hospital 14 days later. For the next six weeks we rented an apartment in San Francisco. During that time I was going to the gym and walking three miles a day. They let me move back home just one day before our daughter graduated high school.

I am here writing this story 1 ½ years later with my lungs and liver in great health. I have had a good run so far with no infection or rejection. The many complications I have are strictly from the immunosuppressant drugs.

Since my transplant I would love to say that I am out there changing the world, but right now I am trying to find my nitch. I have several realistic goals set for myself in 2011 and hope to follow through with all of them. I am now able to do the things I love with great ease such as attending sporting events and throwing gatherings with all of our friends. The most important thing is that I am here with my family & friends. To see our daughters go to college, and watch them grow into the wonderful young ladies they have become. I am excited to see our grandson grow up and am happy to announce that we are expecting a granddaughter in May of 2011.

There are many people I would like to thank for helping me through this process. First and foremost is the young man that made the choice to become an organ donor. I owe him my life and hope one day, to find out more about him; Dr. Mary Ellen Kleinhenz - CF Director, Dr. Charles Hoopes -Lung Transplant Surgeon, Dr. Christopher Freise - Liver Transplant Surgeon also; Kacie Maben, Joe Faulkerson and his gang in Tuolumne for your mad fundraising skills and having the heart to do so. Thank you also goes to all of my friends who supported me before, during and after my surgery; my parents, Aunt Marion and Aunt Pam who helped in my care taking post transplant; my daughters Amber and Kristen; Bekkie - For dropping your life and making the trip from Oregon; Mark and Kathy - For taking us in like family and making your home our home; Jen, I love you and couldn't ask for a more wonderful friend, and of course 'The Great Michael Adams' - for saving my life by becoming my friend.

And saving the best for last, my husband Doug, "You are my savior and my best friend. I could not have made it through this ride without you. Thank you for standing by me then and now and I am so happy that we get to spend a long life together. I love you with all of my heart."

Jeri Dubois, 34
West Point, California
Cystic Fibrosis
Double Lung/Liver Transplant, April 9, 2009
University of California San Francisco Medical Center, San Francisco, California

❧ The Hurricane Kid ❧
By Sam Dunman

Just a little bit about me before the transplant: I'm a Marine. I was active four years, inactive four years, and my job was to refuel aircrafts. I was a light smoker for about six years. After discharge from the Marines I drove a cement mixer for three years. My wife Samantha and I have three boys: Layne (six-years-old), Chandler (four-years-old) and Owen (four months).

My breathing problems started back in 2003 when I wanted to get healthy for my kids and I decided to stop smoking. I went to the doctor for his help. The next day he called and said, "We would like to do some tests." He tested my heart; I thought maybe the smoking did something to my heart. Well, the test came back and my heart was really healthy. The doctor tested my lungs. I still remember the night he called and told me I had pulmonary fibrosis. At that time I thought maybe with some meds it would go away; I was kind of wrong about that.

My wife's mother passed away a month later. Samantha was five months pregnant, with our third child - I started to get sick more and more. The doctor said, "Either more meds or transplant." I think it took two seconds, I said transplant, not knowing what I was getting into. I was 31, and game to get better.

I then scheduled some tests, so I would be able to be listed at Tampa General Hospital (TGH), Tampa. Florida. Well I don't know how you pass for a transplant but I did, didn't even study for it. Three weeks later the nurse called and said, "See you Monday if you don't get transplanted over the weekend." That night Samantha had to work until midnight. She came home, I woke up and said hi, went back to sleep. The phone rang and I thought it was her work calling her back in. I answered the phone... well it wasn't her work, it was TGH, "We have a lung". Next thing you know I had to knock on the neighbors window to wake them up to watch the kids. After the surgery, the surgeon told us, "If I hadn't transplanted you, you would've died in three months." I was like, "Wow, that was close".

[88]

I was in the hospital for 10 days. After the surgery, I was doing really well; off oxygen, almost running on the treadmill (well, a fast walk). I was excited and doing everything I was supposed to do. My dad came to visit from Indiana. A lot of friends came to visit. Our Church was a huge help. I was determined to get better and be back at work in about three to four months. I was doing so good, believed in the Lord, and with His help I could do anything, and I did. I was alive, a modern day miracle.

Six days after being home, I woke up one morning and started to cough, and I felt something weird happen. We went to the hospital, where they removed some mucus. But I remained sick, and complications were discovered. We were in hurricane season in Florida. The next 11 days in the hospital we had three hurricanes. At one point my wife was unable to leave the hospital because all the bridges were closed. (I had my transplant when Hurricane Charley was heading straight for Tampa.) The doctor started calling me the 'Hurricane Kid'.

Just before Christmas, I was able to go home. I was still on oxygen (O2). I was doing everything to get off the oxygen, I was walking, exercising, and my nine-month-old was keeping me busy. But nothing was working; I was stressing, I thought maybe I was doing something wrong all the time and I was frustrated most of the time.

One year later, in August, I was holding my son when I felt something loosen in my chest. I coughed so hard, that I popped my left lung. The doctor had originally said that my left lung (my right lung was transplanted) would just shrivel up into nothing.

I was in the hospital for a month and half, back on the transplant list... this time I'm ready. I knew what to expect this time, we had the kids all set, and my mom was ready. I didn't get to see my wife before the re-transplant because of the long drive, but I did see my mom. October 25, 2005, I received a left lung transplant.

In a few days after surgery I was up walking around still a little weak, but I was able to stand on my own. I was in the hospital for about 15 days. I wasn't going rush this time. I was still on oxygen. I was doing great... once again; the Lord had really surprised me. For this transplant, Hurricane Wilma hit Florida – wow! Two times, one year apart. Finally there was no more oxygen. Well, I'd like to say that was the end, but not yet.

A year later I had go back into surgery to repair my right lung, and of course another hurricane was coming straight for Florida. I figured I was an early warning for hurricanes and the doctor thought the same.

At this point I'd had two transplants, and a lung repair. I was in and out of the hospital.

Two years later I had the flu and it damaged my right lung. (By the way... in those two years there were not any hurricane threats to Florida). A month later I was on oxygen again, frustrated and trying to figure out what my purpose in life was, I still couldn't find it. The doctor put me back on the transplant list for the 3rd time. This time we had a plan, the kids were older, and understood what to do, and I was even more ready this time. I just wanted to get healthy and play with my kids.

My mom kept saying they needed to put a zipper in my chest. The call came after a month on the list, and of course, there was a hurricane heading straight for Florida. Again, we went to the hospital. I was in my room and this lady walks by and asked if I am there for a transplant. She was there with her daughter who had just had a bilateral lung transplant. We started to talk about it and I said I was a pro at this, she asked why and I explained that this was my third transplant. Her daughter Emily had her transplant the day before me.

The day after my transplant, I was up and walking around, I would walk past Emily's room; she was still in bed recovering. Emily's mom would walk over and check on me, and Samantha would walk over and talk to her. When I moved to another floor, my wife stayed in touch with them, and we became friends. I was up walking around doing what I could, every time I passed Emily's room I would wave and say "Hi".

Five days later I was off the oxygen. I had to call my family; I had slept all night without it. I was talking to my oldest son, and told him first. So he says, "Cool with a K". Then my middle son says, "Awesome that's great dad". Then the youngest got on the phone and I told him that, "I am not on oxygen. I don't need any help to breathe" and he said out loud (almost a scream), "All right Dad, I'm proud of you!" That felt really good, I didn't need the oxygen anymore, and I was up, breathing easy and ready to go home, for good this time. The best thing when I got home was Owen (four-years-old at the time) didn't understand why I no longer needed the hose or oxygen tanks. He would keep bringing me my oxygen hose, and when we would go to the mall, he would ask if I needed oxygen tanks, and when I said no, he was proud. It felt really good to be breathing on my own for once. Soon, I was throwing the ball with my boys, swimming, and having a great time.

I had my weekly check-ups, and I was walking the mall every day eating Aunty Annie's pretzels - that was the life! I got to know the lady's at Auntie Annie's and after hearing my story, got lots of free pretzels.

It's been a whole year, and no flu, no rejection, just a little cold here and there. I am feeling really good. Layne has been bowling for four years, his average now is a 110. Chandler and Owen play baseball. The best thing ever is going to watch my boy's play sports, and succeed in the things they do.

I thank the Lord every day I am alive… without Him, my great family, and my beautiful wife, I would not be here today.

Sam Dunman, 37
Holiday, Florida
Pulmonary Fibrosis
#1 Single Lung Transplant (right lung), September 19, 2004
#2 Single Lung Transplant (left lung), October 25, 2005
#3 Re-transplant, Single Lung (right lung), September 29, 2008
Tampa General Hospital, Tampa, Florida

I am here Today and can Say CF has Not Beaten Me
By Curt Dunnet

I have lived with this fatal genetic illness for over 27 years; I have battled physical and emotional issues everyday and have surpassed all life expectancy. I was diagnosed with Cystic Fibrosis (CF) at just three months of age, and it has restricted me from doing many things.

All my life I was subjected to daily chest physiotherapy to reduce secretions and obstructions in the airway, mask inhalation, numerous medications, and have been in and out of hospitals constantly. My quality of life was deteriorating due to severe scarring of my lungs, and reduced lung capacity, which caused my pulmonary function tests (PFT's) to plummet to 17%. I was out of options, and was told the only thing left was to be a recipient of a double lung transplant. I was told I could wait up to three years. It was no easy battle living and waiting for "my call", but I dealt with it.

After 139 days on the list, February 3, 2006, I received my "Gift Of Life", a double lung transplant, which would give me a second chance at life. I was out of bed six hours after my surgery and out of the hospital in 11 days. I felt like a new person, I was able to take deep breaths, which I wasn't able to do for more than 10 years, and no more coughing or mucus. I was able to play the sports I use to; exercise regularly, go hunting, fishing, and now keep up with my friends and family! I even went back to further my education, I was never so happy. Of course there were complications after surgery; such as me dealing with the pain, weakness, shakes, and other things, but to me they are minor setbacks. But of course I recuperated from this.

In 2009, I become ill once again. I had accumulated an abundance of fluid in my abdomen, legs, ankles, feet, and hands. I was retaining roughly 25 pounds of fluid, and was very uncomfortable. Shortly after I was informed I had Ascites, due to the liver disease, cirrhosis, which was caused by CF. I thought I was rather unlucky as 6-8% of people with CF have potentially fatal liver disease requiring liver transplantation. The absolute worst experience in my life was living with this fatal liver disease while on the transplant list. I dealt with jaundice, issues with my bile duct, ascites, severe weight loss, in which I dropped to a frightening 77 pounds; my usual weight being 130 pounds, and was on and off the liver transplant list very often.

Due to persistence, and the good Lord, on January 16, 2010, I received a liver transplant. I knew this was not going to be an easy journey afterwards. I was told numerous times I only had days to live, and went back and forth to the operating room, which put many thoughts into my head, but I was for sure this could not be the end. I fought hard; I had much support and prayers, excellent care from the hospital staff at Toronto General Hospital, Toronto, Canada. I then went to rehab, and underwent extensive physiotherapy for five weeks, and worked hard to regain muscle, and weight.

Because of my liver failing, my kidneys also failed. The doctors had given me the option of receiving a kidney from a deceased donor, or a living donor. My father, Gerald Dunnet went through many tests, and was considered a great match for a donor, after being the right blood type and having 4/6 possible antigens match. The date set for our operation is set for December 17, 2010. I had the "Gift of Life" not once, not twice, but will have a third chance, which I am blessed for. Once this is over, I am looking forward to a bright future; I want to travel, and continue my studies in school, which I had to put on hold because of my liver and kidney issues.

Going through all this; the transplants, diabetes, dialysis, osteoporosis, more tests/procedures than you can think of, and taking 67 pills a day, I can say I have been through a great ordeal! But because I have faith in God, I can stand here today to talk about it! CF has overwhelmed me in many different aspects, but I am thankful to say, I am here today and can say it has not beaten me. Be thankful you have your health, and cherish everything! I have had an enormous amount of spiritual and financial support from numerous people, in which I am grateful for.

There are the few people that sign their donor cards, and this should not be the case. Think of the people you could save if you signed your donor card; you could potentially save the lives of up to eight people. I am alive today because of this! Please don't think hard, sign your donor card.

Curt Dunnet, 28
Miramichi, New Brunswick, Canada
Cystic Fibrosis
Double Lung Transplant, February 3, 2006
Liver Transplant, January 16, 2010
Related Living Kidney Donor Transplant, December 17, 2010
Father Gerald Dunnet, Living Kidney Donor
Toronto General Hospital, Toronto, Canada

 Turning 30 and the Number 3
By Samantha Durrant

It took me a long time to finally work up the courage to be listed for a double lung transplant.

I was diagnosed with Cystic Fibrosis at the age of three and was very lucky to stay healthy and grow up like most other kids (apart from sneaking my pills everyday!). At 21, I went over to live in Europe for a few years and indulged my dreams of travel. I managed to keep quite healthy while travelling and even met my partner while living in Scotland.

By the age of 24, my health started a slow decline and I was becoming seriously underweight. A year later I had a feeding tube inserted which helped me regain weight, and slowed the decline of my lung capacity which had sunk to around 35%.

When my 30th birthday came around I found it a time to reflect on my quality of life. I was spending more and more time on treatments just to get by – I was doing five hours airway clearance and half an hour of exercise each day. After a while I even hired a personal trainer to see if they could help push me harder.

I knew deep down I could not go on like this much longer and my lung function was down to 23%. I was tired all the time and knew I had nothing more to give. It really felt like I was trying so hard to stay alive, that I was missing out on life.

During a hospital admission in June 2009, I told the doctors I was ready to take the next step and get listed. I knew if I didn't give transplant a go I would die wondering, 'what if?'

I found those four days of tests emotional and tiring, but a few weeks later I signed my lungs away. I was told that because I was a common size, height and blood group, I was in a competitive group and could have up to a two year wait for suitable lungs.

Three weeks later I was told my new lungs had come. I was in hospital at the time and surrounded by my support team – Mum, Dad, my partner Mark, and my best friend Deb. The five hours between being told to prepare and when I was told that the lungs were the best match, was the longest wait of my life.

The operation took six hours and went smoothly. I was in intensive care unit (ICU) for three days and whilst I was there I was being filmed for a real life hospital program to show what happens in the ICU of Australian hospitals. Not only did they film me, but also my support team. They were asked about what my life was like with Cystic Fibrosis and their thoughts on organ donation and what it means for all of us.

I was scared about going home – what if something went wrong? Once home I felt more comfortable having my own bed, couch and TV to keep me comfy and catch up on much needed sleep without doctors and specialists coming in constantly.

Transplant gym was hard work, but so rewarding when you reach your personal goals. My goal was to run on the treadmill for five minutes by the end of the program and I did it on my second to last gym session.

After my three-month anniversary, my partner and I started looking to buy our first home, and within three weeks of looking we were lucky enough to have purchased a cute little beach style bungalow. The number three had definitely become my lucky number!

At Christmas I was feeling stronger and I had started thinking about what I wanted to do with the rest of my life. I wanted to work with dogs and knew dog grooming was something I'd love to do so, I booked a course to start nine months post transplant. I was nervous as I hadn't been a student since high school but I loved it, especially the hands on working with the dogs. It went for five weeks and was such a good experience. It really felt like another chapter had opened up in my new life.

By August it was planning time for my 12-month anniversary and I had very mixed emotions. In June, I had sent my donor family a thank you letter so they were on my mind a lot. I was wondering if they liked my letter, scared that I might have opened up old wounds.

On the anniversary day it was a lot more emotional than I thought it would be. Remembering where I was the year before, the emotions, going into theatre, waking to tubes and machines, taking my first breath, the pain and nausea.

I made the most of the day by going on an aerochute flight over the outskirts of Melbourne. It was essentially a lawnmower attached to a parachute that went flying through the air! It was a great experience and something else I could never have done with my old lungs! The next night I had a, '1st birthday party' with family and friends, and even contacted the local paper to do a story for organ donation awareness.

I am so grateful to my donor and their family and feel very lucky to have received these wonderful lungs, and with such a short wait. I want to make the most of this second chance and be the best person I can be and make my donor proud.

Samantha Durrant, 31
Melbourne, Australia
Cystic Fibrosis
Double Lung Transplant, August 13, 2009
The Alfred Hospital, Prahran, Victoria, Melbourne, Australia

🦋 **15 years…Breathtaking!** 🦋
By Angela Eldam

In May of 1990, I was 29-years-old. I was a nurse and the mother of three, planning for my eldest child's kindergarten graduation. My daughter was four months old, I was able to work 40 hours most weekends, enabling me to stay home during the week and be a "stay-at-home" mom. Everything was perfect in the world.

I remember a close friend telling me that I seemed out of breath while carrying my daughter, but I dismissed it reminding her that I had three children, ages five and under and still had my "baby fat". The following month, I felt my left arm go numb. I thought I was going to have a migraine headache, but then it moved up my left neck like an "egg white" had dried on my skin. I suspected it had something to do with my heart. I made an appointment with a cardiologist that we knew.

A heart catheterization was performed and I was diagnosed with Primary Pulmonary Hypertension (PPH). (Now called idiopathic pulmonary arterial hypertension (IPAH).) With my husband by my side and my baby in my arms, he instructed me to "put my affairs in order".

Following several fainting spells, my doctor told me they were caused by the left side of my heart not having enough volume to keep my systemic blood pressure normal. He mentioned a surgical procedure that he could perform to help increase the volume of blood to the left side of my heart by putting a hole in my heart. The procedure is called an 'atrial septostomy', but it too had risks. Fortunately, I had the surgery and it was successful except for a tremendous drop in my oxygen saturations. I had no more fainting spells and was able to take care of my toddler.

After about three years a new drug came on the market called Epoprostenol, it was a miracle! I used Epoprostenol for about 18 months and met three patients also on the drug. We started meeting at a local restaurant once a month. I circulated flyers to see if more patients wanted to come, and they did. We had about 10-12 patients during those first few years. Now we meet every other month, and we have quite a few new patients. I also provide support to patients via telephone or email if they prefer.

In 1995, the week before the Oklahoma City, Oklahoma bombing, I became ill and spent a couple months in the hospital. I had always told my doctor that as long as I could laugh, I wasn't ready for a lung transplant. I stopped laughing, and I was listed for a lung transplant.

I had three "false alarms" before I had my transplant. In the afternoon of October 5th, 1995, it was a go. It was only six weeks to get out of the hospital. Two weeks later was my youngest son's 9th birthday. The physical therapy exercises helped to strengthen my weak legs. I felt that I was stronger; I reached down, grabbed my ankles and pushed myself off the sofa. Then I walked my hands up my legs and stood up. As I was doing this, my son entered the room and said, "That's the best birthday present I could ever get" and we embraced.

After that day, I haven't stopped moving! By January, I was giving my daughter a birthday party with 30, six-year olds without having to stop to rest. One day, my daughter and I were in a hurry at the local supermarket and she told me, "Slow down Mommy, I can't keep up!" I stopped and looked at her and said, "What did you say?" we just burst out laughing so hard that other customers looked at us, but we didn't care. We knew.

I was able to meet my donor's family on my one-year anniversary along with the recipient of my donor's kidney and pancreas recipients. My donor's name was Sarah and she was only 10 days away from her 13th birthday. It's amazing that in her parent's most terrible pain, they chose to help give someone else a second chance. I was allowed to participate in a memorial service for Sarah by singing a solo with her lungs.... it was bittersweet, and I was able to pay my respects at the cemetery. We have kept in touch, spending some holidays together. I call them on her birthday to let them know that she will never be forgotten, and I carry her picture with me always. They know that they can give Sarah's lungs a hug anytime they want to.

I went three years without spending a night at the hospital. I've had a couple of speed bumps along the way with rejection in 1998, and again in 2007, but it was quickly resolved. On October 6th, 2010 it will be 15 years.

I have watched my children grow up. My eldest son is now in Graduate School, the other is a sound engineer, and my daughter is now a junior in college. I have enjoyed baseball and soccer games, school band concerts, vacationing with my family, helping my son move off to college and into an apartment, tending to illnesses and broken bones. All those wonderful things a mother's life affords.

I recently celebrated my 50th birthday and thank God for each and every day. I currently volunteer with 'LifeGift'; our organ procurement organization spreading the word about the new, 'Donate Life

Texas Registry'. You can help to make the decision easier for your family by letting them know your wishes regarding organ donation.

My favorite quote is: *"Don't think of organ donation as giving up part of yourself to keep a total stranger alive. It's really a total stranger giving up almost all of themselves to keep part of you alive."* ~ Author unknown

Angela Eldam, 50
Sugar Land, Texas
Idiopathic Pulmonary Arterial Hypertension
(Formerly known as Primary Pulmonary Hypertension)
Double Lung Transplant, October 6, 1995
Texas Heart and Lung Institute at St. Luke's Episcopal Hospital, Houston, Texas

 The Love of My Mother and Aunt
By Diana Alice Torella-Elwell

Living with Cystic Fibrosis (CF) can either make you or break you....I chose to fight and in the end have won the battle against this horrific illness. What the true effect it has on a person and their family is never known until you live it or with someone who has it. Even then it's hard to really grasp what a person suffers with from day to day.

The first 24 years of my life were filled with a lot of sickness, pain and most of all fighting.... Fighting to stay alive. I always had hope though and a strong faith that God would bring me through. It all stems from my family and the belief that I was a survivor, and we never would give up believing.

In 1996 I went on the transplant list. After still being on the list for two years I was worse than ever. My PFT's (pulmonary function test) were at 17% FVC (full volume capacity) and each thing I did was a struggle, I got to the point that even a shower was work. One thing that I found out about was, living lobar lung transplant, I thought that was amazing, and my parents did too. My blood type being AB+ was the reason why it was taking so long to find me new lungs, so we checked into the living lobar lung transplant.

The response was a good one. My Mom Priscilla, thought she was always B+ so when she found she was my blood type she was my first hero to come forward and say she would be able to be my donor. My other chosen hero was my Aunt Marcia who after being tested told me, "Di, I'm AB+ too"!

We began the process of preparing for the transplant. They had a bronchoscopy, cat scans, x-rays, nuclear x-rays, psychology test, blood work, cardio-pulmonary test, and PFT's. They both passed with flying colors.

The doctor explained it was a 15-hour surgery. Three operating rooms would be set up. He also explained that our lungs are five lobes; three on the right, and two on the left. My aunt was chosen for the right side and my mom would be my left. As she puts it, "Closest to the heart"! Through all of this I still remembered the scriptures I would quote in faith believing it was for me. I received a scripture as a child, in Jeremiah 33:6 "Behold I bring health and cure and I will cure them and reveal unto them the abundance of peace and truth." My promise was going to happen. I hadn't given up on it and God's promise was finally here.

On July 20th 1998, a group of nineteen family and friends walked with me as I was wheeled to surgery at Massachusetts General Hospital, Boston, Massachusetts. As I said my, "I love you" to my loved ones and the thoughts of "I hope they'll be okay, because I know I will. God has a plan", but I could only imagine the fear that was felt by all.

After some time a nurse came to tell my family that the lungs were both in and they were finishing up. The doctors shared that the lungs stood up like mountains. It was a reminder that the promise God gave Dad when I was born that if we, "Speak to the mountain in our life and have no doubt the things we believe will happen" (Mark 11:23). Dad called that mountain, 'Cystic Fibrosis' and never gave up that it would be removed someday! Could this really be the start of a new life? Could all my dreams really be coming true? I always was happy but now it would be even more joy!

I did encounter several complications and my transplant team acted swiftly and expertly. In the hospital my sister Barbara, on the other side of the glass that separated us, would say, "I love you", in sign language to me, and I'd blink as if to say, "I love you too".

Once home, life was good. My mom came over everyday and took care of me, my house and took me out shopping. She always stayed until my husband came home, and had dinner ready. She and dad were my greatest support along with my sister.

I came home with enough pills to fill a fishing tackle box. I was taking 52 pills a day, but; the oxygen, the breathing treatments, physical therapy and most of all coughing and not being able to breathe were gone. Yeah my life changed for good in areas that I so waited desperately for all my life, but I was different in ways that I never expected also. During the post transplant time I divorced.

Due to the early medical complications, and my divorce, I was depressed. My sister said she, "Missed the fighter you have always been and seeing the joy you always had." I took that and used it. I rejoined the "worship team" in church. I took trips like I had never done before. I needed to start living life to the fullest and so I have.

In 2005 I met my husband, and we married a year later. We just celebrated our 4th anniversary. Mike didn't go through everything with me, but he knows the struggle I did go through. He remembers his church praying steadfast for me as the reports were brought to the church that did prayer chains for me. He has been my support, who loves me for who I am, and accepted all me for who I was. Mike and I work in our garden, rake leaves, and shovel. We also did a hike and I surprised myself with the mountain I climbed!! I love my husband Mike and am so thankful to have this gift of life to share with him.

On July 20th 2008, I celebrated my 10-year celebration of new life! We had a big party and I also celebrated my mom and aunts heroic act of kindness. They still to this day do not see themselves as heroes but not a day goes by that I don't think of it. I breathe because they did give me a gift that no one else could...the gift of life.

In November 2009, Mike and I became guardians of our sweet son Matthew. We had always talked about having children and it was always something I had wanted; and it happened. Here a year later I am proving to so many that I am able to do the things that I could only dream of. Today I am blessed with two nieces and two nephews: Jordan 21, Tanner 18, Jacob 10 and Emma 7.

One of my greatest challenges and joys was for the past two years walking for the Great Strides to raise awareness and funds for Cystic Fibrosis. God has blessed me to over abundance, and I am so happy! My birthdays are always one more reminder of how wonderful life is and to never take it for granted. I am excited to see what the next 12 years or even 20 are in store, but I sure know this, "Thank you God for this Gift called LIFE!"

Diana Alice Torella-Elwell, 36
Milton, New Hampshire
Cystic Fibrosis
Living Lobar Lung Transplant, July 20, 1998
Living Lobar Lung Donor: Mother, Priscilla Arlene McNelly Torella
Living Lobar Lung Donor: Aunt, Marcia Ann McNelly Seger
Massachusetts General Hospital, Boston, Massachusetts

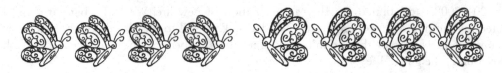

4th Lungiversary
By Trudy Ensminger

The most difficult part of putting my story into words is...finding the words. When diagnosed in 1997 with Pulmonary Arterial Hypertension (PAH) my pulmonary arterial pressure was already 56 (normal is 25), symptoms included low blood oxygen levels, shortness of breath and fatigue. At that time I was not considered for transplant since I was still very functional so I joined an experimental drug study for UT-15 also known as (aka) Remodulin.

As new drugs became available they were added to my regime. My condition remained fairly stable until 2005 when I began a rapid downward spiral. When all approved drugs were exhausted I was listed for transplant. This friends, is a difficult decision to make. My friend Barb, who I met through the Pulmonary Hypertension support group, remained in close contact during this time. She too was waiting for transplant and was my primary support. Both being Registered Nurse's (R.N.'s) it made our conversations interesting at times. I realized that I may die during the transplant or after due to rejection but one thing was certain; I would die soon without the transplant. I have always been a fighter and this time was no different. I decided that if I were going to die...I'd die fighting.

THE CALL:
I've always felt that God walks with me but never as strong as the day I received, 'the call'. By this time Barb had already been transplanted and doing well. On Sept 12, 2006 we planned to meet in Pittsburgh for a transplant support group meeting. Barb felt strongly that I would get the call during the meeting. She was close to being accurate. My husband and I had just made it to Oakland when my cell phone rang. It was Paul my coordinator. There was a donor.

THE WAIT:
I had been listed only five weeks. Could this be true? We arrived at University of Pittsburgh Medical Center, Pittsburgh, Pennsylvania. While we waited for the surgery to begin, we took the time to call friends and family members not only to update them, but requesting prayer. Not only for us but also for the family that was grieving the loss of their loved one.

RECOVERY:
The surgery was about eight hours. I not only had the double lung transplant, I also had a repair of my tricuspid valve and a closure of a hole between my ventricles, both were complications of the PAH. The first thing I remember is my daughter saying, " You're so pink" I think I would have chuckled if I could. It didn't take long for me to realize that I could breathe easy. The struggle for a simple breath was gone. I was so grateful to my donor, her family, the amazing surgeons and God for giving me this gift of life.

HOW LIFE CHANGES:

Pre-Transplant I continued to work full time as a R.N. in Home Health taking medical leave when I was placed on the active transplant list. Looking back I don't know how I did it. With oxygen levels in the low 80's and my cyanotic lips and fingers I woke every morning and went to work. I had sick patients to see. I truly was afraid to stop working...I felt I would sit at home just waiting to die. My husband would joke that I would most likely die with a stethoscope around my neck.

After a year of recovery I returned to work on a limited basis. I soon learned it was difficult to be a nurse while avoiding sick people. I've had several setbacks including several bacterial and fungal infections, episodes of rejection but today I feel better than I ever have. I currently exercise daily, doing Zumba dance and weight training. Thanks to my donor and her family I have enjoyed four extra years of life. I have lived to meet my 3rd granddaughter who is now a one year old. I became a certified Pet First Aid and Cardiopulmonary Resuscitation (CPR) instructor, and have overcome so many of life's hurdles. My life has definitely changed for the better. Although I do have some personality changes and cognitive issues since transplant, every new day is amazing.

I recently celebrated my 4th 'Lungiversary' (as my family has named it) while vacationing along the Atlantic Ocean with family. It was a bittersweet and emotional day for me. As I sat on the beach watching the sunrise, thanking God for this second chance at life I was also praying for my donor's family as they remember their loved one who so unselfishly gave me the gift of life. I think of her often and have printed on my personal checks, "An organ donor saved my life" and a personalized license plate, "2nulngz" (2 new lungs) which has sparked many a conversations about organ donation and transplant. I have just recently become a licensed Zumba and Zumba Gold instructor, yippee!!

Staying healthy after lung transplant is a full time job. Our transplanted organs are exposed to everything in our environment making us more vulnerable to viruses, bacteria and the like. I am now planning to check off another piece of my 'bucket list' as we make arrangements to take a cruise to Alaska. God willing I will be able to realize this goal.

"An Organ Donor Saved My Life"

Trudy Ensminger, R. N., 56
Curwensville, Pennsylvania
Pulmonary Arterial Hypertension
Double Lung Transplant, September 12, 2006
University of Pittsburgh Medical Center, Pittsburgh, Pennsylvania

I Can Breathe Clearly Now- All the Bad Things have Disappeared -
It's Been Bright, Bright Sunshiny Days
By Sonja (Sunny) Ethun

I have read so many fabulous stories in Joanne's first edition that I wanted to include my story in the second book. It's been a rough ride since I was a child. I couldn't figure out why I wasn't able to jump rope as long or walk and run as fast as others without getting a side ache. Actually, I was a tomboy and always enjoyed playing the boys' games like football, baseball, cops and robbers, and hiking in the woods with my brother and all his friends. In high school I wanted to be a cheerleader but couldn't keep up with the other girls during the tryouts. I was not overweight and enjoyed a lot of time outdoors and still do! I also noticed my brother breathing harder through his mouth, and his lips would turn purple when he was exerting himself. Our parents both smoked, as back in those times it was accepted. As teenagers we started smoking also. By that time we were a broken family.

My brother quit his addiction to cigarettes in his early twenties when he married. I continued to smoke, as my husband at the time also smoked. Through my entire life I've been around smokers and was able to smoke at all of my jobs. My brother, on the other hand, worked outdoors in a smaller community where the air was clearer. I worked and lived in the big city in the manufacturing environment with many solvents, cast irons, smoky machinery, welding, and many other metals and plastics. The machines would put a mist in the air that we all breathed in.

Our Mom moved away when we were around ten years of age. She was getting ill frequently and hospitalized some of the time, as she was diagnosed as having emphysema. She died in 1989 at the age of 59 years. There was never a mention of Alpha-1 Antitrypsin Deficiency. I believe it was known a known disease at the time, but she was never checked for it. Our Father passed away at age 76 with dementia and heart and lung issues. But he wasn't as extreme with his lung issues as my Mother was.

About six years later my older brother got pneumonia and continued to get it for five years to the point of hospitalization. As for myself, during that time period I would get colds that were so bad I would need antibiotics to recover. My brother was diagnosed with Alpha-1. Soon after his diagnosis, I was getting sicker, and I asked my family doctor to check me for Alpha-1. She said to me, "What is that?" I told her my brother was diagnosed with it and it's hereditary. She ordered the test and the results were positive, I am an SZ phenotype, same as my brother.

After my brother died, my own lung function dropped to 19%. I used oxygen more and got to the point that I could not walk to the mailbox and back. I contacted the St. Mary's Hospital - Mayo Clinic, Rochester, Minnesota. They had me in for evaluation and I was placed on the lung transplant list. My lung function was down to 13%. To my surprise I got the call within four months.

I still remember I wasn't afraid and I was smiling and waving at my children and their husbands when they wheeled me away. As they put me under, I prayed that God would do whatever was best for me. Through the help of my daughters and friends, everything worked out great as I woke up the following day with "New Lungs!" I can't express how grateful I am to this day, as I'm doing all the things I used to do! I love being outdoors whether it's work or play. Of course there are some side effects from the medications, but not intolerable. I feel like super woman these days!

I've had the greatest pleasure, since the transplant, of meeting my donor's wife, Diane. She lives in the next state and so she came here to visit with me. She lost her husband of 14 years, Dennis, with no warning. I am able to live through him. I currently have a photo of Dennis and Diane that sits in my family room with a red ribbon on it. I am so fortunate to have met her, and to know her story. We keep in touch by phone, as she is a very nice lady.

I would like to say to the staff at the Mayo Clinic and St. Mary's Hospital how wonderful they have been to give me another chance. Also to my friends and relatives a, "Big hug" and thank you for all your help to really make things work well.

A note to all of you who read this story, you will all have your life back, too, if you just, "Believe" and take care of the rest of your body in the meantime. And all of you out there who aren't yet a donor, please, please consider being one as there are so many people just waiting for your gift.

Thank you for allowing me to tell my story of survival.

Sonja (Sunny) Ethun, 62
Elk River, Minnesota
Alpha-1 Antitrypsin Deficiency
Double Lung Transplant, March 1, 2008
St. Mary's Hospital – Mayo Clinic, Rochester, Minnesota

 64-Year-Old Legs, 18-Year-Old Lungs
By Ron Evans

I grew up in northern Kentucky and was hospitalized with asthma before I was five. I had the "average" childhood, but never could really breathe well. As I grew up, I more or less grew out of that phase and wasn't bothered too much, except with allergies. I started having frequent bronchial attacks and bronchitis when I reached the age of 50. I think most of the problem was due to my line of work. My business did a lot of boat interiors and sprayed a lot of paint and glue.

I went to the best lung doctor in Clearwater, Florida. He diagnosed me with Chronic Obstructive Pulmonary Disease (and other chronic lung issues). So we pulled out all the stops to fight the progress but nothing seemed to make a difference. My lungs totally filled up with fluid, and I was rushed to the hospital. I was out for two days and felt lucky to be alive. After 14 days, I was able to leave the hospital, but had no strength and was down to 135 lbs. I had to be on 2+ liters of oxygen 24 hours a day (24/7), which lasted for the next 2 ½ years. I did go to the gym three times a week, as soon as I was able. I needed to be as strong as I could be, to be considered for a transplant. At 62, I was a bit "over the hill" for the normal transplant but we knew that miracles sometimes do happen.

I went to Mayo Clinic Florida, in Jacksonville, Florida to begin the evaluation for a lung transplant. The testing is so thorough they jokingly call it a, "living autopsy". I was accepted onto the transplant list in March 2009.

Then the waiting started. I never knew how long it would take, especially since my blood type is AB-, so my wife and I were shocked, amazed, thrilled and frantic when we received the call from Dr. Francisco Alvarez saying he believed a pair of lungs might be available for me. It was a true miracle. They were waiting for me at the hospital, and I actually saw the helicopter take off to go get the lungs that would save my life...I was about to receive the greatest gift that could be given.

I have a hard time describing the next part because there is no way to explain how beautiful it was to be able to wake up and BREATHE for the first time in years. While the surgery was painful and my recovery is ongoing – the joy of receiving a second chance is beyond description and worth every instant of the challenge.

Now, 15 months have passed. I can do things I never dreamed of being able to do again. I can walk on the treadmill at a fast pace for an hour without breathing hard. I never would have believed that possible, and you wouldn't either if you had seen me before transplant. Thanks to my donor's selfless act and my new lungs, I now have an active life!!! The rehabilitation counselors at Mayo insist that exercise and attitude is a huge portion of a successful recovery and extended success after a transplant.

I don't have to work too hard at being thankful, and a positive attitude just comes with all my appreciation of the new gift. However, the exercise is a bit trickier – these 64-year-old legs have trouble keeping up with an 18-year-old's lungs. I couldn't be more thankful for the miracle that has been given to me, my donor's "Gift of Life". I now encourage friends and family to include organ donation in their advanced directives and to discuss their wishes openly with family members. It is amazing what wonderful ripples of love and joy this one family's act of love and giving has created.

Ron Evans, 64
Clearwater, Florida
Chronic Obstructive Pulmonary Disease
Double Lung Transplant, July 11, 2010
Mayo Clinic Florida, Jacksonville, Florida

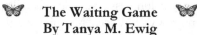

The Waiting Game
By Tanya M. Ewig

They say the waiting is hardest part, and for those of us who happen to be waiting for an organ transplant know matter what organ it is, they are right. I just wish I knew who *they* are and what *their* story is. However until I find out and hope I do find out, I would like to tell my story...I actually start my story as a youngster.

The year: 1976, the place: Milwaukee Children's Hospital in Milwaukee, Wisconsin, the patient: me, the patient's age: 11. I was always sick as a child, starting off with a cold every other month to the ever-scratching chicken pox on every part of my little framed body. My parents finally took me to a lung specialist and the diagnosis was asthma. Enter Dr. Bruns and his team of well-educated physicians. My parents and I were told that my left lung was not cleaning out and filtering the particles of dust balls that were entering my body, therefore I was not getting better and the lower part of my left lung should be removed. Imagine yourself at 11 not being able to go out and play with your sisters and brothers or any of your friends? Not that I had a lot of them; coming from a small town at that time. So I had the lower part of my left lung removed.

Fast forward to 2005, the year that would forever change my mind about organ donation, for that was the year that I was placed on the, "waiting list". I was even told that my illness has a name (Gee, and here I thought I was special when the doctors at Milwaukee Children's Hospital could not tell me). What I have...wait for this...Primary Ciliary Dyskinesia (PCD), also known as Immotile Ciliary Syndrome or Kartagener's Syndrome (KS). It is a rare, ciliopathic, autosomal recessive genetic disorder that causes a defect in the action of the cilia lining the respiratory tract (lower and upper, sinuses, Eustachian tube, and middle ear) and the fallopian tube. (Wikipedia, 2010). So in June of 2005, the doctors and nurses at University of Wisconsin Hospital and Clinics, Madison, Wisconsin, told myself and my mother after a week long evaluation that the odds of being placed on the list was almost guaranteed and I should be receiving the letter in the mail within the week.

Fast forward to the present year 2010, it has been five years and I am still waiting. However I don't really consider myself a waiter, for one thing I don't take food orders or drink orders but I see myself more of a candidate, and I happen to need two lungs before I can be elected to the next level of my life for the better quality of life that we all deserve.

I have such a huge support group surrounding me everyday and I keep myself busy by volunteering for the Wisconsin Donor Network, BloodCenter of Wisconsin and the National Kidney Foundation. I have been job-hunting for a part time job, as I recently obtained my Bachelor of Science in Health Administration. I do need to wear oxygen and I exercise to maintain a good weight but I make a game of it and I bet myself that I can't do that extra sit up, I always end up doing that extra one and I reward myself with a long hot bath with plenty of bubbles!

Waiting can be stressful if you let it be, but I don't. I know that when the time is right I will be getting "the call" and off I go onto the next part of my life.

Tanya Ewig, 45
Milwaukee, Wisconsin
Primary Ciliary Dyskinesia
Pre - Double Lung Transplant
University of Wisconsin Hospital and Clinics, Madison, Wisconsin

The Call
By Amy L. Eyles

I have always imagined the day Death came calling would be overcast. Grizzly gray clouds would hover ominously, struggling against the strength of my resistance to draw me in. The wind would shriek its encouragement through trembling trees, taking crumpled brown leaves along hostage as it screeched across the fields. The sky would split with a rage of thunder and a jolt of lightening as rain pummeled the earth mercilessly. Somewhere amidst the fury of the elements, I would laugh, knowing that it was not enough to make me succumb to Death's visit.

My name is Amy, which means "beloved." I mention this only because it is what I am, beloved. I am 33-years-old; however, my journey began much earlier, when I was age 19. I live in Hamden, Maine, a small but well-to-do community. I had a wonderful childhood. I was always active and never seemed to lack for friends. I am a Licensed Clinical Social Worker who works with children and families at a job I love.

I've often asked myself why someone would stop to read my story. The answer is because it is real. It is not something that happened in a book, or on television. It happened to me. Sometimes things happen in real life requiring ordinary people to rise to extraordinary heights. I am one of those people.

The call came September 27, 2004. Death had been stalking me since my first year of college, at age 18, and it had all culminated in this.

It all originated with one month's worth of birth control pills 14 years earlier, which resulted in shortness of breath and chest pain. I received a diagnosis of Pulmonary Hypertension. Death and I continued to wrestle for the next ten years. I managed to complete college somehow, and to get my Masters degree in Social Work. I was working, until Death got the upper hand. My heart began to fail due to the high pressures in my pulmonary arteries. Death continued to nip at my heels though, as one year later, my heart again, began to fail. I was taken by Air Ambulance to The Cleveland Clinic Foundation, in Cleveland, Ohio, while my parents, wearily, but willingly, packed their belongings.

When I received the call that lungs had arrived, I was eerily calm. I received a bi-lateral lung transplant. Afterward I drifted in and out of consciousness. I wrote a message to my parents on a borrowed piece of paper, "Am I dead?" By the end of November, I was tube free…for the first time in years.

My Pulmonary Hypertension is completely gone, and my heart has returned to normal size and function. I am now running up flights of stairs without getting out of breath. I've found that from the hardships in life, wonderful things happen to change, and shape our perceptions; and we find out just who we're suppose to be. I've learned that our time here is short, and I want to experience all of life, now that my life has been given back to me.

Last summer, I climbed Mt. Katahdin, the highest mountain in Maine, located in Maine's Baxter State Park. I'd done these years ago, while in high school – now 20 some years later, with a new set of lungs. I was amazed that the climb went SO well, and was much easier that what I had remembered…Not that I didn't have the jelly legs and not that I'm without being sore today, but it was amazing! I thought about that 14-year-old girl who gave me the precious gift of her lungs… Pretty sure she never thought her lungs would climb that mountain!

I've got a new horse at a barn near my home and on weekends spend time riding him, as well as other horses at the barn for exercising. I'm able to do everything I use to do, including jumping. My new horse is a retired harness horse (Standardbred racing). I've worked with him to retrain him to ride, and he's doing very well.

One thing is for certain through all of this - every day is sunnier than the one previous.

I always thought the day I would die would be over cast…

Amy L. Eyles, 33
Bangor, Maine
Pulmonary Hypertension
Double Lung Transplant, September 28, 2004
The Cleveland Clinic Foundation, Cleveland, Ohio

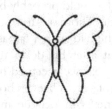

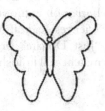

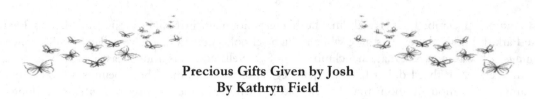

Precious Gifts Given by Josh
By Kathryn Field

On Wednesday, June 3rd 2009, my son Josh was driving on his way back home from the doctors in London, Ontario, Canada. At 5:50pm on Veterans Memorial Highway my cell phone went off in the car he was driving. He and his girlfriend, who was a passenger, tried to find where the ringing was coming from and that small distraction caused Josh to veer the car and he hit the central median flipping the car several times. His girlfriend had minor cuts and bruises but Josh suffered a severe impact to the back of his head and was not breathing. Luckily an off-duty paramedic was passing the scene at the time and gave him artificial respiration. Josh was taken to the London Health Sciences Hospital on Victoria Road, London, Canada and at 6:10pm I had the call every parent dreads.

When we got to the hospital the doctors told us that they had tried everything they could but that there was nothing they could do for Josh and that he was brain dead. We were told that a Trillium Nurse would be coming to talk to us. I asked, "What's a Trillium Nurse?" It was explained to us and after a few minutes she came into the room. Before she could finish her first sentence, we said that we wanted to donate Josh's organs.

He was then taken up to the children's ward. We stayed by his bedside, held his hand and stroked his hair. We knew he had gone, but it didn't stop us talking to him telling how much we loved him and how proud we were of him. All through the night, many of his friends came to say goodbye. On June 4th 2009, Josh went for his operation and his organs went on to help save the lives of six people; heart, liver, pancreas, lungs and both kidneys. Josh was 17-years-old.

My son was a great kid. Funny, well liked and humble. He would probably be so embarrassed by all the fuss he is getting. He had started flying lessons at St. Thomas Airport, and only the Saturday before his accident, he had been voted Prom Prince and he had such a fantastic time that night - he seemed so full of the enjoyment of life. We found out after his death that he had been voted Valedictorian for his graduating year and in October last year we accepted his high school diploma and made the valedictorian speech on his behalf. He got on with everybody he knew and could always be counted on for a shoulder to cry on. He was never in a clique and would equally talk to the football team star player or the shy, quiet person at the back of the room.

The worst thing that anyone can do to a grieving family is to not talk about their child. Doing this today is what we love to do - it keeps Josh's spirit alive. I make no excuses for wanting to talk about my son at whatever chance I get. To spread the word about organ donation is very important to us. Earlier on in the year I was lucky enough to talk about this cause on the radio for the London Health Sciences Radiothon. Josh's school, East Elgin Secondary in Aylmer, has raised money by selling "Just Donate" bracelets in Josh's memory. They have organized alumni soccer and basketball matches all in Josh's name, and all to raise money for organ donation awareness.

Back in April during national organ and tissue donation awareness week, we were lucky enough to be part of a giant living green ribbon on the school field with 952 people. On Josh's 19th birthday, on August 20th 2010, close friends organized selling personalized organ donation car magnets, with all profits going to Trillium Gift of Life.

Up until Josh's death organ donation wasn't something we had really thought about. We are originally from England, and I carried an organ donor card in the United Kingdom, but we never thought that we would need to make a decision regarding our own son. It has only been since then I have researched and found out more about the donation process and the chronic lack of donors.

I read a great quote the other day, which said, "Transplants not only save lives, they recapture productive lives". That is so true. Many people know the difference that having a transplant means to their lives. Life altering is very probably an understatement.

We didn't know how the recipients would feel about contacting us - we thought perhaps they would feel awkward if they went first because our son had died, so we decided to break the ice and write first. A couple of months after Josh's death we sent letters to the recipients because we wanted them to know about our son. What he was like, his interests and his plans for the future. We have received the most wonderful letters in return from those recipients who are truly grateful for another chance at life and the fact that they care so much about the precious gift given by Josh, gives us such a boost. It is wonderful to read that all these people were in critical condition with their illnesses and that by receiving part of my son they now live full lives again. When someone tells you in a letter that they were confined to a wheelchair and were on oxygen and since receiving my son's lungs they have now improved so significantly that they are back at work and can do whatever they want, or that the woman who was so ill before receiving Josh's pancreas has now gotten married and even did a dragon boat race, we can't help but feel so proud of Josh that he has allowed all this to happen.

We are positive people and we wanted to celebrate our son. Knowing that he lives on in others gives us such comfort. We will never get over his death for the rest of our lives, we miss him every day, but knowing the change that he has made does give us a great deal of comfort. So, as Josh did in life, dance as if no ones watching, sing as if no ones listening, love as if you've never been hurt, live as if you've got nothing to lose.

Kathryn Field, Donor Mother
Son, Josh Field, Organ Donor
Belmont, Ontario, Canada
Josh Field, June 3, 2009
"Forever 17"

Sometimes, Life Takes a Very Unexpected Turn!
By Geoff Foley

For the first fifty-five years of my life I was an extremely healthy and active individual. I worked twelve-hour days at my management job, traveled all over the world, and lived a generally very busy, albeit stressful, life. My life outside work revolved around family and friends, and a collection of hobbies for which there was never enough time.

However, in late 2002 I began to feel a little out of breath with even modest exertion, and more fatigued than usual. I mentioned this in passing to my primary care physician who thought it was probably nothing but said, "Let's get an x-ray of your lungs just to be safe". Following my x-rays and as I finished dressing, the technician came back to my cubicle and said, "The radiologist wants to see you". I had a feeling that my life was about to change. My instincts were right. "Your lungs look like hell", was the blunt message the radiologist gave me and indeed my life has never been the same again.

Soon afterwards, I learned that I had something called Idiopathic Pulmonary Fibrosis, or IPF for short. A quick search of the Internet revealed all I really needed to know about the disease. There was no known cause, no treatment or cure, and a life expectancy of perhaps eighteen months to two years. For someone who had never had anything much worse than a headache or a mild case of 'flu', this was devastating news. This wasn't part of the plan I had laid out for my life. It especially wasn't part of my plan for the "golden years" with my wife and family.

There was however, one ray of hope to cling to, a lung transplant. And so I began the process of evaluation for a transplant at The Cleveland Clinic Foundation, Cleveland, Ohio. By 2005, with my health declining rapidly I was approved for a double lung transplant. Within about a week, perhaps because I was both very sick and also in need of lungs much larger than the typical transplant candidate could utilize, I was blessed to "get the call" to inform me that suitable lungs had become available.

The "Gift of New Life" came to me through a double lung transplant on April 20th, 2005 when I received the largest pair of lungs the Cleveland Clinic had transplanted up to that time. I was in the intensive care unit about three days and out of the hospital in another nine.

The gift of life is an extraordinary gift to receive, and now five years later, I still have a sense of wonder at how incredibly fortunate I have been. A transplant has given me further precious years to spend with family and friends. It has allowed me to witness another of my children get married, and to see the birth of a second grandson. There has been great joy even in seemingly small things, like being able to watch our eldest grandson get on the school bus for his first day of kindergarten. It has allowed me the pleasure of seeing the excitement on our grandchildren's faces when they come over to play with "Bup" and with Grandma.

Life of course has changed in many ways. After working for a year post transplant, I have become a retiree. It's a retirement that is much different than I had anticipated twenty years ago. My interests in woodworking and gardening have been relegated to fond memories and replaced with activities that pose less risk to my precious new lungs. There is a drug regimen to follow with absolute discipline (about fifty thousand pills consumed to date). There is the constant effort to avoid viral and bacterial infections that can threaten rejection of my transplanted lungs. I practice almost religious adherence to the use of anti-bacterial hand cleansers and to hand washing whenever my hands have been shaken, and whenever I have handled doorknobs, phones, remote controls, shopping carts and so forth. There is the frustration when I discover that the person sitting in the pew next to me in church, or behind me in the supermarket checkout line, has the mother of all colds and may well share it with me unaware of the implications that may carry. There is the sheepish feeling that comes from being the only person on an airplane using a surgical mask to avoid infection by one of the many and varied viruses being efficiently circulated through the aircraft cabin (and wondering whether my fellow passengers are imagining that I have some dreadful communicable disease!). Most of all however, there is a new appreciation for the simple act of breathing without effort, and being able to complete life's most mundane activities without benefit of an oxygen line.

Yes, life does sometimes take an unexpected turn. For me it was a turn off the paved highway on to a dirt road that didn't show up on any map. However, at the end of that dirt road I found a miracle, the gift of new life. This was a miracle made possible by the wondrous generosity of my donor family, by the skill of an extraordinary team of doctors and nurses at the Cleveland Clinic, through the loving care of my family, and by the grace of God. Today, with that miracle in hand I am back on a paved road, albeit a slightly different one from the one I was traveling before. I am truly blessed.

Geoff Foley, 63
Fairport, New York
Idiopathic Pulmonary Fibrosis
Double Lung Transplant, April 20, 2005
The Cleveland Clinic Foundation, Cleveland, Ohio

Because I Can
By Kerry Geron

After 27 years of living a very healthy and active life I started coughing with exertion and exercise, getting sick frequently and having each sickness go straight to my chest and linger there until briefly feeling better before the next cold.

I lived with Idiopathic Pulmonary Fibrosis (IPF) for over 10 years. It went undiagnosed for about four years due to uncaring, disinterested doctors focused on insurance billing rather than my healthcare. After diagnosis, we focused on treating the symptoms as there was, as is, no treatment or cure for IPF. I did everything I could to take care of my overall health and remained as active as possible. I was relatively stable for about four years then my lung function declined quickly. After evaluation, I was on the transplant waiting list for nine months. I did not relocate for transplant and that was one of the deciding factors in choosing my hospital. One of the most difficult parts of the wait was the realization of how dire my situation was since I was listed 2nd in the state. There was also the consciousness that for me to receive a transplant someone was going to die. I was overwhelmed by the entire concept of transplant.

After finally admitting I needed oxygen, I started on 2-4 liters with a Portable Oxygen Concentrator and home concentrator, but quickly increased liter by liter until I was on 10 liters. My biggest issue was diffusion, no matter the amount of oxygen pumped into my lungs; it just wasn't passing through to oxygenate my blood and body. Being out of breath affects and limits everything. I had no therapies or treatments. I exercised to stay in the best condition possible and took cough suppressants and expectorants. I did not take steroids or any other prescription medication for my lung disease (since there were no effective treatments) so I presented in the purest state of the disease without any additional complications or prescription side effects.

From what I'm told, the surgery took over seven hours. The donor lungs were hard to fit into my very small frame and my "wiring" was opposite how a normal person's is supposed to be and they had to work around it, making it difficult and the surgery longer. I lay on one side for an extended period of time so blood pooled causing more post surgical pain and my recovery more difficult. I was on the ventilator an extra day. However, once off I was up and walking and doing all my exercises on or ahead of schedule. I felt great and was set to release early. I blew away prior records on the 6-minute walk test.

I feel very lucky to have the advances of every transplant ever performed before mine. I have told many recipients that we owe the donors and donor families our lives, but we should also honor every recipient. The doctors learn from each and every one of us, and those that follow benefit without question. I feel blessed to have had a double thoracotomy rather than the older clamshell method and no ribs were broken in the process. The incision scars on my back are barely noticeable, but I am proud of them and call them my angel wings.

Since transplant I can again take care of my household cleaning, cooking, yard work, gardening, and errands and move about the entire house and stairs easily. I can shower and wash my hair without struggling for breath. I again enjoy walking, yoga, core classes, working out with weights and playing with my children better than ever before. I started bicycling six months after surgery and it has become my new love. I bicycle throughout the week usually 45-60 miles and up to 35 miles in one ride. My husband and I did a fundraising bike ride 10 months after transplant for the Pulmonary Fibrosis Foundation in Chicago raising over $5K (and I am doing so again this year). We were able to attend local family gatherings again, traveled to California (where I was born and raised) seven months after transplant, the bike ride in Chicago, Florida for Spring break. We attended the 2010 National Kidney Foundation (NKF) Transplant Games in Madison, Wisconsin where I competed in 5K cycling, 20K cycling, 1500m racewalk, bowling and a 5K walk.

With my renewed life, I have done fundraising and worked to raise awareness for the Pulmonary Fibrosis Foundation, public speaking at local hospitals regarding pulmonary fibrosis and Organ Donation, volunteer work for my daughters' soccer club, volunteer for my children's school garden, school library, and with Louisville's Second Chance at Life and Kentucky Organ Donor Affiliates to educate and promote Organ, Eye and Tissue Donation. I have shared my journey with my very large group of supporters and welcome any outlet that helps me spread the word about IPF, self-advocacy, positive attitude, health, exercise, wellness, and the amazing gifts that come from Organ, Eye and Tissue Donation.

Having a terminal restrictive lung disease and being constantly and increasingly short of breath affects absolutely every aspect of life. There is not a single thing that has not improved, become more enjoyable or a new possibility. I can again live my life without a continuous battle, without the fear and panic that comes with the coughing attacks, sickness and struggle for every single breath. I breathe deeply and easily and take such pleasure with each breath. I can play in the snow in winter and the heat of the summer and travel.

I can laugh with my husband and at my kids without fear that it will lead to a coughing attack and struggle to recover my breath. I do have to make sure I have my anti-rejection medication every 12 hours, but I don't have to calculate how many tanks of oxygen I have to pack in the car, how long I can be out, how much I can do without running out of air. I am no longer tethered to a leash around my house or feel like my ears and nose are getting yanked off when the tubing gets caught on a cabinet, door or stepped on by my family or myself. My nose no longer bleeds from the drying effects of the supplemental oxygen and we no longer hear the drone of the concentrator. I am not stared at and judged by complete strangers who assume I did this damage to myself. I no longer have to explain what I have, what it is and that, "No, I would not get better" and that there is no treatment and no cure for Pulmonary Fibrosis. I proudly do share my story with everyone so that I can continue to spread the word about my mostly unknown, under publicized and incredibly misunderstood disease. I am here and I plan to live my life and get the most out of every single day. I plan to be here to experience absolutely every moment of my children's incredible life.

I am thankful for my wonderful husband and love him more every single day. I want to give back to the people and organizations that I have gained so much from. I want to honor my donor and his family by the way I live my life. I do what I can because I can and to do anything less than the best I can do, is to sacrifice the gift of life and the second chance I have received.

I am eternally grateful to my donor and donor family and will continue to express that and honor them to the best of my ability. I do now live a life forever connected with my donor, and with me he lives on. I wrote my donor family a year after my surgery and felt so blessed to receive a reply. I have learned about my donor and am so grateful to hold that part of the puzzle. I hope to stay in contact always and that someday they will want to meet my family and me. In learning about my donor and talking to other recipients and donor families I have decided that all the "coincidences" and "commonalities" just can't be a fluke. There must be a reason for everything and for our lives to have become intertwined.

I sing the praises of the doctors who have made the difference in my life and helped me in this journey. I have learned that you know yourself and your body better than anyone else. I know that you must demand the best treatment and care, never settling for anything less. I know that attitude and perception make all the difference in how you live your life and the outcomes that you help create. I realize the importance of creating the best environment for you, both physically and mentally. I know that surrounding yourself with the best and having a great support system gives you strength and raises you up. You need to educate yourself and be a full participant in your healthcare. You need knowledge, optimism, support and faith.

Kerry Geron, 40
New Albany, Indiana
Idiopathic Pulmonary Fibrosis
Double Lung Transplant, December 18, 2008
Clarian Health-Methodist, Indianapolis, Indiana

Donovan's Transplant Journey
By Beth Gobeil

November 8, 1988 is a day that is engraved in my mind with a clarity that only life-changing news can bring. The news my husband, Laurier and I received that day concerned our two-month-old son, Donovan. We found out he had Cystic Fibrosis (CF). This news would be hard for any parents to receive, but for us, it came at a time that was already fraught with anxiety. Laurier's brother Colin, only 25-years-old, was dying of the same illness.

Donovan's arrival, on August 26, 1988 was a joyful event, a firstborn son to join our family of two little girls. The name "Donovan" means warrior, we later learned. How did we know it would be a name so fitting for our son, who had a lifetime of battles ahead? Days after Donovan's birth, his uncle Colin left for Toronto, to be assessed for a double lung transplant, which was at that time was in its infancy, a risky and very new therapy for end-stage Cystic Fibrosis.

It was just two months after Colin left for assessment, that Donovan was diagnosed, symptom-free at that point, and our lives were turned on end. Six weeks after Donovan's diagnosis, we grieved the loss of his uncle Colin, who passed away while on the transplant wait list in Toronto, Canada.

During Donovan's elementary school years, he developed a love of nature, and wrote stories about eagles, which fascinated him. By age 10, he had a cough that lingered, starting with morning chest physiotherapy, and reappearing with exertion during the day. We soon realized that we rarely had to call Donovan's name; if we waited a few minutes Donovan's cough would reveal his whereabouts.

When Donovan was in grade nine, his lung function plunged to a new low, qualifying him to have a wish granted by The Children's Wish Foundation, and our family enjoyed a trip to Cairns, Australia, where we snorkeled the Great Barrier Reef with Donovan, who had always wanted to see this wonder of the world.

Donovan graduated with distinction from high school in 2006, finishing the last few months at home with a tutor. He moved with a friend to Saskatoon, in Saskatchewan, Canada, ninety minutes from our home, and rented an old house inhabited by several young people. It was a time he had dreamed of, stretching his wings in the adult work-a-day world, just like his friends, a time he cherished, however short-lived.

In 2008, Donovan's CF doctor suggested he travel to Edmonton to meet the lung transplant team. We interviewed with Dr. Justin Weinkauf. Shortly after, Donovan was admitted to the hospital, gravely ill. After a week in Saskatoon's Royal University Hospital, where we anxiously paced the hallways near the intensive care unit (ICU), Donovan was airlifted to University of Alberta Hospital in Edmonton, Alberta, Canada. He was officially placed on the transplant list sedated, and unaware he was barely hanging onto life.

On September 13, 2008, Donovan got his second chance at life. I rejoiced in my heart that this chance was being given by grace to our family…at the same time I said a prayer for the donor family, knowing that wherever they were, this was most likely the worst day of their lives. Dr. Nitin Ghorpade, a handsome and pleasant man with a lovely smile, met us after surgery, and said it had gone without a hitch, and that Donovan was stable in the ICU. Tears streamed from my eyes as I hugged this man who had saved our son; then our family and friends who had supported us throughout the day joined our celebratory "circle of love".

Donovan's chest, which had heaved so mightily with each breath in the previous days, seemed to barely move at all as he was now breathing with ease, with new lungs! His fingernails were the next things I noticed---a beautiful shade of pale pink, not the oxygen starved blue to which we'd grown accustomed. Donovan's respirator was removed in three days and he was out of the ICU in six days. He had a lot of work to do, and he faced the challenge with silent determination. Finally, he became an outpatient, twenty-three days post operation (post-op).

Donovan's first post-op pulmonary function test was 60%, then up to 70% and finally into the eighties, and beyond. Each day, while exhausting for him was a new milestone met, and it was a joy to witness the miracle of every one! Donovan crossed the threshold of home, some six months after driving away to the hospital in respiratory distress, not knowing what awaited him. He had climbed many mountains, and his homecoming was like standing on a summit, waving a flag of victory!

In the year and half since his homecoming, Donovan continues to thrive and embrace life with "used lungs." He has worked at summer camp, resumed his hobby of taking gorgeous photographs, learned the new sport of long-boarding, and perhaps most dramatic, has begun running. On Father's

Day 2010, I watched in awe as Donovan completed his first official 5K race, in 29 minutes. Two months later, he entered another 5K race, shaving off five minutes from his previous time, then, to celebrate the two-year anniversary of his transplant, on September 13, 2010, Donovan completed a 21.1 Km. run: an entire half-marathon!!! His time was an incredible 1:55 (with two stops to check his blood sugar!!!)

Watching Donovan recover from what we can only describe as a miracle has indeed been like watching a beautiful butterfly emerge from a cocoon. Life, we know, is as fragile as those delicate wings, which are most beautiful when they do what they were designed for, and that is to fly. Donovan has yet to decide on a direction for his "flight" and many options await him. While his peers were making their life plans in high school and afterward, Donovan was fighting a battle for his life, unsure of what was ahead in the next week, or even the next day! At the moment, he is a typical 22-year-old, working in a local mall, selling cell phones and taking a night class, while contemplating career choices, including post-secondary school. He relishes his independence, and is happy to be alive, hanging out with his great circle of supportive friends, enjoying life a breath at a time!

Donovan has now run four half-marathons, and dedicated his most recent run to those who are struggling with CF, to those awaiting transplant, to those who have lost their battles, and to his donor family, to whom we are deeply indebted. His donor family has given him his very breath, and whatever direction his "wings" may take him, we know it is their very brave decision that has allowed him to fly.

Whenever I see a butterfly, landing gently on a flower, perhaps momentarily, perhaps lingering there then lifting off, spreading multi-colored wings and soundlessly taking to the skies, I am reminded of our transplant miracle, a life lost, a life given back, and my heart is filled to overflowing.

Beth Gobeil, Mother to Son, Donovan Gobeil
Donovan Gobeil, 22
Saskatchewan, Canada
Donovan, Cystic Fibrosis
Donovan, Double Lung Transplant, September 13, 2008
University of Alberta Hospital, Edmonton, Alberta, Canada

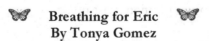

Breathing for Eric
By Tonya Gomez

My name is Tonya and I was born with Cystic Fibrosis (CF). Diagnosed at six months of age; my mother could not figure out what was wrong with me. She took me to every doctor in the area. They continued to diagnose me with pneumonia. My mother had different instincts than the doctors. She finally got an appointment at The Children's Hospital in Columbus, Ohio. The minute the doctor looked at me, he knew I had Cystic Fibrosis. Once the appropriate medications were administered, my health began to turn around. I was breathing better and digesting foods more efficiently. Two years later, my brother, Eric was born. He was diagnosed with CF immediately and treatments began. My brother lost his battle with CF at the young age of six. I cannot imagine the grief my mother endured in losing a child. 30 years have passed, yet the pain never ends.

I grew up being very private because I knew that I was different than other children. I was afraid of being made fun of. Only my closest friends knew my secret. I was always careful not to bring attention to myself. I decided to twirl baton in junior high and became a majorette in high school. That was the most attention I could stand. I was always afraid of developing coughing spells at the most inopportune time. It never failed; when all was quiet, whom do you think started to cough? Yours truly! It wasn't just a cough. It was a full blown, "Are you okay? Maybe you should stop smoking!" type cough. I always dreaded being in large quiet groups.

High school graduation was such an accomplishment for someone who wasn't expected to live past her teen years. As I grew older, treatment regimens for CF improved. Aerosol tents came to an end and so did the "morning dew". I was off to college. Coming from a small town, The Ohio State University was a major culture shock. I fell in love with the campus immediately. I lived in a suite with five other girls and it became difficult to hide the fact that I carried a life threatening illness with me daily. I learned to cope, and though I was not perfect, I took the best care of myself given the situation. During that time, I was involved in the study of a drug called Pulmozyme and fortunately, it turned out to be a life-changing drug for CF patients.

Another accomplishment in my life came about. I graduated from college! I originally wanted to become a nurse. After spending so much time in the hospital and getting poked so many times, I thought I could place the intravenous antibiotics (IV) line with my eyes closed! I learned that was not the field for me. I ended up in nutrition. Life after college was confusing. I spent some time trying to 'find myself', taking different jobs and enjoying my life

I received an internship, became a registered/licensed dietitian and decided it was time to become an adult. I found a real job and met my husband. Telling him about my illness was not as difficult as I thought it would be. I also forewarned him that I might not be able to have children due to my illness. He was okay with this. After we became engaged, we found out we were pregnant. 7 ½ months later, our miracle baby boy, Eric (my brother's namesake) was born healthy! God gave me the gift of a child that I didn't think I would have. He also allowed me the experience and privilege of motherhood. My life couldn't be better

As time went on, my lung function began to decline. In 2003, my worst fear became a reality. I needed a double lung transplant. I was told I might be waiting two years. Because of my petite size, I would likely need a child's lungs. I waited five months and one week. The call from The Cleveland Clinic Foundation, Cleveland, Ohio came on May 25, 2004, telling me that there may be lungs available.

I had a limited amount of time to get there. I lived 2 ½ hours away. I was in the middle of making my son, Eric, scrambled eggs. I had not showered for a couple of days and knew that if this surgery was a "go", I may not shower for many more days. I told the nurse I needed to make some phone calls and get a shower. So many emotions, so many questions: Would I ever see my family? Would I see my precious son again? I needed this transplant so I could see my son grow!

Well, my transplant was a success and I am here today to tell you about it! My surgeon said the lungs were a perfect fit. Working in a hospital, I knew about surgery reports. I asked the nurse if I could see mine. I wanted to know everything that the surgeons had done to me. This is when I found out that my lungs came from a ten-year-old boy. My husband and I were silent and began to sob. I needed a child's lungs and I received a child's lungs. What I never wanted to experience, what my mother experienced so many years ago, now another family was experiencing that same grief. And I was alive because of it. Only transplant recipients and their families can understand what I am talking about. Only the donor family can understand the grief. I finally realized that God had His plan and it was going to happen because it was His plan.

I am thankful that I do not remember most of what occurred after the surgery. Modesty is not a commodity! People say, "How did you handle it"? I tell them, "I was asleep during the hard part"! After getting out of the hospital and beginning the road to recovery, I could not believe how much energy I had. I wanted to do everything! The greatest thing: Breathing! My lung function had declined to 19% out of 100% prior to surgery. I will never take it for granted, like many people do, what it is like to breathe. I do things now because I can. I have the energy to keep up with my son and enjoy life with my family.

My lung function is well over 100% now and I make sure I take the best care of myself. I have many future goals in life, and my next one is to see my son graduate from high school.

I believe everything happens for a reason and God is not done with me yet. I fundraise for cystic fibrosis and take every opportunity to promote organ donation. I hope to inspire as many people as possible to become organ donors. I have participated in the United States Transplant Games and have even won medals. That is just the bonus.

I, like many others, participate in these events because WE CAN! I have met my donor family. They are truly wonderful and have suffered a great loss. I believe it gives them comfort in knowing that I can now raise my son and that their son left a legacy in me; and others that he was able to donate to. So far, I am the only recipient my donor family has heard from. As long as I am alive and the Lord will allow, I will continue to serve my purpose here in this world.

I am a registered organ donor and when my time is up on this earth, I will offer the same gift that my donor family offered me. Miracles do happen, and I am living proof. I want to give hope to those waiting for transplants, but also to CF patients that think their life may be short lived. Nothing in life is ever guaranteed. Our plan is mapped out for us. Life is good. You just have to live it!

Tonya Gomez, 38
Archbold, Ohio
Cystic Fibrosis
Double Lung Transplant, May 25, 2004
The Cleveland Clinic Foundation, Cleveland, Ohio

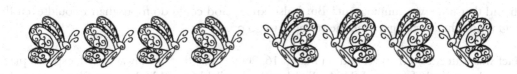

Flappy the Butterfly
By Alfredo Goodyear

It was a cold morning in February as I sat sipping my cup of tea, staring out my kitchen window when I saw it flutter by. It caught my attention immediately, and I thought, 'No it can't be a butterfly', after all the temperatures in the cold Newfoundland winter's in Canada don't allow for butterflies flying around. I kept watching until suddenly it fell, and after a short while froze onto the icy ground. My husband went outside picked up the frozen butterfly and brought it into the warmth of our home where it came back to life and after a while started flapping its wings. I named it 'FLAPPY'; we kept it protected from the cold for two weeks until it lived out its lifespan.

That little butterfly, that day, made me appreciate all the more my new "Gift of Life". I was diagnosed with Pulmonary Fibrosis in 2005 a disease, which had three years earlier claimed the life of my 52-year-old brother.

At first the disease didn't seem to interfere much with my life apart from maybe shortness of breath upon performing certain activities. I kept working as a seasonal worker at our local fish plant, until my health started to decline. My breathing became worse, even simple everyday chores became difficult and life as I knew it was completely changed.

By the end of summer things had gotten so bad I had to relocate to Toronto, Ontario, Canada, where I was listed for a transplant at Toronto General Hospital. Coming from a small outport community in Newfoundland, Canada, with a population of less than one hundred residents, was needless to say quite an experience. I was very fortunate to have family and friends in Toronto who were more than willing to help us in any way they could, that plus the overwhelming love and financial support from family, friends, and community helped ease the burden and made the journey a whole lot easier to bear.

Settling into our new apartment and getting used to city life was quite interesting to say the least. I was very blessed to have some of my family members with me at all times for support and encouragement. My life as well as my support person's took on a whole new routine of regular clinic appointments and physical therapy. I waited on the transplant list for 5 ½ months during which time there were many challenges. There were times when the journey got quite rough. But despite the challenges there was never a time when I lost hope. My faith in God and encouragement from family and friends kept me strong.

My health deteriorated very rapidly to the point where I had to be hospitalized until if, and when donor lungs became available. It's then when my faith could not wavier. I knew the condition of my health and that time was running out. But I also knew God could do more than I could even think or imagine and that's what gave me the strength to go on.

The fact was, I needed a miracle, and on March 16, 2009, a day that will always hold a special place in my heart, that miracle happened. Lungs had become available, God had answered my prayers, and even though I was overjoyed, it tugged at my heart to know that somewhere some family's heart was breaking. The surgery lasted for about 10 hours, it was a complete success and today I feel very blessed indeed to share this story with you.

It's difficult to explain to someone how hard it is not to be able to breathe without being on 100% oxygen, but it's even more difficult to put into words or describe the feeling to be able to breathe on your own again without it. What a blessing!!!

I will be forever grateful to Dr. Andrew Pierre and the rest of the Toronto lung transplant team for dedicating their lives in such a special way to help others live. Their skill and expertise, their care and concern for others is beyond measure.

I've heard it said before you can never know the joy of being on the mountaintop without first walking through the valley, and through this valley experience I now look at life in a different perspective. I've learned to treasure the important things in life and not sweat the "small stuff". I now take out lots of time to spend with family and friends, life is too short to let the time pass you by, the moments and days seem to go by so quickly. Share things with each other and have lots of laughs together. Breathe easy and cherish each new day, everyone is so precious.

Just as that butterfly found itself in our front yard that morning and was given a second chance, in life so was I. My heart overflows with gratitude and love towards my donor family for their selfless act of love that day.

No pen can or ever will be able to write my thankfulness towards them in words, but they will be etched upon my heart forever. To anyone out there who may be waiting on a transplant list, hang in there and keep believing and when you do receive it, give God thanks, flap your wings and soar into the future with renewed hope for you have truly been Blessed!!!

"Be An Organ Donor and Give the Gift of Life!"

Alfredo Goodyear, 51
Newfoundland, Canada
Pulmonary Fibrosis
Double Lung Transplant, March 16, 2009
Toronto General Hospital, Toronto, Canada

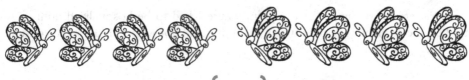

11 Years, 4 Months & Intend to Keep on Going
By June Gorecki

Wow! Who would have thought? Here it is 11 years later, and I am still alive! It was 11 years and four months ago when I coded on the table after my new lung went into shock and my body was rejected it.

Miracles do happen. But you have to fight to stay alive for the rest of your life. I am so lucky. I was able to see a new grandchild born, six grandchildren graduate from high school and two of my grandchildren graduated from college and my oldest granddaughter got married.

It is so very important to take your medications and listen to your doctors. My doctor told me that I would know my body more than anyone else, even doctors, and he was right. He also told me I would learn my medication so well, better than anyone else, and that came in handy. Twice when I was in the hospital, the nurses brought me the wrong medications. I asked them to check my medicine list again; when they did, I got an apology, and they asked how I was so sure that I was brought the wrong medication. I think transplant patients get a little more respect. A lot of people do not realize that we are different.

Everyday, I still thank God and my donor, Geoffrey Widen, for my second chance at life, and I never ever fail to talk about organ/tissue donation to anyone who will listen. I will go on for as long as God allows me to, as He does have a purpose for me yet.

When I am done on this earth, I have asked my family to let my donor family know, and to have a memorial service to remember any of the good things I have done…and to let any of the bad things I have done go with me as well. I do not want anyone to cry over an empty shell. Remember, fight to stay alive - the rewards are well worth it.

June Gorecki, 69
Montgomery, Illinois
Chronic Obstructive Pulmonary Disease
Single Lung Transplant, June 17, 1999
Rush-Presbyterian/St. Luke's Medical Center, Chicago, Illinois
Read June's Lung Transplant Story in the 1st Edition of Taking Flight

The Most Important Birthday
By Howell Graham

I was born on February 20, 1962, the day John Glenn; United States Marine Corp astronaut circled the globe for the first time. My mother says that no one cared if she gave birth to a kangaroo that day since all doctors and nurses were glued to their TV set watching the momentous orbit. My father and grandfather are Marines; this "first" was doubly exciting for our family.

But I have another birthday...the one that means more to me than my actual arrival in the world. It is October 8th and this year...2010...I celebrate the 20th anniversary of that event which literally gave me a new life, a spectacular second chance.

Diagnosed at age two, there had been some red flags up until that time. I was sick a good deal, but mostly with digestive problems. My mom read a featured monthly column in McCall's magazine called, "Everything You Wanted to Know about..." and featured different diseases like measles, rheumatic fever. This month the topic was Cystic Fibrosis (CF) and the bells went off.

The doctor confirmed the fears and told my parents that I would not likely make it to first grade. They refused to accept this and began an all out campaign to keep me as healthy as possible...postural drainage, a percussive exercise to help expel the thick mucus in my lungs, done several times a day. Antibiotics, plus enzymes to help digest food, and a mist tent, fashioned from bent pipes, which supported a heavy plastic cover. It looked like an oxygen tent but allowed antibiotics to be inhaled through a tube attached to a respirator. My father bent the pipe frame, and my mom made the tent by sealing the edges with a warm iron. After 13 years using this contraption, experts said the tent was doing more harm than good and was discontinued.

Growing up in Charleston, South Carolina, I did the usual activities: swimming, tearing around the neighborhood bicycling, and was the left fielder on the Dixie League Baseball Team in Mt. Pleasant. We had a sailboat and I spent countless hours out in the salt air learning the specifics of sailing the Charleston Harbor. The years went by. I had long passed first grade... the initial date the diagnosing physician at Camp Lejeune had given me.

I came to the University of North Carolina in Wilmington, North Carolina and fell in love with the coastal city and the opportunities I had to continue boating. After graduation, I got a job in real estate. By 1990, my health had deteriorated significantly and breathing difficulties became a constant. When I lay in bed, I could hear my labored breathing. The everyday events like taking a shower or fixing my breakfast cereal and toast, made me breathless. Activities like boating and water skiing were out of the question now. My energy was gone, and the days were becoming long sessions of inhalation therapies and trips to the doctor. The fatigue level now outweighed the stamina level.

My Chapel Hill, North Carolina physician, Dr. James Yankaskas, talked with me about being a candidate for the new double-lung transplant procedure that had just started to be performed at Chapel Hill. The statistics were less than glowing: a fifty-fifty percent chance of surviving the surgery, not to mention the post-operative risks of rejection and infection. It was a grim decision, but my life at that point was miserable. I knew I had to take the chance I had been offered.

My parents and I moved to an apartment in Chapel Hill for several months. I did a good deal of physical therapy to build up my stamina during this time. When the beeper went off...no cell phones back then, we were ecstatic. The call had come. Dr. Thomas Egan, my transplant surgeon who pioneered the brand new double-lung transplant program at Memorial Hospital in Chapel Hill, had gotten a call and was flying down in a private jet from North Carolina to Pensacola, Florida, where a physician's son had been fatally injured in a motorcycle accident. He had to make sure the lungs were in good condition and that I would have the best chance possible. It is interesting to realize that my new lungs were from Pensacola. I had been born in Tallahassee, just 200 miles down the road but had never been back to Florida since we moved away when I was six months old.

Again the waiting. Some of the young people I knew from the CF clinic came by to wish me luck. I realized that their hopes were riding on me too. The success of this operation could make a difference in their lives in the future. I was prepped for the operation in anticipation for Dr. Egan's report that the lungs were good and waited for the news from my surgeon. Dr. Egan called from Pensacola just before boarding the plane with my new lungs in a cooler. His words were relayed to me; "Everything looks good. Tell Howell, ... it's a go!"

The operation took about 13 hours. Splitting my chest from side to side horizontally with an impressive incision, Dr. Egan cracked the ribs to make an opening to remove my diseased lungs and replace them with my donor's freshly procured lungs. I only know that I woke up in intensive care unit (ICU) with a beautiful dark-haired nurse hovering over me as I drifted in and out of the haze. Then the scenery changed abruptly. My beautiful brunette was gone and a burly male nurse was adjusting the machinery I was hooked up to. I remember a distinct wave of disappointment...I think now that this must have been a good sign!

The weeks of recovery in the hospital were a blur. I remember being walked down the hospital corridor only hours after I got to the ward and was in my room. It seemed I had a hundred tubes and wires coming from all sorts of places but my parents and I shuffled determinedly down the hall. It became a daily ritual until I built up to four or five strolls each day, someone pushing the poles and machines, while I trudged on.

The physical therapy in this rehab phase was extreme but I was willing to do whatever it took to make this thing work. We all had a goal of getting home to Wilmington before Christmas and we did.

Since then, my life is more than I could have ever dreamed it would be. I became a partner in my real estate appraisal firm, met a wonderful and beautiful girl...a dentist who knowing the risk took a chance on me too and became my wife. We are still here in Wilmington with our two Labradors, and a great little 23-foot Scout named Nine Lives II. We cruise around the marshes, take the dogs for outings on Masonboro Island and enjoy life with our friends and family.

Only months after we got home from the transplant surgery, I took the Boston Whaler I had at that time out into the ocean…it was the perfect day but extremely windy and rough. But it soon became too warm for my shirt, which I pulled off. Still too warm. I stood and dived into the ocean and realized as I was surfacing that I had made a strategic error. The boat had caught the wind in the Bimini top and the current swiftly moved it out of reach. I knew better than to be that foolish. I tried to swim after it but it quickly glided away from me parallel to the beach. I knew not to panic. I treaded water for over an hour. I was four miles out from the beach. I could not even see land. The Whaler was long out of sight by now. I treaded water some more and thought about my dilemma. My only thought was that Dr. Egan was going to kill me for wasting my new lungs by sinking to the bottom of the ocean.

I heard something slapping across the waves. I saw a guy on a windsurfer sailing some fifty yards away. I yelled for help. But he could not see me due to the three to four foot waves. I yelled again and saw him heading toward me. He pulled me aboard and we headed back to shore. I seem to be beating the odds again. My boat was retrieved some three miles distance down the beach at Figure Eight Island.

I didn't tell my parents about this incident for months. When I finally did, there was a long silence, "Dr. Egan would have killed you! Are you kidding? He would have had to stand in line behind your daddy and me!"

I have tried to be an advocate for promoting organ donation and to correspond or talk with anyone who needs any advice or encouragement about cystic fibrosis or transplant surgery. I know how much it means to have someone to turn to when you think no one really understands, and how debilitating and discouraging the disease is. Struggling to breathe is difficult to understand until you've been there.

I am still in survivor mode. I have, in the latter part of these past twenty years, pulled through a ruptured appendix where I developed sepsis ("miraculous", Chapel Hill said) and colon cancer. Am I grateful? More than I can tell you. I am grateful for Dr. Yankaskas for keeping me afloat through some pretty dark times in my teen and young adult years. I am grateful to Dr. Egan for his amazing skills in an equally amazing surgery. I am grateful to the generous parents who gave the gift of their son's lungs in the most devastating circumstances… and gave me a future. I am grateful to my family for their dedication and support, and to my wife, for her loving patience and continued understanding, and mostly for just putting up with me.

Twenty years and I am celebrating my second birthday, and my twentieth year out with a vengeance. They say I am one of the longest surviving double lung transplant recipients in the world…it's amazing! And my boat named Nine Lives II? I still have the boat and I think I still have a few of those lives left. I thank God for getting me this far.

Howell Graham, 48
Wilmington, North Carolina
Cystic Fibrosis
Double Lung Transplant, October 8, 1990
University of North Carolina Hospitals, Chapel Hill, North Carolina

Transplant, Baby and Blessings
By Tammi Green

When I was 14, I was diagnosed with Pulmonary Fibrosis and given five years to live. Well, I just turned 45, thanks to a great pulmonologist in my hometown and a great team of doctors at the University of Pittsburgh Medical Center (UPMC), Pittsburgh, Pennsylvania.

My local doctor treated me and I responded well to medicines until my mid 20's, that's when he suggested I consider lung transplantation. I chose UPMC and went to be evaluated. I was accepted into the program before we boarded the plane home.

When I was 27 I got "the call", and had a single lung transplant. The first year was hard! I encountered some setbacks, illnesses and rejections. I was one of the first patients put on the inhaled Cyclosporine program at its inception. After the transplant the doctors told me, "The first year you are going to ask yourself why you did this, it is not going to be easy, but after that first year it will get easier." …And it did! I got better, stronger more active!

After a few years, I met and married a wonderful man and had a beautiful baby boy who is happy, and healthy, and the light of my life!

In 2007 my lung started to fail and I was put back on oxygen. My doctors asked if I would consider re-transplant. "Of Course!" I had a family to live for! A family I needed to be active for, that needed me! I needed new lungs! So I went in to be re-evaluated, and was accepted into the program again.

In September 2010 I was given the 'GIFT OF LIFE' for a second time, a double lung transplant! The recovery was harder this time, but well worth it…I just spent Christmas at home with my family without oxygen!

Tammi Green, 45
Walkerton, Indiana
Pulmonary Fibrosis
Single Lung Transplant, November 1993
Re-Transplant, Double Lung Transplant, September 2010
University of Pittsburgh Medical Center, Pittsburgh, Pennsylvania
Tammi Had a Son, April 1999

Never Quit!!
By Kent Griffiths

"Kent, Kent, are you okay?" Captain Jon was looking down at me while I lay on the deck of the tug 'Dolphin'. I was preparing to go on deck for my watch. I passed out. This would be the first of many times to come. I was sent to the emergency room at Piney Point, Maryland. The tug and oil barge could not be moved until I returned. The doctor told me I was in excellent condition as far as he could see, except for my lungs. I explained to the doctor that I had pneumonia several times and that I was still recovering from the last one. I was advised to see a pulmonary doctor.

We returned to the New York harbor, Penn Maritime Shipyard. It was the last day of my three-week hitch. Before leaving the yard, I was ordered to see a pulmonary doctor and bring back a, 'fit for duty letter.' I had just moved to Indialantic, Florida, to be closer to my youngest and her mom. I figured I'd start a guide service on my off time from the tug.

I made an appointment with a pulmonary doctor. The doctor studied my test results, and I was advised that I had Pulmonary Fibrosis. He seemed a bit somber. I just wanted to get what ever medication he was going to give me and my 'fit for duty letter' and get out of there. The doctor advised me that this thing had gone pretty far, and that in his opinion I had two or three years to live. He said the only advice he had was to look into a lung transplant. That day I gathered my four daughters and told them. My girls all jumped into this thing with both feet, along with a few friends and family members. If it weren't for them I never would have come this far.

After three days of intense testing at Shands Hospital at The University of Florida, Gainesville, Florida, I drove to Cedar Key, and had clam chowder at Tony's Famous Cedar Key Clam Chowder and checked the area out. I loved it. About half way back to Gainesville I saw a 'for rent' sign in front of a little cracker house with huge beautiful oak trees all around. The owner was doing some work on it, I told him and his wife my story and we were able to make a deal and I moved in a few weeks later. I was listed at Shands in 2008. The day I was accepted into the program, my caregiver my daughter Brooke, was accepted into the respiratory therapist program at Santa Fe College in Gainesville. My daughter Brooke graduated four months before my transplant. Today she has a position at Shands. I will never be able to thank her enough.

I did lots of sight seeing. I'll bet I've seen more of north Florida than most of the folks up there. I got in two or three fishing trips before it was just too much for me. I would put several oxygen tanks in my forward compartment connected to 50 feet of tubing hose. There was an old pigpen in the back yard. My landlord gave me permission to put two pigs in. My neighbor Lamar sold them to me for $25.00 each. They were babies. Two pigs turned into eight then one day when I was walking out to feed the pigs, I passed out. By this time I was on about six liters of oxygen at all times and 10 liters from a mask whenever I fed the pigs or when taking a shower. (This was one of the hardest things.) Oh! The things we take for granted.

I joined the support group at Shands that was just starting. Two weeks later I received a call. "We may have lungs for you, come on in." After a few hours they sent us home. There are so many factors to deal with; it all has to be perfect to work. It's weird; I was almost relieved as well as disappointed when told to go home. The mind works in mysterious ways when you know time, as we know it, is running out!!!! By this time my little cabin looked like an oxygen factory. On my front porch was a big stainless steel tank of liquid oxygen, as well as one in the living room, an oxygen concentrator, and at least 20 small bottles of oxygen on the porch. I had two hoses hooked up to me.

One day, I was having coffee and watching television and the phone rang. It was one of the logistics people that coordinate everything in regards to transplant. He asked how I was doing, and my heart dropped. He said, "Today just might be your day! Go ahead and get your stuff together, advise your caregiver, and make sure you have a ride, just in case. We'll be in touch." That was it. I prayed and waited. Another call, "Why don't you go ahead and head this way." As I was leaving I looked at my little cabin and wondered if I'd ever see it again.

The parking at Shands is a real challenge. It's terrible! I walked to the side of the hospital. No lobby, no receptionist, no security, just the door I was told to knock on. I knocked! A young man with red spiked hair opened the door. The kind of kid you might run into at Gator's on Saturday or Sunday, watching the game, and eating chicken wings and having a cold Budweiser. He had a bed right there at the door. "Come on, get up here", he said. I said, "I can't. If I lie on my back I'll start coughing real bad."

The last thing I remember is him pulling me up on that bed and reading, 'Anesthesiologist' on his lab coat. I received my bi-lateral lung transplant, September 22, 2009.

I came to about 15 hours later, with the ventilator in place, wires all around me, and an early complication. Dr. Maher Baz seemed concerned when he told me. I put my faith in him, his staff, and God, that I would make it. Guess what? 10 days later the tube came out and I was sent to a regular room. God Bless Dr. Baz!!!!

I stayed with my daughter Brooke for a month. Then they cut me loose!!!!! From that day on it's been non-stop! The only problems I have are those that I create. Sometimes I just go way too fast!! So I stop, breathe, eat, sleep, and pray, then just move on. Today I go to graduations, tee ball games, and take my grandson fishing and hunting and just love being alive.

I'm a miracle, I'm Blessed, and I'm Grateful!

Live, Laugh, and Love!

Kent Griffiths, 56
Chiefland, Florida
Pulmonary Fibrosis
Double Lung Transplant, September 22, 2009
Shands Hospital at The University of Florida, Gainesville, Florida

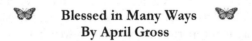

Blessed in Many Ways
By April Gross

When I was 1 ½ years old, I was diagnosed with Cystic Fibrosis (CF). The doctors told my parents that I probably wouldn't live past the age of 12.

I grew up a lot healthier than most people with CF. I took enzymes every time I ate, and my parents did the daily chest percussion on me until I was old enough to run on my own for airway clearance. The few times that I did get sick while still living at home, I only had to take oral antibiotics.

Once I got out on my own I didn't take the best care of myself and had my first hospitalization at the age of 20, and was given intravenous (IV) antibiotics to treat my infection. After that, I was hospitalized once every couple of years or so and treated with IV antibiotics. I had a pneumothorax in 1998 and wasn't hospitalized again until 2003. At that time, I was diagnosed with CF related diabetes. From then on I was in the hospital usually twice a year. I was still able to keep up with my husband and do house and yard work. I started using oxygen at night and when I exercised. I was spending almost two hours a day trying to keep the infections at bay. In 2008, my husband and I went on a great vacation since we knew the time for me to seriously consider lung transplant was getting close.

I completed the transplant evaluation at the University of Minnesota Medical Center, Minneapolis in Minnesota, while we waited for the University of Iowa Hospitals and Clinics, Iowa City, in Iowa, lung transplant program to become accredited. I was listed at University of Minnesota, and by this time my FEV1 was down to 18%. I was on oxygen 24 hours a day (24/7), and it was a struggle to do basic things like dressing myself…even something as simple as walking was difficult. Luckily, I am married a wonderful man who kept everything going while still working full time so I could do my three breathing and vest treatments a day.

After University of Iowa received their accreditation, I decided to go on the waiting list there. I only had to wait three days for the phone to ring with "the call" to come to the University of Iowa. I was the 20th person at the University of Iowa to have lungs transplanted. I was begging to go back to work after three months.

Ever since then, my life has been like a dream. Rarely do I even feel like I have Cystic Fibrosis. I met my donor's family in April 2010, and learned that my gift of life came from a beautiful young lady who suffered a brain aneurysm, her name was Lisa Darling and she was only 14-years-old. Since then my husband and I have participated in several running events with Lisa's family. Most recently, I ran the Dam to Dam, a 20K held in Des Moines in Iowa, each year, with my husband and Lisa's father Greg. It was such an emotional experience for my family and me, and for Lisa's family.

I have no limitations now, as my current FEV1 is 120%. I am physically active everyday, as I'll never take advantage of this wonderful gift I have been given. I have been blessed in many ways and am so grateful to share my story with others.

April Gross, 39
Woodward, Iowa
Cystic Fibrosis
Double Lung Transplant, March 20, 2009
University of Iowa Hospitals and Clinics, Iowa City, Iowa

 My Flight With New Lungs
By Cheryl Guillory

My name is Cheryl. My journey began three years ago on May 18, 2007 with the devastating diagnosis of Idiopathic Primary Pulmonary Arterial Hypertension (IPPAH). After a childhood of constant weight struggles I was finally able to get control of my life, get married to my soul mate, adopt the worlds most amazing little boy and give birth to two beautiful daughters. What else could be better, right?

Well after battling IPPAH for two years, things had gotten so bad that my husband would come home three times a day from his business just to check to see if I was still breathing. How he dealt with this emotional upheaval I'll never know. Not being able to care for my three children or even myself was one of the worst feelings in the world. Denial, denial, denial....That is how I survived.

Then in November 2009 things went from bad to worse. I began to be hospitalized frequently almost every week for fluid build up. I'd go in for a few days, and then go home only to turnaround and go right back. Trips to the hospital in New Orleans, Louisiana, from Duson, Louisiana were about two and a half hours each way. For someone unable to breathe this seems like an eternity and then some. The medical paraphernalia and medication was exhausting to say the least. Intravenous (IV) medications of Vasodilators to help keep my pulmonary arteries open, and oxygen concentrator at four liters per minute (LPM). My children suffered more than they should have in a lifetime of suffering. Constantly scared that "Mommy" was going to die. This hurt beyond all hurts.

ULTIMATE DEATH! There is no known medical cure, only the hope that organ transplantation will stop the disease. This is what they proposed to my family and me. A bilateral LUNG TRANSPLANT, but again, it's not that easy. The medical hurdles that I had to jump through were mind-boggling. But everyone that's been through this process knows exactly what those hurdles are. How we all made it through that, I'll never understand. Especially since we didn't have the strength to do the "normal" everyday task of LIVING.

The day was February 3, 2010, only 47 hours and 15 minutes after being listed, my pre-transplant nurse coordinator called, and she said, "Cheryl, what are you doing?" My response was, "Just finished cooking supper, and about to eat." The next words out of her mouth were, "NO! Don't eat, you need to come to New Orleans, we have new lungs for you." I was stunned to say the least. February 4, 2010, I was wheeled to the surgical suite. The last thing I remember from that moment was, "Please just let me wake up!" Next was another new chapter in my journey.

Waking up from anesthesia was one of the most glorious feelings of my life, right up there with giving birth to my two daughters. It was a strange feeling, being conscious yet unable to speak, move or even open my eyes. I can only guess that it was a few hours before I was finally able to let the doctors and nurses know that I was indeed awake.

The next eight months were filled with new and challenging moments, therapies and clinic visits. I've had minor glitches in the process but otherwise a wonderful journey. I have been blessed to have no evidence of infection or rejection, and except for the occasional bump in the road; I've continued to make remarkable strides. I continue to love life and all of its joys and sorrows. I've lost many friends to this disease over the short, three years, too many for my liking.

One other wonderful gift I've been given just in the last couple of weeks....I have had contact with my Donor's family. This yet another chapter and I'm so looking forward to meeting them in person. I've had this quiet, sweet connection to my donor for almost nine months now, and have had to come to grips with the horrific circumstances that lead to her death, and my ultimate receipt of. "The Gift of Life". She was a remarkable person, and has one of the most caring families. Yet there is another connection that I never saw coming....My lung donor was a twin! How amazing to have a living link to my donor, as close as her twin sister.

This is a fabulous journey that I do not intend on ending any time soon. I now volunteer for Donate Life Louisiana, and Louisiana Organ Procurement Agency (LOPA). I now volunteer at my children's school, and I'm living my life as any forty-year-old wife and mother of three should....with each and everyday....one at a time. To my family, my donor's family, my transplant team, and nurses....THANK YOU! Because of you all, I am alive.

The greatest HERO

I never knew....
Was the ORGAN DONOR

Who saved
My LIFE!

BE a HERO, BE an ORGAN DONOR

Cheryl Guillory, 40
Duson, Louisiana
Idiopathic Primary Pulmonary Arterial Hypertension
Double Lung Transplant, February 4, 2010
Ochsner Foundation Hospital, New Orleans, Louisiana

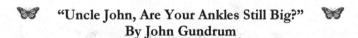

"Uncle John, Are Your Ankles Still Big?"
By John Gundrum

My name is John Gundrum, and I am 52-years-old. I was diagnosed with emphysema in 1994. I developed this from working for my family roofing business, which entailed working with and around hot asphalt fumes for roughly 20 years. I had to stop working in 2005.

In 2006, I was rushed to the hospital because I could not breathe and my oxygen saturation was at 72%. The normal and preferred oxygen saturation is 100%. That is when I stared oxygen 24/7.

I was in and out of the hospital 19 times. I started the process for getting on the waiting list for a double lung transplant in 2007. It took a year to get listed. One of the biggest problems was that I was single and the transplant center was afraid I could not take care of myself, but I showed proof to them, I had support. The biggest support was my nephew Jeff and his wife Brenda. Without them I could have never been able to be transplanted.

On September 20, 2008 I got "the call" and went to the University of Michigan Medical Center, Ann Arbor, Michigan and received my double lung transplant. It was so awesome. I was in surgery for about 12 hours and I stayed at the hospital for eight days, and then went to Jeff and Brenda's house for six days.

My favorite part of staying with Jeff and Brenda were that their three children, Gianna, Trevor and Braden were there when I would wake up and they would ask, "Uncle John are your ankles still big or can you get your shoes on today?" due to my feet being swollen. I went home after that and a lot of friends helped me with shopping and other errands. It took about a month before I could bring my two dogs home.

It has now been two years since the transplant, and I am doing great. I attended the Transplant Games in August 2010 in Madison, Wisconsin, with my girlfriend, Chris. We had a great time and I was happy to participate in my events, bowling, golfing and table tennis. I met Joanne Schum at the games and many wonderful people at this amazing event. A highlight for me was going to the Lung Gathering and meeting the longest living double lung/heart transplant recipient, Cathy McGill.

I would also like to thank my donor family because I would not be writing this if not for them. I hope someday to have some contact with them. MY life has changed in many ways because of the transplant. I can get out and do things; I can walk my 'real' dogs, instead of my 'third dog tank'. I also thank Joanne for all her hard work in writing this book.

John Gundrum, 52
Ann Arbor, Michigan
Emphysema
Double Lung Transplant, September 20, 2008
University of Michigan Medical Center, Ann Arbor, Michigan

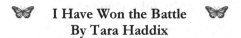

I Have Won the Battle
By Tara Haddix

When I was first born all seemed well but very soon I began wheezing. My mom knew something was wrong with me but the doctor kept telling her she was just a new mother, and I was fine.

One day I was rushed to the emergency room of the local hospital. They suspected water on my lungs, but it turned out there was no water on my lungs. They were not sure what was wrong with me. Finally one of the respiratory doctors had an idea, "Test her for Cystic Fibrosis" (CF). My parents had never heard of CF and had no clue what it was or what it meant. I was tested and it came back positive.

During an 8 ½ week hospital stay, my doctor came in and talked with my parents. He told us that I was dying. He also told us about a new procedure that was being done for people with CF at the hospital down the street, a double lung transplant.

On the morning of December 23, 1991, we received a call from the lung transplant coordinator, Mary Pearl, at The Cleveland Clinic Foundation in Cleveland, Ohio. Mary said we have a possible donor. Stay home and don't go anywhere. My grandparents came over, and so did Santa and Mrs. Claus. They were planning on coming over on Christmas Eve to bring my sisters and me gifts but with the good news they decided to make the trip from the North Pole a day early. We sat around waiting for the phone call. At least opening gifts from Santa helped the time pass. We had such a good community, that they donated gifts to my sisters and me so that we could have a good Christmas that year.

The phone rang. Everyone froze. We knew this was it. We would soon find out if I was going to get lungs for Christmas. My dad answered the phone and after a short conversation he hung up the phone and looked at all of us and said it's a go. So we hurried off to the hospital.

I was on oxygen for a little while after I was off the ventilator. I was so used to being on oxygen that when the doctors wanted to take me off of it, I freaked out! They didn't want to cause more problems, so they left me on it. But they didn't tell me that every time a nurse would come in my room they were turning it down, until they had no oxygen going into me at all and it was just room air. So the next time they tried to take me off of it and I said, "No", they told me I hadn't been using oxygen all day. I couldn't believe it. So I let them take it off me, and I COULD BREATHE!!!!! It was the best feeling in the whole world.

I have accomplished so much in my life because of my organ donor, Christina. I graduated high school, and I was able to meet my nephews and niece. On November 29, 2003 I married my husband Kevin, and he has been there for me through all my health problems. If I am in the hospital, he is by my side. We share our love by being involved with our church, where Kevin is the assistant pastor. We also both performed in the Wizard of Oz at our church, where he was the scarecrow and I was a munchkin. (Amazingly, my organ donor played the same role as a munchkin, nine months before I received her lungs.)

There have been challenges along the way but nothing too hard for me to handle. I have battled Cytomegalovirus (CMV), Methicillin-resistant Staphylococcus Aureus (MRSA) and even End Stage Renal Disease and have won. Although I still have Cystic Fibrosis in the rest of my digestive system, my new lungs have taken care of my biggest problem. Everyday I battle with my health, but every day, which I just get out of bed, I have won the battle.

Tara Haddix, 30
Brunswick, Ohio
Cystic Fibrosis
Double Lung Transplant, December 24, 1991
The Cleveland Clinic Foundation, Cleveland, Ohio
Related Living Kidney Transplant, July 24, 2001
Related Living Kidney Donor, Mother, Linda Bell
University of Cleveland, Cleveland, Ohio

What a Ride!
By Tony Hamel

Today, February 25th, 2010 I went in for my **_nine-year_** check up on my single left lung transplant. It was very good to say the least.

This has been an amazing and blessed trip I have been on since I found out that I needed a lung transplant to survive. I was 51 when I got that information and I was devastated. 51! I was young and they said my life expectancy was about five years at the most without a transplant. At this point my FEV1 was 17%. That was the worst day of my life.

I had to have a transplant from smoking for 38 years and always believing I was bullet proof. Well, I wasn't. At 45-years-old I could play football and run with the kids all day long. At 52, I struggled to walk up a flight of stairs with supplemental oxygen.

My transplant was February 10, 2001. The "gift" I was given has allowed my wife and I to do so many things we wanted to do. Mostly we have traveled. We went to Hawaii, Mt. Rushmore, Colorado, San Diego and spent many wonderful weekends at our cabin on Lake Texhoma. I am able to get down on the floor with my grandkids, and I truly enjoy being a granddad.

After transplant, life became so precious. I never realized just how fragile I could be. I was always strong but my lifestyle and smoking cost me dearly. Not only in pain and mental suffering, but also in financial suffering. It was a hard lesson that God taught me.

I have my own web site about my transplant and why I had to have that transplant. My goal is to try to reach those who struggle with smoking and help them or let them know they can quit before they get to where I was.

Because I was not careful enough when traveling, especially flying. I am now in chronic rejection. I should have worn a mask!

At this point in my life, I am not a candidate for another transplant. I am 62 and have had several viruses. Since a re-transplant is not an option for me, I will be getting stem cells. I believe this is my best chance for extending my life.

The worst part is the Food and Drug Administration (FDA) does not recognize them as beneficial, and they are very expensive. You have to go out of the United States to get them, but I have nothing to lose at this point and I have been researching stem cells for the last four years and as far as I am concerned this is my next move. I will be keeping up my web site with the progress of the stem cells. I have already had one injection of stem cells (not embryonic cells) but umbilical cord blood cells. The results have been amazing. Since March 2009 to the present, my FEV1 has increased 7%. I will be getting more stem cells this late March or April and am very excited about what could come my way. My life has been truly blessed.

My web site has many pages including a dedication page to my donor. I know who he was. I do what I can to honor him and to the glory of God.

Tony Hamel, 62
(a.k.a. "Tony in Dallas, Keep on Keepin' on)
Dallas, Texas
Chronic Obstructive Pulmonary Disease, Emphysema
Single Lung Transplant, February 10, 2001
University of Texas Southwestern University Hospital – St. Paul, Dallas, Texas
Read Tony's Lung Transplant Story in the 1st Edition of Taking Flight

 New Lungs and a New Kidney are just Two of the Gifts God Has Given Me
By Christy Hamilton

I was diagnosed with Cystic Fibrosis (CF) when I was four-years-old. My lungs were not affected at that time, but I was having malabsorption problems and unable to gain weight. My physician told my parents that I would probably not live past the age of 20, and gave them instructions on how to take care of me.

My childhood was normal, despite having to take medication with each meal to absorb my food, and antibiotics to prevent infection in my lungs. My parents let me get involved in any sport or activity that I wanted. Pseudomonas aeruginosa (a common bacteria found in the lungs of people with CF) was first found in my lungs at the age of 16. I increased my nebulizer use, and continued to do aerobics to help reduce the secretions in my lungs.

Attending school for fashion merchandising, I had hopes of becoming a buyer for a retail store after graduating from high school. Later I decided that I wanted a more rewarding career and attended a community college to take pre-nursing courses. It was then, at the age of 23 that I was first hospitalized with a lung infection. In my second year of nursing school, Glenn and I were married. I graduated in 1995 with a Bachelor of Science Nursing degree.

Six months after graduating, I gave birth to a beautiful, healthy baby girl. Casey is such a blessing to Glenn and me, because I never knew whether I would be able to have children or not.

After recurring infections, we found out that I had a mycobacterium in my lungs. Dr. Daniel Howard informed me that we needed to consider evaluation for a lung transplant. It was something that I knew one day would come, but deep down I had hoped I could beat this disease and not have to consider a transplant, at least not at this age.

Dr. Howard referred me to Barnes-Jewish Hospital in St. Louis, Missouri to be evaluated for a transplant. I was placed on the waiting list but was told there was a two-year wait. Dr. Howard then referred me to Duke University Medical Center in Durham, North Carolina.

I had a large number of antibodies in my blood that made me incompatible with 96% of the population. This meant that it would be very hard to find a cadaver match for me, and that I should consider a living-related, lobar lung transplant. In other words, they would start testing family and friends who would be willing to give up a lobe of one of their lungs. They immediately found a match with my Mom's brother Joel. About 40 family members and friends were tested. We were overwhelmed at the generosity of these people who were willing to do this for me. Even more wanted to be tested, but didn't meet the requirements that were set for donors. These included being taller than me (so the lobe would be of adequate size), the age of 55 or younger, being in good health with no medical problems and being a close friend or relative to me (for ethical reasons).

While all of these people were being tested, I was going through treatment to try and lower the antibody level in my blood. I had to have plasmapheresis treatments three times a week at Duke. This treatment is where they remove your blood and separate the plasma from the whole blood to try and remove the circulating antibodies in the plasma. Each treatment lasted about two hours. I then had to get a gamma-globulin infusion, which lasted another two hours.

Dr. Scott Palmer knew that we needed to find a second donor quickly. My transplant team decided that my Mom should be tested. She wasn't tested before now, because she is three inches shorter than I am. She was a match. They determined that her lungs were actually large for her size. This was a blessing, because it meant that her lobe would be of adequate size. The surgery took about 7 ½ hours. My Mom and Uncle's surgeries took about two hours.

During surgery, the surgeons removed both of my diseased lungs and replaced them with my Mom's left lower lobe and my Uncle's right lower lobe. They had to turn the lobes sideways in my chest cavity so that they would fit properly. I now had two beautiful pink lobes that were oxygenating my blood perfectly.

48 hours after surgery I walked from the intensive care unit (ICU) to my room on the step-down unit without oxygen. I had about 10 different IV medications running, so the pole that the nurse pushed along beside me looked like a Christmas tree.

Glenn was by my side, and being one of my 'nurses' for the next three weeks. The only break he took was when my sister Renee was there. He was then able to spend some time with Casey, since her visits to my room had to be limited due to the risk of infection; she was in kindergarten at the time, and there was no telling what type of infections she had come in contact with.

Glenn would make me walk even if I didn't feel like it, which was most of the time. He really pushed me, so that my recovery would be faster. I thought at the time, a marathon for him would have been easier than my few laps around the floor. After 16 days, I was discharged from the hospital just a few days before Christmas. My mother-in-law had decorated the entire house.

A lot has happened since February 2002. First of all, my lung capacity exceeded what they thought it would, so that has been great. I have also been able to keep my weight up for the most part. Because of the prednisone that I have been taking since transplant, I have severe osteoporosis in my lumbar spine. I had my first acute pneumonia due to pseudomonal infection in February 2006. Intravenous (IV) antibiotics and nebulizer treatments have taken care of it. Because of diabetes, high blood pressure, and the anti-rejection medications, my kidneys failed, and I had to have a kidney transplant in November 2008. My wonderful Mom also donated the kidney! We are both doing great since surgery.

Glenn and I are divorced, and we are both remarried. I was married on Valentine's Day, 2006 to a wonderful man named Jason. We met at church and had a very short engagement. Casey is so happy to get a step-dad, and Jason adores her. Casey also adores her step-mom, and thinks it's pretty cool that she gets double presents, double vacations, and double holidays.

Sometimes it's easy to ask, "Why?" when bad things happen, but in the end, God always reminds us that He is in control and that things will work out for the best.

I know that there is a purpose in everything and that we go through adversities to make us stronger, and closer to God. I can only hope that the trials that I have gone through have made me a much more compassionate and loving wife, friend, mother and daughter. God has been good to me and blessed me with so much. New lungs and a new kidney are just two of the gifts He has given me.

Christy Hamilton, 40
Mooresville, North Carolina
Cystic Fibrosis
Related Living Lobar Lung Transplant, November 12, 2001
Related Living Lobar Lung Donor, Mother, Gail Hubbard
Related Living Lobar Lung Donor, Uncle, Joel Walker
Related Living Kidney Transplant, November 10, 2008
Related Living Kidney Donor, Mother, Gail Hubbard
Duke University Medical Center, Durham, North Carolina

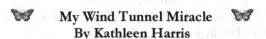

My Wind Tunnel Miracle
By Kathleen Harris

The life I thought I'd be missing has continued on since my double lung transplant on July 10, 2006. A perfect stranger has given me an awesome gift and I thank and pray for her and her family every day. I will honor her by taking care of myself. I will try to be a good person, help others, and give back when I can.

I have Cystic Fibrosis (CF), but wasn't diagnosed until age 40 (along with my older sister and younger brother). A few years before transplant my health began to deteriorate. I lost weight and I was on oxygen 24/7 for several years. I couldn't do much of anything I had before – no tennis, no nights out, no normal household chores etc. I didn't want to accept the transplant option at first, but after much prayer, I began to realize that God had placed me on this path and I had to embrace it.

When I was originally diagnosed, Johns Hopkins Hospital, Baltimore, Maryland had no CF adult treatment program so I was treated by Dr. Lucas Kulczycki at Georgetown University Hospital, Washington, D.C. and by Dr. Milica Chernick at National Institute of Health, Bethesda, Maryland. I am deeply grateful for their support, guidance, and care during those difficult times.

In the meantime Johns Hopkins created an Adult CF Clinic and I began treatment there in 1998, shortly after my sister, Peggy, passed away from CF. Dr. Michael Boyle and the entire staffs of doctors, nurses, nutritionists and therapists were wonderful to me. They supported me in every way and, towards the end, kept me alive and encouraged me to consider transplant.

My husband of 47 years, Richard, my children, Karen and Christine, and my grandsons, Joey, Mark, and Patrick, were all very supportive. That support and their love were appreciated so much! At first we considered relocating to Duke University Hospital, Durham, North Carolina area to arrange for the transplant there, but Dr. Ashish Shah, who had performed numerous successful transplants at Duke, transferred to Johns Hopkins. We were thrilled to be able to have a great transplant surgeon at the Johns Hopkins Hospital that we knew, and loved, and to get to stay home during all the pre and post transplant events.

I was listed for transplant on my 63rd birthday. In just three days, I was called in because lungs had become available. This was the first of three attempts. As we had been cautioned, sometimes the lungs are just not, "right for you". On July 10, we got our third and final call and, in a five-hour surgery, Dr. Shah transplanted my new lungs.

After about a day in intensive care, I was placed in cardio-pulmonary surgical recovery unit and before long, they got me up to walk. It must have been quite a sight with three or four nurses carrying the boxes from my six tubes and my husband following behind with an easy chair. Of course I couldn't go too far, but what a thrill! My first feeling was that of a wind tunnel blowing in and out of me. I realized for the first time that it had been many years (maybe never) since I could really breathe freely. Amazingly, I had no supplemental oxygen!

In just seven days I was ready to go home. I had walked all around the unit nine times the night before. I looked good, felt good, and had received the necessary training with regard to my medications, contacts etc. My kidneys acted up at the last minute and my stay at the hospital was extended for two more weeks. Finally I got to go home.

I had the love and prayers of many friends, my church, and my extended family including my sisters, Patsy and Mary Ellen, and my brother, Gary, who were so caring.

I continue to have the guidance and support of the Hopkins transplant team of doctors and nurses headed by Dr. Jonathan Orens. The nursing team especially Susan Miller, Terry Cook, and Sharon Allen kept up constant communication with me to be certain that I was getting all I needed. I am forever grateful for that care even when I didn't want the bronchoscopies or the Coumadin etc.

I have resumed doing household chores, have been able to enjoy a few trips with my family, and my husband and I are planning to spend a month in Florida this winter. I have a number of medications, but no oxygen. I've seen two of my grandchildren go on to college and the third one act in a number of high school plays (yes he wants to be an actor).

I'm so grateful for these blessings, and I intend to be the best I can be with the Lord's help and my faith without which I would not be here. A special thanks to my husband. His love and support have been awesome. He saved my life. Again, thanks to everyone who had any role in helping me get through this difficult time. You know who you are. May God bless you all!

Kathleen Harris, 67
Bowie, Maryland
Cystic Fibrosis
Double Lung Transplant, July 10, 2006
Johns Hopkins Hospital, Baltimore, Maryland

 Sky and Telle's Love Story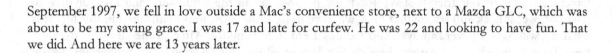
By Shantelle Harris

September 1997, we fell in love outside a Mac's convenience store, next to a Mazda GLC, which was about to be my saving grace. I was 17 and late for curfew. He was 22 and looking to have fun. That we did. And here we are 13 years later.

Our love story isn't typical. It is one filled with more depth, intrigue and adoration than most. This I know. We have traveled, loved and been each other's rocks. Each other's strength and solidarity. My name is Shantelle and I met Sky through mutual friends back in high school. Sky has Cystic Fibrosis (CF) and just underwent a double lung transplant. We are still in recovery but can't wait to restart our life and have a baby, travel more and share our story.

About us? Where to start... Well I'm a tall, lovable, comedic gal who fell in love with her prince charming. Sky would pick me up from work at lunch on his motorcycle when I lifeguarded. Whisk me away for adventurous weekends doing motocross, and hold me in his arms under the stars every chance he got under the falls in Jamaica and in Cayman Islands. Everywhere. We are destined to share our souls. Now and always. Sky once wrote to me that our love is like iron or steel, always and forever. His character and zest for life is unmatched. His charm, intelligence and character, grabbed my heart from day one. He's such an all around great guy! Mr. Popular. Everyone's go-to friend! Yet at times we were ostracized for how we lived and loved, probably because at times it was so fast and fierce and without abandon. Through this we realized people were jealous of our bond. They didn't understand our bond, as they weren't fighting a terminal illness. Yet we got though it all together and realized that what we had was rare. That it was special. Different, life altering! Not just teenage love, real love. Unbreakable!

We often from a young age had to fend for ourselves and got through our hardships together. I moved out at the age of 17, after my parents divorced and Sky took me in, under his wing...from that day forth. Struggles ensued. We felt robbed at times because of how we had to watch others enjoy, "the simple things", where as we had to strive and push that much harder. Not sure if Sky's CF played a part in that but we were always painfully aware that every little stress could cause sickness, hospital-time and eventual loss of lung function. So little things to us were not so little.

Daily stresses had a significant impact on our future. And, our life together, work, play, having babies. But the most amazing thing is that, through it all, Sky never let CF define him.

We have gone to school, bought our first home, traveled to many different countries and been a part of many amazing things. When we went to Key West one year we had to sleep in our car, as we couldn't afford the luxurious hotels in the area. Sky woke me up just as the sun was rising and put a beautiful flower in my hair that he had picked from the side of the road where he had gone to get us freshly squeezed orange juice. He told me how beautiful I was and then we took off to a nearby resort to lie in their hammocks and pretend we were locals.

Another amazing memory was when Sky spent all day waxing our car and making it just right for my prom. Flowers, fresh roses, and balloons. Then a few weeks later when I turned 19, Sky took me outside just after midnight on my birthday and told me he was having the time of his life and gave me a Gold Giorgio Armani watch. Oh yes, my man has style! But material things don't matter to us. It's not what's important in this life. Perhaps this was another lesson we learnt very young. While we have seen a lot of our friends strive for these possessions all the while suffering loss, divorce or whatnot, we sit back and realize that love, what we have, is the most important thing in this life. It is what we will have forever...always. And for this I am truly thankful. After all the struggles over the years fighting health crisis', career changes, family turmoil etc. our blessing was knowing this lesson and knowing that we had love, above all, to see each other through.

It is our love that has gotten us to today. In April, Sky entered the hospital. Things got progressively worse and then in June the doctors said he probably wouldn't make it through the night. He wasn't even listed for transplant at the time so a, "Do not resuscitate order" was put up. That night we swore we would get through it, that Sky would get listed...that we'd get our second chance. Sky held me in his arms and asked to have a dance. He told me we would dance like that again on our anniversary, which was in October. At the time it seemed a distant dream...not one of reality. We fought hard. So hard. Endless sleepless nights, chest physiotherapy, crying and just holding each other, promising we'd never be apart or let the disease take hold. We were gonna fight this! And that we did! Sky got his new lungs September 22nd and I got my love back, our dreams and prayers were answered and I got my dance. October 10th, our 13th anniversary we got engaged!

Dreams do come true. Believe. Love can see you through. Sky and I, if anything, are proof of this. I am proud of him, of our unbreakable bond, of our enduring and everlasting love. We will always have this. Forever... And always...Just like Sky always said...XO

Shantelle Harris
Fiancé of Sky William Hillier
Oshawa, Ontario, Canada
Sky, Cystic Fibrosis
Sky, Double Lung Transplant, September 22, 2010
Toronto General Hospital, Toronto, Canada
Sky William Hillier, Died December 20, 2010
"Forever 35"

Have Lungs! Will Travel!
By Zoie Harris

I was born 23rd December 1971 in the mining town of Broken Hill in New South Wales, Australia. As soon as I was born I was tested for Cystic Fibrosis (CF), because my brother had died nine months earlier of CF. the result came back positive, and my parents were devastated because I looked chubby and healthy.

Throughout my childhood I did things that normal kids do (and more) with the addition of clinic appointments, hospital admissions, many tablets and treatments. I used to joke with people that I couldn't eat because I was too full from tablets. When I turned eight, hospitalizations became common place for intravenous antibiotics (IV's). I started going into hospital every three months for about two weeks at a time in Adelaide, which was about 550km away from our home. I hated the needles and missing school. Each time I went back I felt like I'd missed out on something – school activities, parties etc....

I moved to Darwin – to the tropics – in Northern Australia. The weather in Darwin suited my CF as I avoided the winter colds and flu but I still went into hospital regularly or did home IV's. I tried to keep up with tennis, netball and volleyball, but these did become harder.

Accepted to Northern Territory University to attain a degree in Psychology, I joined the university volleyball team and traveled to Kupang - West Timor to compete in a Youth Exchange. My 2nd trip overseas was to a CF conference in Vienna, Austria in 1990. I went with one of my best CF friends Anne-Marie, and we visited London, Paris, Frankfurt, Venice and Salzburg. Subconsciously I was ignoring my CF and having a great time going out, drinking and night clubbing. (Not a great recipe for health success and many of my CF friends weren't so lucky, including Anne-Marie) It was on campus that I met Mitch, whom I would later marry and spend nine years with.

In 1995 I spent six weeks in the hospital. My lung function had deteriorated to about 28%. It was then that my doctor suggested that I go through the tests for lung transplantation. One good thing that happened for the year is that I completed my Psychology degree which was an achievement in itself.

On August 2nd 1997 - in hospital - whilst I was watching live coverage of Stuart Diver (the only survivor) being pulled out of the Thredbo ski resort disaster in which 18 people were killed, I received 'the call', nearly two years after being listed. I honestly think the nurses were panicking more than me. I calmly called Mitch and asked him to pack our suitcases as we were going to Melbourne. We flew to Melbourne aboard a Royal Flying Doctor Service flight. I was still calm and never really got nervous; it was everyone else who was the problem! My transplant went well and had a few complications.

Since my transplant I have completed my Masters in Social Work, divorced and remarried in 2003. My husband Scott has had a kidney transplant and understands the need to keep fit and healthy, and keeps me motivated. He is very sporty and loves cycling and swimming. Scott shares my love of travel and we have done three major overseas trips – two of them to World Transplant Games in

Kobe, Japan in 2001 and Canada in 2005. I have also attended six Australian Transplant Games; my main event was tennis.

Last year while on a seven week trip, taking in San Francisco, California; Miami, Florida; a Caribbean Cruise; Orlando, Florida; Las Vegas, Nevada; Vancouver and Whistler, Canada; Alaskan Cruise; Seattle, Washington; Hawaii, then home to Oz (Australia), the 2nd day in San Francisco I developed chicken pox. Needless to say we made it to Whistler, Canada before I ended up with renal failure, and chicken pox in my eye and had to be flown home. I was devastated that I missed the Alaskan Cruise but grateful that I made it home in one piece. I also have an appreciation for the Australian Health Care system (Government funded Health Care) after costing our travel insurance company nearly $60,000 Australian Dollar's (AUD) in medical expenses. It has however put an end to my tennis days as I can no longer see the ball until it hits me in the face!

The other traveling highlight for me was a three month summer camp in Hunter, New York where I met many people from different countries and looked after some great kids with disabilities that really make you think, "My life is not all that bad after all!" I am now working part-time in a busy hospital Emergency Department as a Social Worker, and I am a foster carer looking after two wonderful boys aged three and four. They certainly keep us busy……. I have my anonymous donor family to thank for my life and my adventures since my transplant and I am hoping there are more to come.

Zoie Harris, 38
Adelaide, South Australia, Australia
Cystic Fibrosis
Double Lung Transplant, August 3, 1997
The Alfred Hospital, Melbourne, Victoria, Australia

Worth the Wait
By Megan Herdegen

I had been waiting for a year and a half (six years if you count the years I was inactive) by the time I received my, "Gift of Life". I was ready to throw in the towel, "When will it be my turn?" Well, on July 18, 2007, my turn finally came. I "got the call" in the middle of the night and six hours later, I was in recovery.

When I woke up, I took the biggest breath that I had taken in years. It was the strangest sensation that I have ever felt. The lungs felt like they were too big because I could feel my whole chest expand, and I haven't felt that in a long time. I was up and walking around in about five days. I stayed in the hospital for 16 days because I had a few minor complications.

When I came home, I was as good as new. I can't even describe what I felt. It was like I was high all the time because I was getting so much oxygen. All my life, I thought that it was normal not to be able to breathe deep. Now I could do it whenever I wanted to. It was unreal. I never knew someone could feel this good. 19 days after my transplant, I was taking walks around the block.

Two months after, I took part in a three-mile walk for the Respiratory Health Association, Chicago, Illinois.

But the best part of not having the trache and having new lungs was that I could talk again!! I still had the trache in, but it was capped. My three-year-old nephew had grown up without ever hearing my voice. The first time I talked to him, he didn't know what to think. He just laughed the whole time!

They kept the trache in for two months after the transplant. Once they felt that I was not in any danger of needing to be placed on the ventilator again, they removed it. The next step was removing all of the equipment from my house. That was a bittersweet day. I was happy to see it go but at the same time, it had become such a part of me that I was a little nervous about letting it go. After the last tank left my house, I celebrated. I was finally free!!!

My life was now better than I could have ever dreamed. I was walking miles everyday. In February of 2009, barely a year and a half after my transplant, I once again took part in a fundraiser for the Respiratory Health Association and I climbed all 94 flights of the John Hancock Building in Chicago. I did in it in one-hour and 18 minutes!

I could now chase after my 5-year-old nephew. I could take him to the park and not have to sit on the bench and watch him play. I could read to him. I could watch him grow up. I could go anywhere, anytime, without having to plan ahead. I could get a real job, go back to school, and get back into dance, theater and singing. I went from having no options at all to having too many to choose from. I had been given a 'do over'. I could now live the life that I have wanted to live since I was three-years-old. Best of all, I could be there to watch my nephew grow up.

I would not have this chance if it weren't for that selfless person who gave me the best gift he could give. He didn't just give me my life back; he gave me my nephew's as well. I have yet to get in touch with my donor family. All I know is that he was 24. I hope and pray that one day; they will want to get in touch with me so that I can thank them in person for giving me this beautiful, new life.

Megan Herdegen, 31
McHenry, Illinois
Unknown – Form of Fibrosis
Double Lung Transplant, July 18, 2007
Loyola University Medical Center, Maywood, Illinois
Megan Wrote This Story, October 14, 2010
Megan Passed Away, October 18, 2010
"Forever 31"

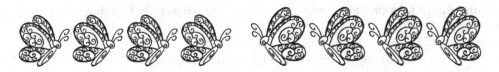

To My Wife, Without Whom Life Would Not be so Interesting
For Better or Worse, in Sickness and in Health
By Geoff Hillary

You would think the task of being a caregiver could be daunting, but it's actually just a frame of mind. It's a chance to better and closer connect in many different ways with your spouse. For me, a guy, it's a chance to learn a whole new way of life. The days of coming home to a cooked meal, or of having clean pressed clothes in the closet, became a thing of the past. My wife was ill for several years before she received her double lung transplant, and almost eight years on she is doing remarkably well. Comparatively, pre-transplant she was in a wheelchair, on oxygen 24 hours a day (24/7), weak, tired and struggled to get through the day doing very little. Now she is traveling around the world and enjoying the new life she has been given. Me, I had to go from breadwinner to bread maker with very little training. Being a caregiver is a time to understand what's really important in life, and to work around the insignificant issues. Here's what I mean:

Laundry
Do you ever read those tags on the back of your clothes? The ones that say cold wash, dry flat, cool iron, or the others that say, wash with similar colors, tumble dry low heat. Modern technology has created a whole host of fabrics and dyes that will stand up to nuclear radiation, so to tell me that I have to separate blues from reds, or cottons from polyesters is a hokum. Here is how to do laundry. Find the washing machine! Fill with whatever clothes are in the laundry basket to some reasonable level. Add washing powder – about a handful, or if liquid, two glugs. Assume that the water level, heat and spin cycle settings are correct. Turn on. When the machine stops, transfer everything to the dryer. Throw in a dryer sheet. Hit start. It couldn't be any easier. When the dryer stops, empty everything into the basket, transfer to drawers or hangers, repeat next week or as often as needed.

Ironing
This is a fairly short section; nothing needs ironing. My mother-in-law irons sheets, go figure. If you find something that mentions the need for ironing, and it's already clean, give it to a charity shop and purchase something similar (see next section) that says, "Do not iron" or "dry clean."

Shopping
As a guy I generally don't like shopping, even for myself. As for going with my wife, forget it, there is not enough time in the day. Have you stood there and seen your wife pick up and examine every item on a rack? They are the same color, same size, same style, and yet every one of them has to be looked at front, back, and inside. Believe me, inspector 13 has done this for you at the factory and got paid for doing so. If it were faulty it would have been rejected already. For most guys, it's much easier. Shoes are just an example. The last four pairs of dress shoes I have bought were identical. Same size, same color, same maker, same store. I didn't need to browse, I didn't need to try them on,

and I didn't even need to know if they were on sale. I just said, "Give me a pair of those; size 11", in whatever color I needed, and two minutes later I was on my way home.

That gets me to the point – shopping when my wife was in a wheelchair. She would say something like, "Can you take me to XYZ store, I need to buy a new, (fill in the blank)." She didn't say, "I need to wander every store at the mall looking at everything there is." It was always specific, one store, one item. We would load up the wheelchair and head out. No stopping to look at a rack of this or a pile of that, head straight to the relevant place, pick a color, a style, and the size, that's a wrap for the trip, and off back to the car. Arms outstretched trying to grab at something didn't' work; asking to go to some other section didn't work, and forget going to another store. You have total control, you are the driver of the bus and it goes where you want it to go, and that's shopping for a day.

Housework
It's not hard to run the vacuum cleaner round the carpets once in a while, but it would be easier to get a Roomba (autonomous robotic vacuum cleaner) and let that chore take care of itself. As for dusting, well there is no point in picking anything up to dust under it, if it stays put, who would even see if there is dust there. Any large flat surfaces – cover them with a cloth of some sort, a tablecloth, or even a drop cloth and if anyone shows up at the house, tell them you are decorating. Windows, well the outsides are washed when it rains, so there is only the inside to worry about, that's half the work.

Cooking
Peas in one pot, carrots in another, potatoes in another, and meat in a dish, invest in a slow cooker, it's all going on the same plate, invest in a slow cooker, one pot feeds all. Paper plates and plastic utensils and just throw away when done, it's easier than washing a whole host of crockery. You get to eat what you want, when you want it, and cooked the way you like it. No coming home thinking you are having roast beef to find out you are having hot dogs. You are the chef de jour. All these savings in cost, time, and effort easily transfers to allowing extra time to take your spouse shopping!

Vacations
Forward planning is critical. Flat and level anywhere you go, and it doesn't necessarily have to be scenic. Don't try pushing a wheelchair from the Falls to the Skylon Tower in Niagara Falls. It seems like a 45 degree incline and once you have started uphill you can't stop because you will never get going again and you can't turn around and go back or you will lose control and your spouse will become the fastest human in a wheelchair. Go to Ocean City and do the boardwalk instead. Go to New York City – too many pedestrians? No problem. Your spouse takes her cane and hits anyone on the ankle if they are in the way. Go to Disney, it's an automatic to the front of the line if you are in a wheelchair. Forget the little kids and those who have stood there in the relentless sun winding round and round – a wheelchair gets you the next opening.

Conclusion
There is more than a grain of truth in everything I have written here. It is a daunting task to work around a loved one being sick, but it isn't a chore, it can be funny, it can be thrilling and, it can be time spent getting to know the other side of your spouse. It's hard work, it's rewarding, and it did eventually come to an end in our case when my wife received the gift of life. Would I wish it had

never happened, sure, but it did, and I wouldn't change what we both went through. The good times, the bad times, and the adventures we had. To those who are still trying to resolve how they will cope, believe me, it happens somehow. Just don't worry if a piece of clothing gets ruined, or if dinner is late. Enjoy the time planning for a brighter future together when things won't be stressful.

Geoff Hillary, Husband of Maureen Hillary
Maureen Hillary, 60
Easton, Pennsylvania
Maureen, Alpha-1 Antitrypsin Deficiency
Maureen, Double Lung Transplant, November 29, 2002
University of Pennsylvania Medical Center Philadelphia, Philadelphia, Pennsylvania
Read Maureen's Lung Transplant Story in this Edition of Taking Flight

From Oxygen to High Octane!
By Maureen Hillary

Within a period of six months I went from being in a wheel chair and on oxygen for several years, to dancing at a Bruce Springsteen concert, walking on the beach, flying back to see my mother in England, and generally living and loving life again. All of this made possible by my being the grateful recipient of a new pair of lungs from a 22-year-old, anonymous young man and his family. I have written to them about six times and they have sadly never written back, but people grieve in very different ways.

Try breathing through a straw for years and you'd realize just how wonderful that simple act is for me. In fact I love life and enjoy every extra moment that God has given me through the twin miracles of organ donation and lung transplantation.

I started having difficulty breathing in my early 40's. At the age of 45, I finally went to see a pulmonologist who diagnosed me with Alpha1-Antitrypsin Deficiency. We went to the University of Pennsylvania Medical Center, Philadelphia, Pennsylvania. Thank you Dr. Argassoy! I was put on the waiting list.

Thank God for my husband, Geoff, who did everything for me while trying to hold down a full time job, which involved a tremendous amount of traveling. He cooked, cleaned, washed and tried to iron…I'd cringe while watching him work his way so slowly through his shirts!

Finally on 'Black Friday', November 29, 2002 my call came. We grabbed my bag...it had been packed for three years, called my mother in England, and headed down to Philly with Geoff driving in a record 80 minutes! Now I want to tell you something special. I'm a natural worrier and my immediate reaction was pure panic. However, within a couple of minutes, this amazing sense of peace came over me and stayed with me all the way to the operating table...a higher power certainly stepped in and sustained me through that journey. I would like to think that this would also happen when one reaches the end of life.

I spent 16 days in the hospital, where although I could barely move, I announced to my doctors that I was going to do the Rocky Run on the last day of my compulsory three-month rehabilitation. I am now told that they didn't believe for one minute that I'd be able to do it.

The hospital and the Gift of Life program are both building transplant houses, which will make it much easier for future transplants and their families to get affordable accommodations. This has become one of our pet charities.

Rehab finally finished on St. Patrick's Day, and I had Geoff drive me over to the Art Museum where I donned my boxing gloves and wearing my Guinness Tee-shirt, I ran up all 90 steps of the Art Museum pumping my arms in the air triumphantly at the top! To this day my transplant doctor uses this picture at the end of his lectures to tell his students and colleagues that this is the reason he stays in Lung Transplantation...a fact, which makes me feel very proud. The Philadelphia Gift of Life Program on a recruiting pamphlet also used the picture for the 2004 Transplant Games in Minneapolis.

I cannot say that it has all been plain sailing. There have been bumps in the road. I have joined Team Philadelphia and have participated in the 2004 Transplant Games in Minneapolis, the 2006 games in Louisville, Kentucky, and the 2008 games in Pittsburgh. The Games themselves are an amazing experience, and for Geoff and myself probably the most emotional event which we have ever attended. We have made friends all over the country that I keep in touch with by E-mail.

At the Transplant Games, one meets hundreds of fellow transplant recipients and most importantly many, many donor families. We treat every one of them as if they were our own donor family; hugging them and thanking them for their generosity. We listen to their stories and cry with them, but most importantly we are living proof that their loved ones did not die in vain. They are there cheering us on through all of our sports and you'd be surprised at some of the athletic prowess shown by a lot of our fellow transplantees.

Organ donation gave me a second chance at life; a life which I really appreciate and celebrate each and every day. After nearly eight years I still have an FEV1 of over 100%; it was 13% at one time! Since then I have probably done more and seen more than most people do in a lifetime. I have not wasted my special gift at all!

I fly back to England regularly to see my mother, daughter, sister and the rest of my extended family. I have been to Italy, and on three cruises; Alaska, Bermuda and the Baltic Capitals including St Petersburg, Russia. I also fly regularly to visit our three sons in Oregon, Colorado & Texas. I once had a fear of flying but no longer, as God had his chance to take me and he chose to let me live.

I regularly attend Broadway shows, Rock & Classical concerts and just about every event to which I am invited. My friends are absolutely amazed by my energy and enthusiasm for life.

I also try to repay this wonderful gift I have been given by doing volunteer work at our church and for other organizations. I do Meals on Wheels, volunteer at our Senior Center, and try to help other pulmonary patients keep up their spirits. My enthusiasm to help my fellow pulmonary and heart patients at my local rehab center has made them give me the title, 'The Queen of Rehab'; I think that my English accent might also have some bearing on that LOL!

I've spoken about the need for Organ Donation, participated in the Transplant Games and actually won a bronze medal in table tennis! I do walks for charity, including our annual Donor Dash in Philadelphia, the 24-hour Cancer Relay for Life, and raise money for the Transplant House currently being built near the Hospital of the University of Pennsylvania.

For this wonderful new life of mine I have first to thank Geoff, my wonderful husband and caregiver of many, many years. Thank you to my very adept surgeon, Dr. Alberto Pochettino. Thank you also to my transplant pulmonologist of the past nine years for his caring and compassion, Dr. Vivek Ahya; now Medical Director of the Lung Transplant Department and named as one of America's top docs! Then last but certainly not least my Transplant Coordinator, James Mendez, who is never too busy to talk to me on the phone, answer my E-mails and generally take care of my well being.

If you are considering lung transplantation go for it; it is so much better than the alternative!

Maureen Hillary, 60
Easton, Pennsylvania
Alpha-1 Antitrypsin Deficiency
Double Lung Transplant, November 29, 2002
University of Pennsylvania Medical Center Philadelphia, Philadelphia, Pennsylvania
Read Husband Geoff's Story in this Edition of Taking Flight

❦ Remembering Bob: The Best and Worst of Y2K ❦
By Laura Hoekstra-Bettig

Back in 1996, Bob's pulmonologist/cystic fibrosis (CF) specialist informed us that Bob was in "end-stage" lung disease and should be evaluated at Loyola University Medical Center, Chicago, Illinois, for a bi-lateral lung transplant. He was given an "average" life expectancy of two years based on the results of his breathing tests. We were nervous and scared to hear such a diagnosis. And, after meeting with the medical director for Loyola's transplant program, we were troubled by the news that Bob was "still too healthy" to even be placed on the waiting list. It wasn't until January of 1998, one week before our daughter Elisabeth was born, that Loyola accepted Bob and placed his name on "The List."

We were told it would be a 12-15 month wait for a suitable donor. That later changed to a 15-18 month wait. And, as our experience went, a 28-month wait was more exact, including the disappointment of one "false alarm" where the donor organs were not suitable for transplant. In May of 2000, we received the call from Loyola. They had a donor that matched Bob. We were told nothing more than that the donor was out of town and the transplant team needed to travel to assess and recover the lungs.

We drove to the hospital in a thunderstorm and later learned the med flight was almost grounded due to the storm. But on that Memorial Day weekend, God answered our prayers and worked a miracle of healing through a 6 ½-hour operation, allowing Bob to leave the hospital six days later breathing on his own without his oxygen tank.

Our elation lasted for two months as we watched Bob recover and return to some semblance of his "old" life, even installing a water line to our refrigerator, hooking up an icemaker, and working with a friend to rig up a battery-backup for our sump pump! But in late July, he experienced what the doctors called a "speed bump" on the road to recovery. In August that speed bump turned into a major complication and Bob died suddenly.

We were devastated. What we had hoped for, a long and fulfilling life after transplant ended all too quickly. Bob was 43-years-old, our daughter was only two-years-old; he had everything to live for. For many years I struggled, wanting to share our story with others waiting for transplants but fearful they would be discouraged by the final chapter in Bob's story. But I gradually came to realize that Bob was still given a priceless gift when that donor family chose to donate their loved one's organs. He received a pair of incredible lungs, lungs that worked right from the start, never needing the heart-lung bypass machine during surgery!

Instead of slowly dying from diseased lungs that forced him to breathe with the help of a ventilator, Bob was given the gift of three months of life breathing with new, healthy lungs. During that time, our family's faith grew and we experienced such joy and gratitude. While it is true that he did not ultimately have the extended lifespan that we had hoped for, our hearts will always marvel at the wonder of life…the gift of life shared through organ donation.

On Sunday, December 17, four months after Bob's death, my daughter and I stood before our church family to read that week's advent reading and light the Shepherd's candle. I will never forget how the candle was very slow to light…and for several minutes after we sat down, its flame barely held out. As I watched it, I knew that my heart felt just like that dimly lit candle. I wanted so desperately to feel some joy in the celebration of Christmas but, inside, my heart was flickering between light and dark, hope and despair. As we sang the final hymn, the flame of that advent candle suddenly began to blaze brightly. Through tears, I thanked God for the symbolic reminder that He had the power to heal my heart and keep my hope alive.

Going through the transplant experience with Bob taught me the real meaning of life and love; family and community; patience, faith, and hope. I wouldn't trade those lessons for anything. Bob will always be my hero for the way he faced life and death; with strength, determination, inspiration and courage.

Laura Hoekstra-Bettig, Wife of Robert Hoekstra, 43
Belmont, Michigan
Robert, Cystic Fibrosis
Robert, Double Lung Transplant, May 28, 2000
Loyola University Medical Center, Chicago, Illinois
Robert Passed Away: August 15, 2000
"Forever 43"

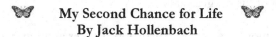

My Second Chance for Life
By Jack Hollenbach

In looking back now, my first indicator that something was wrong occurred while on a weekend fishing trip, at Apache Lake (outside Phoenix, Arizona). I remember climbing up an embankment from the water to the car and being seriously out of breath. Friends asked if I was all right, and I joked that I was getting old. This attitude led me to return to school and finish my degree when I had decided that toting a toolbox was too much after 25 years, and I was going to get into Project Management.

I went to the doctor's office for my annual physical; the look of concern on the doctor's face, and his sending me to see a colleague that afternoon (my first pulmonary doctor), was another indicator. He would not let me leave his office that afternoon until we had an oxygen supplier at my house to meet me. I was diagnosed with severe Chronic Obstructive Pulmonary Disease (COPD). There was shock on my coworker's faces the next day when I came in wearing a cannula with an oxygen tank in tow; I had never had a sick day in my time there. I continued to work for several months until my boss Bill came into the office one day, looked at me and said I did not look well, I should go home. I protested a bit, but left and went home, turned on a movie, ("An Inconvenient Truth" ironically) and fell asleep. When I awoke I could not breathe – I called 911.

I went into Good Samaritan Medical Center in Phoenix, Arizona weighing 165 pounds, and came out at 125 pounds, two weeks later. I was so weak I could not cross the room without stopping to catch my breath. My doctor recommended a lung transplant; needless to say the thought scared the hell out of me! My family came to the rescue. It seems that University of California San Diego Medical Center in San Diego, California (UCSD) had been having very good results with their program. My sister teaches there, and she got me an appointment to see the transplant doctors.

My father came out the day after I was discharged from Good Samaritan, took one look at me and started packing a bag; we left the next morning for San Diego. I still remember cranking the oxygen up as we drove through the mountains and thinking that I had never noticed the air being thin before. Sure your ears would pop, but it was no big deal before . . . amazing the things we all take for granted.

I still remember meeting Dr. Gordon Yung for the first time. It was quite an effort to walk into the clinic and make it to the exam room; I had to stop several times to catch my breath. They wanted me to do a six-minute walk to see how far I could go. The six-minute walk is a measure of distance you can walk, in the allotted time. As I stood up from my wheelchair my saturation level dropped so fast that they terminated the test. I remember thinking, "Oh great, I failed that portion – there goes the transplant…"

Soon after, I received a call telling me I was on the waiting list for a double lung transplant; no score was given to me at that time, but they did say I was high on the list. The next day, Stephanie Osborne, the Lung Transplant Coordinator called me and asked what I was doing, and if I'd be interested in getting a new lung. My father and sister were with me, and we spent several hours speculating on what would happen, what life would be like and how things would change. Dad left the hospital to feed and walk my dogs, and he took along my clothes and oxygen tank, as I would not need them anymore. After a while a nurse came in and let us know that the lung was not viable for transplant, and I could go home…only, I had no clothes, no oxygen, it was now 10:00 p.m. and I was starving! Lesson learned: you ain't transplanted 'til you're transplanted-keep your stuff with you 'til then.

It was four months until I received the next call, during that time I had participated in Pulmonary Rehab, which was two hours twice a week, one hour of instruction - how to live with our conditions; one hour doing exercises. When I started I was barely able to maintain 0.7 mph (miles per hour) on the treadmill for five minutes (this was after walking daily at home in preparation for this) with oxygen. By the classes completion I was up to 1.4 mph and I could go for 20 minutes! BIG IMPROVEMENT!

Then on August 2, 2007 – the phone rang. Stephanie again asked me what I had planned for the day; they had been given the opportunity for a donation of two lungs if I was interested. I had to scramble, as there was nobody at home with me. Unknown to me, my surgeon had flown to Las Vegas, inspected and 'harvested' the lungs and was en route back to San Diego when I was called.

I remember being placed on the cold table and being put out. Next thing I remember is waking in the intensive care unit (ICU), having a doctor ask how I felt and not being able to speak (I was still intubated). I was in ICU for a week. One day the nurse asked if I wanted to 'get rid of the cannula'; I kind of panicked, I'd had it for so long, so I asked if I was ready. She informed me the oxygen had already been off for a day. The doctors were very conscious and worried about infection. Visitors had to wear a cap, gown and mask, plus some booties and gloves when they come into the room.

I learned that my surgeon, Dr. Michael Madani, had had a long day; he flew to recover my lungs in Las Vegas, returned and preformed my transplant, catnapped, and then did another transplant the same day. Talk about high-pressure occupation!

I was in the hospital for another few weeks before returning to my father's home. Several weeks later, we were evacuated from our home because of the wildfires that ravaged the San Diego area. My transplant team thought it best that I get as far from the smoke as possible. We spent the following weeks in Palm Desert, California; I would get up, go to the gym in the hotel, wipe down the equipment and walk for 30 minutes at three miles per hour (mph) – unbelievable! I would check in every other day with my coordinators as to local conditions and my condition.

It has been a fantastic few years now since I had my transplant. Yes, there have been 'bumps in the road', I've been hospitalized twice – but overall life has been good! This past fall I took my dog and went camping and hiking in the Redwoods of Northern California, something a fellow transplantee inspired me to do, and I did it in his honor.

I am an active volunteer with the Project Management Institute, San Diego Supplier Development Council, UCSD Heart & Lung Transplant Support Group, Carmel Valley Library and Transplant Buddies.

Jack Hollenbach, 54
San Diego, California
Chronic Obstructive Pulmonary Disease
Double Lung Transplant, August 2, 2007
University of California San Diego Medical Center, San Diego, California

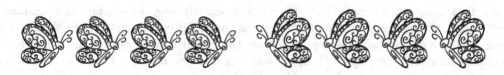

From Spectator to Participant in Life Again
By Gill Hollis

A few years ago, I attended a wedding with my husband, Peter. It was a family wedding, of a sort. I don't know if there is a term that describes the relationship of the bride Susie, to me - but we are related. One night in February 2004, Susie and I received life-saving transplant operations in next-door operating theatres. She received the heart and I received a lung from the same donor. So we all had much to celebrate at that wedding.

My lung problems began in 1987, when I was in my early twenties. I'd always been fit and healthy, so it was a shock when I suffered three lung collapses in six weeks, soon after a trekking holiday high in the Indian Himalayas. Having just started my first job in London, I ended up in hospital there. Nothing specific was diagnosed, but I underwent some fairly brutal surgery – a partial pleurectomy. Essentially, I was patched up and sent on my way.

Five years later, after some more lung problems, I was told I had the chronic disease Lymphangioleiomyomatosis (now known as LAM). At that time, very little was known about the disease. With no Internet, the only sources of information were textbooks with one-line entries along the lines of, "...a very rare lung disease which affects women and is usually fatal within 10 years." Oestrogen is thought to play a part in LAM, so I was advised not to have children. I was told that my prognosis was uncertain, but that there was no treatment and no cure. Certainly, a lung transplant was not considered an option at that time. It was a devastating diagnosis. I was 27-years-old, had recently moved to Edinburgh to a new job which I loved, and which involved a lot of trans-Atlantic travel, and had just started seeing a boyfriend, Peter, who was later to become my husband. Until then, my future had been a place of opportunity, ambition and optimism. Now, it was a dark place where uncertainty and danger lurked. And yet I had been told to go ahead and live my life as normal.

In practice, however, the disease progressed through slow attrition. I grew increasingly breathless, and required more surgery after further lung collapses. It was in 1995, before another operation, that the possibility of a transplant was first raised with me. This was fantastic news; finally, I was given some hope that my future might hold something other than the ultimately terminal march of the disease. In the meantime, though, I was being forced to give up my favourite activities one by one. And it was not only me who was affected; my world was shrinking, but so was that of my family because we couldn't do anything together. By summer 2003, I was on oxygen 24 hours a day; eating and sleeping were difficult; and showering and dressing in the morning took hours. I'm naturally an energetic and sociable person, but was unable to be either. I was finally put on the transplant list in 2003. By then, my physical symptoms were at least matched by the psychological impact of my situation; I was deteriorating rapidly, and was terrified that my call would not come in time.

However, I was lucky. In February 2004, I received a new left lung. In general, the operation went well and thanks to my donor, her family, the team at the Freeman Hospital, Newcastle-Upon-Tyne, England, United Kingdom, and the support of my family and friends, my life since then has been absolutely transformed. Leaving the hospital was extremely emotional – I felt like a new woman. Three weeks after the operation, I was able to walk outside for an hour, and was weeping with gratitude and amazement.

Of course, there have been setbacks, but the best piece of advice I received was that I should expect a roller coaster ride post-transplant, particularly in the first year. Even if the medical team cannot predict the exact nature of such setbacks for each individual, being warned in advance to expect problems certainly helped me deal with mine when they inevitably occurred. My own blips included two episodes of acute rejection in the first months and, more recently, a struggle to eradicate a bout of the water-borne disease cryptosporidium.

But the benefits have far outweighed these problems. My quality of life is excellent. It is wonderful to live a normal life again: going out for supper with friends, working, walking to the cinema, going on holiday, playing with my young nephews. I even appreciate being able to do my own supermarket shopping! I am able to indulge my love of sport again too; since my transplant I've been kayaking, skiing and golfing, and have even learnt to roller blade. Earlier this year, my husband and I traveled to New Zealand, where we completed the arduous one-day trek, The Tongariro Crossing. In summary, I am a participant again, rather than a frustrated spectator. It is a complete miracle.

Ironically, I think my illness and transplant have allowed me to achieve a better life/work balance than I otherwise might have not had. Having spent my career in the financial sector, I now mix freelance consulting, and writing with work for charities associated with organ donation and my underlying disease, giving talks and writing articles. Currently, I also chair the research and support group LAM Action. Together with exercising, and spending time with friends and family, life is busy!

Soon I will celebrate the seventh anniversary of my transplant. But while it will be another happy milestone for Susie and me, it will also be a sad anniversary for my donor family. I wrote to them soon after my transplant; it was the most difficult letter I've ever had to write, but also the most important. I can't thank them enough, but hope that my letter – and those from Susie and other people who benefited from their brave decision – helped them in their loss.

Gillian (Gill) Hollis, 45
Edinburgh, Scotland, United Kingdom
Lymphangioleiomyomatosis
Single Lung Transplant, February 11, 2004
Freeman Hospital, Newcastle-Upon-Tyne, England, United Kingdom

[153]

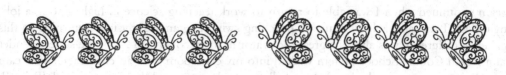

Dreams
By Mike Horgan

Have you ever dreamed about – "What if?" My dream began on July 24, 2000 in the safe confines of Jackson Memorial Hospital University of Miami School of Medicine, Miami, Florida, under the expert artistry of Dr. Si Pham's team of surgeons. I dreamed of a normal healthy life. I was looking forward to living the dream after fighting back the deadly effects of Cystic Fibrosis (CF) for 39 years. The last few years had been a nightmare as this disease had taken its toll on my family, friends, body and my spirit.

I had once lost hope of realizing my dream after United Health Care rejected my coverage for this center that would allow me a support network, and allow me to fight the end stages of Cystic Fibrosis close to home. Instead they asked me to take a transplant at a hospital on the other side of the state of Florida. The prospects of having my wife quit her job and act as a required support during the waiting period was defeating. I would rather forfeit my opportunity at a new set of lungs than to put my family through any more. After some media coverage Jackson Memorial and United Health Care made an agreement and my optimism soared.

I waited eight months on the list complete with a beeper, medical support and hope. I looked forward to the pager ringing through the pain of lungs that would fill with fluid and sleepless nights filled with fear that I wouldn't be able to breathe if I fell asleep. After all, I had to labor to get the newspaper and every breath required effort. CF sufferers understand this feeling. I enjoyed swimming for therapy and comfort, pulling from my experiences as an athlete, to make it through each day. Everyday was harder than the day before, both at work and at home. Down to one hundred and thirteen pounds, but not down to my last breath.

Over ten years have passed. The initial months of recovery, on and off hospitalizations and complications are now behind me. Over ten years of celebrating life with my wife, of 25 years, Jennifer, and my now seventeen-year-old son, Stephen. My friends think my wife is a Saint for not only putting up with me before and during, but even more so after. My real heroes have assisted me along the way. My heroes are not sports stars who demand millions and then act entitled but Dr.'s Pham, Fertel and Sandra Gerity who are tirelessly dedicated to saving lives.

My dream started when I came back to my family. My wife no longer has to worry about our future and witness me suffer and vent my frustrations about Cystic Fibrosis. She now has a husband who is not out of breath and can work. My son now has a father who is there for his teenage years unlike mine who abandoned his first family. I get to see my son approach his adult years, learning how to drive. My son was named after one of my two brothers who succumbed to Cystic Fibrosis and he had honored the name with academic and athletic successes.

My dream continued when I was able to return to work teaching science in high school, a job that was my calling. I was also able to return to coaching swimming and exercising. Returning to this job and making a difference was always a great motivator in my recovery. In 2008, the superintendent of the Palm Beach County School System walked into my classroom with an entourage. With cameras rolling and pictures snapping he handed me balloons and announced that I was named, 'Palm Beach County Teacher of the Year'. 21 years of sacrifice to this great profession were validated. I still cannot believe this ever happened except when I pinch myself I can feel it. This was a great high that balanced some of the lower points in my medical history.

Following my return to work my dream took on more of a selfish side; the purchase of a boat and adventures on the high seas. I could now fish, snorkel and cruise adding to my experiences as a marine biology teacher. Smelling the salt air and watching the sunrise and sunset is spectacular, but the bonding with my wife on the oceans is priceless. I was able to catch and release a fish larger than myself similar to Hemingway, (Alluding to the book, "Old Man and the Sea", Hemingway was noted to be a big game fisherman.) in my case it was a 450-600 pound mako shark and battled hundreds more. Sharing the great wonders of the sea, and the animals that live in it with my friends, and family has been rewarding.

Recently my dream took on a blissful moment. On March 14, 2010 our swim team the Lake Lytal Lightning won the Junior Olympic Swim competition held in Coral Springs, Florida, the home of Dara Torres. This was the first victory for a Palm Beach County team in the meets' 40-year history. I was pushed into the water, in the tradition of victory for this sport. We were all in the pool smiling, some crying and celebrating the hard work it takes to be champions.

As I floated in the water, content, I reflected back to July 23, 2000 and the beeper sounding as I exited the finals of a swim competition. I remembered a friend and fellow coach, an ex-Olympian, took it upon himself to watch over me. He hurried me off the deck to travel to the hospital, which was 30 minutes away. I went back to the cold steel gurney and the bright lights of the surgical room and the quiet confidence that I would make it, from the nursing staff. I went back to the holidays and months spent in hospitals. I reflected on the sacrifices of the donor's family for the gift that was given. I remembered my two brothers who never had a chance for a transplant before this cruel disease took their lives. I floated silently at peace hoping to never wake from this dream.

Mike Horgan, 49
West Palm Beach, Florida
Cystic Fibrosis
Double Lung Transplant, July 24, 2000
Jackson Memorial Hospital University of Miami School of Medicine, Miami, Florida
Read Mike's Lung Transplant Story in the 1st Edition of Taking Flight

❀ I am Going to Lead an Extraordinary Life! ❀
By Evlyn Hossack

Hello my name is Evlyn Hossack and I received a heart and double lung transplant in July 2008.

I was born in 1983, in Perth, Australia, the youngest of four children in our family. I was born with three things wrong with my heart. I had patient ducts, transposition of the main arteries and a hole in my heart. When I was nine months old I had an open-heart surgery because the pressure in my lungs was too great.

I lead a semi normal life growing up going to primary school, high school and started to work, The only thing different was I would get out of breath very fast when I did any type of exercise, and I had to see my childhood heart specialist once a year.

In 2005 I went on holiday to United States of America for two weeks and when I came back I had flu like symptoms. So I went back to the general practitioner (GP) and she did an electrocardiography (ECG) on me and told me my heart was failing and I needed to go to Royal Perth Hospital Emergency Room, East Perth, Western Australia, immediately. I had so many tests done, blood test; computer tomography (CT) scan, and many more. My family and I were told I had pulmonary hypertension (a lung condition which is high blood pressure in my lungs) and that I needed a heart and double lung transplant.

I was put on oxygen 24/7 and medication to see if it would reduce the severity of my condition. I was on the transplant list for around six months and then I started to improve so the team removed me from the list as I was too well for a transplant. After being taken off the list my life started to improve each day. I was doing really well and the doctors were even talking about taking me off oxygen.

Then in September 2007 I got pneumonia. The doctors decided to put me back on the transplant list. On the night of the 19 July 2008, my sister, mum and I were sitting down to have dinner when my pager went off, saying I had to ring my nurse. I phoned her and she told me they had found a donor and I needed to come into hospital as soon as possible. It was the most incredible news I have ever heard in my life. I arrived at the hospital and the only other thing I remember was saying to everyone who came in, "You are going to wake me up aren't you?" I was wheeled to the operating room with my family surrounding me. The feeling is indescribable; it was a mixture of fear of so many things that could go wrong, yet joy of knowing my life would be so much better when I woke up. I felt my heart pounding and butterflies in my tummy. I was so nervous and excited at the same time.

The operation took six to eight hours. When I was in intensive care, I kept lifting up my left leg. All I knew was there was a really weird sensation on my lower legs. I found out later it was air pillows, which were there to help with my circulation! Once the breathing tube was out I was so amazed that I was able to breath without struggling. I was then taken to the ward where I was taught to breathe properly. For 25 years I had done shallow breathing. I needed to be taught how to breathe using my whole lung (still forget sometimes). I also had to learn to walk again as I was taking really small steps "nana steps" they were called. I was in hospital for 17 days with nurses, doctors, physiotherapists and my family coming and helping me in my recovery. I could not have done it without them.

I am now 27 months out of transplant and I am living a "normal" life. I have a full time job, I have travelled to the World Transplant Games in 2009 and my next big thing is to travel to Europe for the 2011 World Transplant Games in Sweden (my events will be ten pin bowling and squash), and travel Europe while I'm there.

My major passion in life is to live every day to the fullest. I try different things at least once and travel the world to see how different cultures live. I don't want to waste any of my extra time and I want to always be learning. I fought so hard to stay alive, and life is way to short that I am not going to lead a "normal" life; I am going to lead an extraordinary life.

Evlyn Hossack, 28
Perth, Western Australia
Pulmonary Hypertension
Heart/Double Lung Transplant, July 19, 2008
Royal Perth Hospital, East Perth, Western Australia

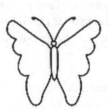

Hard Knocks to a Grateful Life
By Sandra Howard

I was still in my 30's, suave, looking sexy, smoking and waking up in the mornings coughing my insides out "to get my pipes open". I was totally unaware that Chronic Obstructive Pulmonary Disease (COPD), (an umbrella term for several lung diseases) claims one in every five smokers and that it's the 4th leading cause of death in the United States of America. I thought I was out of "condition" because I got out of breath so easily. It wasn't until I was in my 50's that I went to the doctor with a bad cold; not my first by a long shot. He said I had asthma.

Well, for the next 10 years I learned to HATE asthma. I took medicine for it but breathing became more of an effort. Finally, I thought (because of insurance issues) that I might be eligible for disability. My primary care (PC) agreed but wanted to send me to a pulmonologist. That dear doctor told me I didn't have asthma, I had emphysema. He gave me a few days for that to settle in, and made an appointment for both my husband and me to see him. I got home and told my husband that the good news was that I didn't have asthma. The bad news was that I had emphysema. We both thought it couldn't be too serious because I was not skinny, and drawn, but way over weight. The doctor cleared up that image for us in our next meeting. Not only did I have emphysema, I had severe emphysema.

I was enrolled in pulmonary rehab, one of the best things that can happen to people with breathing trouble. And for a few years I felt pretty cocky. I was still able to do almost anything, just slower. I had joined several "lists" on the Internet and got myself educated pretty quickly about my disease. One of the main things I learned was that I needed to be in charge of my disease. My medical caregivers needed to be more like "consultants".

We were traveling around in our motor home in those years and found that my blood oxygen saturation would fall when we were at altitudes over 2,200 feet. But that wasn't so bad. Then we found I needed to keep my oxygen turned up at night while I was sleeping, still not too inconvenient. By the way, it is not unusual to need supplemental oxygen at night; we aren't breathing very deeply at night, so it's common to drop in oxygen saturation. Then I got pneumonia, and went on oxygen 24 hours a day (24/7). I thought it would just be for a little while until I got better. But with lung disease you don't get better. You can delay the deterioration but you can't stop it all together.

I remember the first time I tried on the cannula (the nose hose) and my eyes got pretty misty. The first time I wore it out in public must have been pretty silly looking. I was accustomed to walking away from my cart to look at something, but now I was on a seven-foot leash. Twaa-ang! And I wasn't a fast learner. Some people get really self conscious when they need to wear oxygen in public, but I knew already that if I wasn't exchanging enough oxygen it would damage my other organs, and that was more important to me than my vanity!

I met several other "lungers", first through the Internet and then, in person. That was a real comfort to be with people who understood where I was. One of them said he was going to try for a transplant. Whoa! And he did. Then another friend got listed and three days later was taken by ambulance to the hospital with pneumonia. She woke up four days later with new lungs. Talk about a way to cure pneumonia!

Under the able care of Dr. Fischer, I started the process of lung transplant evaluation and was placed on the waiting list. I hoped to make it to 65 before getting transplanted, but on May 4th, 2008 (Sunday, Irrigation Festival), the phone rang. It was "the call". I thought I was pre-packed and pretty much ready to go, we stood around looking stupidly at each other. They took me to pre-op hours later, but the lung was still up in the air on a plane, flying in from Alaska.

I must have been out of surgery sometime on May 5th. I was awakened much later in the day, in fact, into the night. In the following days, I was euphoric. Although I didn't get off oxygen for a couple of days, life was immediately better.

My 'new-to-me' left lung had come from Alaska; a beautiful 19-year-old boy injured in a car accident by a drunk driver. He was on life support for six days before his mother let him go and generously gave his surviving lung to me. I still get pretty teary eyed when I think of her courage, and what a huge difference that gift has made in my life. It's a second chance. Since then, his family and I have been in contact and refer to the lung as "ours". We honor Ryan on his birthday with chocolate chip cookies, as his mother would have made for him.

So, from my brand new life point of view: If you are having trouble, getting winded easily.... get tested. And if you test positive, then test to see if it's environmental or genetic. If you smoke, don't. I know it's hard to quit but it's so stupid to put that stuff in your body. That also goes for the times you should be wearing a mask to protect yourself. I know they are uncomfortable, but it's soooo stupid not to wear it. If you get diagnosed with a lung disease, it's not the end of life.... there is life after being diagnosed. Also important is for everyone to get flu shots as much as possible. Not only are you more protected, but also you help protect the medically vulnerable.

And finally, organ donation is so important. Please sign up to be a donor, let your family know that you have done that. If you have to make a decision like my donor's mother, know that you are giving life to another, in a very real sense.

While my freedom is so appreciated, one of the most important things to me from the transplant is the exquisite appreciation of life. Somewhere, somehow, joy and hope are so closely related.

"The highest tribute to the dead is not grief but gratitude"
Thornton Wilder quoted in: The Oklahoman.

"Creativity requires the courage to let go of certainties", Erich Fromm

Sandra Howard, 69
Port Angeles, Washington
Chronic Obstructive Pulmonary Disease
Single Lung Transplant, May 8, 2008
University of Washington Medical Center, Seattle, Washington

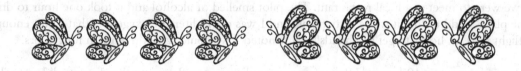

🦋 All for Jeremiah 🦋
Bobbi Huebner

My story is one that has allowed me to keep living for my son Jeremiah, who is now 11-years-old. In actuality he is the reason I had BOTH of my lung transplants. Spending time with him and being able to take him to Disney – what a truly amazing gift.

I never smoked, never any lung problems, but I went to the emergency room to be treated for bronchitis. I was sent to Shands Hospital at The University of Florida, Gainesville, Florida and told the shocking news. One, I had Idiopathic Pulmonary Fibrosis. Two, I had one year to live. Three, I needed a lung transplant and four; I had to lose 45 pounds to get listed. That is quite a list.

My sister Emma Jean played a large role and truly I couldn't have done this without her support. My first step was moving in with my sister in Panama City, Florida. Then it was a "weighting" game.

"First set of lungs", February 9, 2006 we received "the call" at 1:00a.m. Angel Flight was contacted and we were to meet at a local restaurant. The pilot smelled of alcohol and it took one hour to drive to the plane. Add to that it was a bitty plane, and I was on 15 liters of oxygen. If that is not enough, the flight took six hours to get to Shands!! Duly noted – we could have driven it in four hours.

The surgery was over 10 hours. Having some complications and anxiety that I never did as well as everyone had hoped; the doctors eventually relisted me. An infection had me hospitalized at Shands, and on November 2, 2006 the nurse walked into my room and said, "Are you ready for your new lung? You're having your lung transplant today." Great news! I was home in two weeks.

Though I have never been in touch with either of my donor families, "I thank God for them; I wish I could give them a hug".

Home schooling my son, scrap booking and being an avid reader are my present day fillers, and enjoyment. The joy of being with son is my biggest reward.

Overall, I am much closer to God and would not change a thing and my motto is, "Don't Sweat the Small Stuff".

Bobbi Huebner, 51
Lynn Haven, Florida
Idiopathic Pulmonary Fibrosis
Double Lung Transplant, February 9, 2006
Re-Transplant, Single Lung Transplant, November 2, 2006
Shands Hospital at The University of Florida, Gainesville, Florida
(Story written by Joanne Schum)

Just Breathe
By Catina Jackson

To breathe seems like such an easy thing to do for most people. For me it was almost impossible.

In 1996 both of my legs had swollen up from the knees down. I just thought it was either the knee-highs I had one were too tight or I had eaten too many salty items. I was wrong. I was diagnosed with end stage emphysema at the age of 43. My heart was also enlarged due to my lungs being in such bad shape.

The first step was to get on oxygen and stop smoking. I believe my oxygen level was at 72 % as opposed to 100% like most people. Okay, so there I was on oxygen 24 hours a day (24/7). I smoked very little but still I was afraid I could not stop. I did of course stop. I had no choice. The outlook at that time was very grim. I am sure my doctors did not think I was even going to live very long.

Well I remember going to sleep at night those first few weeks putting my life in God's hands. I would close my eyes and not be sure I would wake the next morning. The oxygen helped tremendously. Once I got my fight back I decided I was going to see at least one of my children graduate high school. I just want to mention that in 1978 I had lost my infant son after he had undergone heart surgery at the age of 19-days-old. That my friend, is a heart breaker. Needless to say I was all about my children.

By 2004 I was unable to get around walking and needed a wheel chair for the most part. I fought this whole illness with all I had. It was amazing what I was able to do on oxygen. When I think about it now, I laugh. I was a fighter. Eventually, my oxygen saturation was very low, even on the oxygen.

I went to a new pulmonologist who actually saved my life. He told me I needed a lung transplant, possibly a heart/ lung transplant. The Cleveland Clinic Foundation, Cleveland, Ohio was contacted and I was on my journey to receive a transplant and a new life. I went to physical therapy for at least two months to be eligible to receive a transplant. On August 29, 2005 I got my new lungs. I was so tickled that I was going to get two new lungs. Usually people of my age, at that time, only received one lung. I am not sure why I received two lungs, but I wasn't going to question their decision. Again I say, "God is good".

The whole process went very well for me at Cleveland. I was back home in 10 days. I started my new life. I was free!!!! I could move again. No oxygen tanks or tubing in my way. I do remember my legs felt heavy and it was a little difficult to climb stairs but who cared. I added dancing to my regular exercise program. I could move the top part real well and my hips, but my feet weren't getting the message. That all worked out in time.

There were bumps in the road the first year. I had wonderful post transplant coordinators. I remember Keith, a post transplant coordinator said, "You have some rejection going on. You can get all worked up or we can just change the medications and solve the problem". It's funny I never felt bad at any point when I did have issues going on with my new lungs. I trusted them that much. I did get to see both of my daughter's graduate high school and college. Now I am looking to take Zumba lessons. God is good.

My post transplant life has been spent, doing for others. I have three brothers and three sisters who I have always looked after in one-way or another. Did I mention I am the oldest of seven siblings? We are very close. My mother had all seven children in nine years and there are no twins. Both of my parents are gone. Both died of cancer. My father died in 1980 at the age of 54 and my mother in 1998 at the age of 72. They were incredible role models. I mention that because not only did my sisters and brothers help with fundraisers and whatever, but also all their friends supported me. My thoughts were to give back to them and at the same time show them how well I was doing and that God is good. I would say I am a miracle. I am not sure why God choose me and what exactly he wants me to do but I always give the credit to God.

I am very aware of keeping my appearance and my physical body in good shape. I want people to see the results of organ donation and transplantation. It is amazing how many people's lives we touch without even knowing. I serve as an example of organ donation. That is one of my goals. To have people become donors. To save a life. I cry each and every time a person tells me they are now registered to be a donor because of me; knowing that I may have given another person a chance at a new life. I believe all survivors should be united. If you have overcome any life threatening illness or event, you are a hero. I walked in the Breast Cancer 5K fundraiser and met many survivors. It is funny how I did the walk for a very beautiful friend who handled her cancer with such poise and grace. I have so much admiration for how she handled the whole thing. She laughed and told me she looked to me as her inspiration. Life is good.

I have spent a portion of my post transplant days planning weddings, birthday parties, showers (baby and bridal) and fundraising events. I am so fortunate to have had the chance to be part of and coordinate my own daughter's and my "adopted" son's wedding. I am even luckier to see my second daughter marry in the next year.

I am starting my sixth year out from my transplant. I never thought I would get this much more incredible time on this earth. I have to say even now I am looking at life differently. I feel even a stronger conviction to reach further. I almost feel like wearing a tag on my clothes that reads 'transplant survivor', to the gym I attend, the parties I attend, the charity meetings I attend, and really any interaction with new people I want them to see what can be possible.

Fight the fight, walk the walk, just breathe.

Catina Jackson, 57
Albion, New York
Emphysema
Double Lung Transplant, August 19, 2005
The Cleveland Clinic Foundation, Cleveland, Ohio

🦋 Moments That Take My Breath Away 🦋
By Kimberly Jackson

My life started out with pneumonia at birth, and growing up thinking I had severe asthma. I was in my late 20's when I went to University of North Carolina Hospitals, Chapel Hill (UNC) where Dr. James Yankaskas discovered through a biopsy of tissue taken from my sinuses that I had a lung disease called, Primary Ciliary Dyskinesia (PCD). The disorder is also called Kartagener's Syndrome, except with Kartagener's you can have what they call, Situs Inversus (reversed organs). I am one of six children. I have sisters that are twins (Regina and Ren'a) who also have the same lung disease, except Ren'a has Situs Inversus. They are both on the list now for double lung transplants at Chapel Hill, but for now they are inactive, as they are doing well.

I participate in a lot of research with Dr. Peadar Noone at UNC Hospitals on our disease because it is not widely known. As a matter of fact, my old lungs are part of a study now.

Before my transplant my life was very difficult. I had to wear oxygen 24 hours a day, I had to do breathing treatments every four hours, chest physiotherapy, and I had to have intravenous antibiotics to fight infections in my lungs, ears, and sinuses. I was having severe episodes of hemoptysis; therefore I was an inpatient at UNC Hospitals for about four months before I received my donor lungs.

Dr. Thomas Egan did my double lung transplant on July 27th, 2000 and my whole life changed. I could breathe again!! Praise be to GOD!! I remember Dr. Noone coming into my room right before I was taken off the ventilator, and holding an x-ray, and telling me that they were a beautiful set of lungs. Now thanks to my donor family, the Lord, and my doctors I can breathe without coughing and fighting for every breath.

I also want to thank my family and friends for all their support during and after my transplant. My husband David and I have been married for 17 years now, and after my transplant we went to Hawaii for the honeymoon we never had. We had so much fun that he took me back a couple years later. While we were there, we swam with trained dolphins and we took a tour in a helicopter over the island, and some of the Maui waterfalls. The entire island was breathtaking.

Because of my lung disease I could not have children. Due to the dramatic change in my health condition, I decided that I would love to be a mom. So after my surgery we started talking about adoption. We contacted an adoption agency and began our search for our special child.

On January 28th 2004, we became the proud parents of a baby boy! We love him very much, and he has brought so much joy to our lives. We took our son Andrew to Walt Disney World when he was four years old. We had a great time, and we are going to take him back again this fall (we can't wait). We go to the beach at least once a year at Emerald Isle because that is where Andrew's grandmother lives. We also went on a cruise with his Grandparents to the Bahamas, St Thomas, and St. Maarten last year. It was so beautiful and hopefully we will do it again someday.

Andrew is in the 1st grade now and we love being parents. There is so much happiness to write about. I just love living my life to the fullest, and there is not a single day that I don't forget what a blessing it is to be alive. I do have regular check-ups, and, I take a lot of medicines, but I am happy and breathing so much better than before my miracle.

Both of my parents were alive when I got my transplant, but sadly they both have passed away because of cancer. I do look forward to seeing them again, as well as a brother and sister, (that both died before my transplant) one day, when the Lord finally calls me home. When I get to heaven I going to thank my organ donor. I will tell them about the life they gave me, and how much I enjoyed it because of their gift.

Life is short; spend it with the ones you love. There is a quote that I really love, it goes, "Life is not measured by the breaths that we take, but by the moments that take our breath away." I love the Lord, and I thank God everyday, for all of my blessings. I love my family, but most importantly, I have the opportunity of being with them today because of the selfless, generous actions of the donor's family, and the medical team that performed my transplant. Under the knowledge and direction of God I have been given a second chance at having just a normal life.

Kimberly Jackson, 44
Vale, North Carolina
Primary Ciliary Dyskinesia also known as Kartagener's Syndrome
Double Lung Transplant, July 27, 2000
University of North Carolina Hospitals, Chapel Hill, North Carolina
Kimberly Adopted a Son, Post Lung Transplant
Read Kimberly's Lung Transplant Story in the 1st Edition of Taking Flight

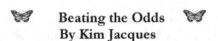

Beating the Odds
By Kim Jacques

My name is Kimberly Jacques and I received a life-saving heart and double lung transplant 14 years ago. To tell you how I got to this point I have to start at the beginning. I was born on January 3, 1980, as a preemie with a multitude of health problems. While it was obvious that my lungs were very underdeveloped, it didn't even occur to my doctors that there might be something wrong with my heart.

People have been throwing statistics my way ever since I entered this world. I should have died at birth, become blind, become deaf; mentally retarded, died during infancy, or not survive to see my teenage years. Transplant statistics say that a heart/double lung transplant is the most rarely performed, least successful surgery, and to make it past five years is a miracle. I've beaten them all. I'm still here, I am 14 years post transplant, and recently entered my fourth decade of life.

When I was 2 ½, my doctors thought I'd be doing better since, I was still on oxygen. A cardiac catheterization revealed that I had inoperable holes in my heart. I was diagnosed with, Eisenmenger's

Syndrome. Once I was diagnosed, my doctors, "tip-toed" around what type of surgery I may need. It was determined I needed a heart and double lung transplant.

At the age of five my parents decided a move for our family of four, as I now also had a younger sister, from Boston, Massachusetts to Tampa, Florida to see if see if the warmer climate might help me. It worked, and I ended up having a normal childhood. I was able to grow up in a great neighborhood with many kids my age. I was also an above average student in school, and I was active in Girl Scouts, and in my church.

In June of 1994, I went to my cardiologist for my yearly check-up. It was the first day of summer vacation and I was antsy to go get the check up over with, and go on with my summer, but fate had other plans. After several visits to St. Louis, Missouri, throughout 1994 and 1995, it was decided that my family and I would need to move there to wait for my transplant. We moved to St. Louis in the spring of 1996, and during the early hours of June 14th, I received the call I'd been waiting for. The organs I needed had become available!

Since my transplant, I've been able accomplish so many things. I graduated from high school, and received an Associate's degree in Science. I have had the pleasure of watching my sisters grow up and graduate high school and college. I was able to welcome numerous cousins into the world. Two of them (Harry, 13 and Madeline 12) are now old enough to know all about my transplant journey, and are equally thankful that they got to grow up with "Cousin Kim."

Since 2002, I have been an active participate at the United States Transplant Games proudly representing Team Florida. At the 2006 games, I won a bronze medal in the 1500m-race walk, and at the 2008 games; I won a silver medal in the same event. Though I didn't medal at the 2010 games, I'm still happy that I had the opportunity to compete in my events. Besides, there is always 2012.

I created a Team Florida group on Facebook for the games, and am a member of various transplant networking websites. I am able to offer advice and support to those on the waiting list and give them insight on what lies ahead in the post transplant world.

I am so grateful that my donor family said, "YES" in their moment of tragedy and I'm proud I've been able to give this heart and these lungs such a good home.

Kimberly Jacques, 30
Tallahassee, Florida
Eisenmenger's Syndrome
Heart/Double Lung Transplant, June 14, 1996
St. Louis Children's Hospital, St. Louis, Missouri

Living for the Moments that Take our Breath Away
By Christena and Kevin Jones

July 17th, 2010, Kevin and I finally became husband and wife. Yes, I say finally even though we are only 23 and 21. Yes, I say finally even though we have so many lessons yet to learn and so many life experiences to embark on. I say finally, because neither Kevin nor I were supposed to make it to this day. If our parents were truthful with themselves, they'd probably admit that they could not imagine that their children ever enjoying a normal life, graduating high school or attending college, and they definitely didn't envision their children getting married. You see, Kevin and I both have cystic fibrosis (CF) and we are both transplant recipients. While we might have those two things in common, most of the rest of our lives have been a bit different.

Kevin was born in 1986, and before the age of one, he had been diagnosed with cystic fibrosis. He mainly suffered from malnutrition and digestive issues and by the time he was two-years-old, Kevin had cirrhosis of the liver. From that point on, Kevin frequented the hospital a couple of times a year for lung infections and visceral vein bleeds. Even during his years spent doing treatments, intravenous antibiotics (IV's) and receiving blood transfusions, Kevin tried to maintain his active lifestyle and enjoyed taking part in outdoor activities such as four wheeling and hunting.

Unfortunately, by the time he had reached his 10th birthday, it became eminent to both Kevin's doctors and family, that he needed a liver transplant. After the rigorous testing involved with transplant evaluation, Kevin was listed at St. Louis Children's Hospital at Washington University Medical Center, St. Louis, Missouri for a liver transplant. He continued to live in Kentucky. After nearly two years of waiting, and continued declining health and lack of adequate transplant offers, Kevin's physicians considered a relatively new and radical idea; Kevin would be placed on the double lung transplant and liver transplant list. Knowing cystic fibrosis was a chronic lung disease his doctors knew that a lung transplant would be in Kevin's future, even if he got a liver transplant.

On November 11, 1998, Kevin received his lifesaving double lung and liver transplant. He was only the third person in the St. Louis area to have that transplant combination. Kevin had some rough times post transplant, but luckily, Kevin's tenacity and zest for life couldn't keep him down, and by the summer of 1999, he had returned to his hometown and begun truly living his life. After Kevin's transplant he was able to focus on all the things he was passionate about. Being from a small farming town, Kevin learned the ropes of how to tend to his family farm. He became an avid hunter and fisher and enjoyed spending the rest of his free time four wheeling and hanging out with his friends like everyone else his age.

I was born in 1988. I was diagnosed with cystic fibrosis soon after birth. I was born with a blockage and it was an immediate red flag for CF, unlike Kevin, I had severe lung problems from day one. My very first hospital stay was at the age of six months, and following that, I was regularly admitted to the hospital for lung infections two to three times a year. I was swallowing pills by the time I was two, I could tell you all the positions for chest therapy by the time I was three, and I was helping flush my own IV's by the time I was four. I grew up knowing that this was my life. I still enjoyed 'normal' childhood things, but they always had a medical aspect. All of my favorite baby dolls went to surgery with me. Each one got IVs and broviacs. I had more bags of medical supplies to play doctor than I had Barbie dolls.

As I grew older, my hospital visits became more frequent and lengthy. Throughout middle and high school, I would spend multiple weeks in the hospital, followed by multiple weeks on home IV's. Since I couldn't take part in sports, I put all of my efforts into my schooling and I took pride in knowing it was the one thing I could control and determine the outcome. By my sophomore year in high school, shortly after I turned 16, I had to quit school. I couldn't even walk to the dinner table without getting into horrendous coughing fits that left me without any oxygen or strength to eat. In the spring of 2005, my family and I traveled to St. Louis Children's Hospital in hopes of finding some answers. After the weeklong extensive testing, we received a call that I had the highest score for my blood type on the lung allocation system, and I was to relocate to the area immediately.

We moved to St. Louis, and just one week later I got the call and received my double lung transplant on June 13, 2005. My immediate recovery was much less interesting than Kevin's. I felt amazing right away, and I wouldn't let anything hold me down. I was out of the hospital in 11 days. I joked that it took less time for me to recover from a transplant than it took for me to have a CF tune up.

Shortly after, I was able to move back home to Kentucky. Once home, I returned to high school. I caught up with the two semesters I missed and rejoined my classmates in the middle of junior year. I was able to attend my prom, get a job and drive. I finally was living the life of a teenager. In 2007, I graduated from high school in the top seven of my class with a grade point average exceeding 4.0. I couldn't believe I had accomplished so many dreams I never thought I'd ever even have the opportunity to attempt. I set off for college that year and I lived on campus nearly two hours away from my family. It was during this time that my life changed in a completely unexpected way.

By now I'm sure you are wondering how Kevin and I ever crossed paths. It's amazing that it actually took us this long, really. We both are from Kentucky, but we lived nearly two hours apart. We always saw the same CF doctor and went to the same hospital. Our families knew of one another, but we'd never really met.

While I was living in St. Louis post-transplant, Kevin and I were introduced briefly, but I joke that we were more interested in talking to each other's parents than actually talking to one another. Unfortunately, the meeting wasn't very impressive to either of us, and we never thought a thing about the encounter again. But then a mutual CF friend mentioned his name around Christmas 2007. I naturally thought I should look him up on Facebook and add him as a friend. It was purely as a 'one CF /transplant friend to another' type thing at first. I quickly realized that Kevin's profile stated he attended the same university I did, and I simply suggested we should meet for lunch between classes. He 'commented' me back, informing me that he did not go to that school anymore, but he would gladly make the two hour trip to take me to dinner. Needless to say, we did go on that dinner date, and it ended up being more than a 'friend' thing.

Most people assume that Kevin and I were a match made in heaven because we had so much in common with cystic fibrosis and transplants, but the truth is, the only benefit we gained from those commonalities was the fact that we could bypass the awkward "... so I have cystic fibrosis and I had a transplant..." conversation that was always the prelude to every other relationship. We could skip that and go right to the 'normal' dating process. We talked about our hobbies, our goals and our lives, not about our lives as CF and transplant patients.

I fell in love with Kevin because he was everything I wasn't. He was free, had such a beautiful spirit, and he showed me a refreshing passion and zest for living. I was generally uptight, cautious and had a plan for everything. While I always lived by, "Life is not measured by the breaths you take but the moments that take your breath away," Kevin actually enforced that in my life. I quit planning everything and began enjoying more, living more and actually breathing more. I learned things I never thought I'd care to learn, like four wheeling and learning how to hunt and I began to love this life he showed me. When he asked me to marry him 1-½ years after we first started dating, there wasn't any question.

Our life together hasn't been easy. On top of regular couple issues, we've dealt with some pretty devastating periods of time. The first year we were together, I was diagnosed with chronic rejection. I'd never been sick, not even had a cold since I'd been transplanted, and out of nowhere, it felt like my lungs were going to give out at any moment. Kevin was sick at the same time with pneumonia, so we couldn't be there for each other. Shortly after I was successfully treated for the rejection, Kevin was admitted to the hospital and he began dealing with rejection. I couldn't be with him during this time, because I was still so vulnerable from the rejection treatments I'd recently received. Miraculously, Kevin's rejection was treated and we were able to get back to planning our life together.

We've endured the frustrations of insurance, doctors and medical bills but we've tried to keep it from overshadowing our happiness. Kevin and I know our futures will not be easy and parts won't be fun. We have a lot of living to do and a lot of things left to learn, but we both agreed, that we didn't want to live another day, or learn another thing, unless we were hand in hand. We don't know what to expect from day to day. We've seen the ambiguity of transplant and know that nothing is a certainty but we are living for the moments, especially the ones that take our breath away.

Christena and Kevin Jones, 21 and 23
Knifley, Kentucky
Christena and Kevin, Cystic Fibrosis
Kevin, Double Lung and Liver Transplant, November 11, 1998
Christena, Double Lung Transplant, June 13, 2005
Christena and Kevin both Transplanted at
St. Louis Children's Hospital at Washington University Medical Center, St. Louis, Missouri
Christena and Kevin were married July 17, 2010

Lacy: The Win/Win Transplant
By Carol Joyce

Lacy is the name I gave my newly transplanted lung while laying in the hospital bed, September 18, 2004, in drug-induced semi consciousness. It's remarkable how many things swirl around in your head under those conditions and since my mind was already playing games with me, I decided my thoughts were going to be as pleasant as I could think to make them. And oh my, it is absolutely amazing what a little imagination can do and that is how the name Lacy was born. To me the name "Lacy" gave the mental image of light and air, a name that would encourage easy, breezy breathing. It had a pleasant sound and was much nicer to say than "my donor lung" when referring to my transplant.

Pre-transplant I had been praying for many months, that my unknown lung donor was having a stress free, wonderful and fulfilling life. I am aware that people die every day and that some choose to be organ donors so I convinced myself that those "HEROES" who made that choice wanted to better someone else's life by donating their organs when they passed.

I was very much indebted of my new chance at life that I was anxious to contact the donor family to let them know that their loved one's right lung was with someone who would take excellent care of it. I wrote a beautiful and sensitive letter of appreciation but never heard a word back. To tell you the truth, I was disappointed but I understand that people must find closure in his or her own way and I was just going to have to accept this amazing gift of life and deal with it. My way of doing that was to promise myself to always take the very best care of my new lung, to be compliant about taking my medications and to follow the guidelines of avoiding exposure to illnesses. Those were the things I knew I could control. I also adopted a silly little ritual. Every time I washed my hands I sang (in my head) "Happy Birthday to Lacy". What the heck, the girl had celebrated birthdays for years, and since I didn't know which day to celebrate, I covered them all. I celebrated her life every day because if not for her I would not be writing this missive. I hope Lacy's family knows how much I loved her for her "Gift of Life." to me, but I know God knows.

The transplant doctors and nurses at Johns Hopkins Hospital, Baltimore, Maryland, my husband Jim, devoted children and grandchildren, family members; loyal friends and prayerful congregation at church were the people who helped me get my hat back on and helped me keep it straight. That was a very big job! Each one of them at some point played an important part in helping me through my illness, pulmonary rehab, doctor's visits, surgery, post surgery and recovery. I have met countless wonderful people since my transplant and am blessed beyond words. I must mention at this point, as ridiculous as it may sound, even the computer played a major role in getting me through my struggles to breathe and recovery from surgery. The computer was my lifeline to the outside world and allowed me to feel a vital part of existence in spite of my fatal illness.

Once I recovered from the initial surgery, two rejection attempts, and a bout with Cytomegalovirus (CMV), I gained strength and hope for my new and improved life.

One thing you get to do when you have been told you are dying is to think, over think and re-think about so many things and I certainly had plenty of time to do just that. I had always been an active person prior to my illness. I was a busy hairdresser for 27 years, taught Sunday school, worked with the youth group and helped with my nine grand children as much as I could. I wanted more than anything, now that I was so much better, to give back. I had been accepting help from others for what seemed like such a long time I felt it was time to pay the piper.

I started by having monthly dinners for my family of almost 20, and did that successfully for over a year but the family schedules started conflicting and after a while it got too complicated. I do feel I was able to show some of my appreciation for the many wonderful things my family did to help me during my illness and afterward.

In spite of the fact I could no longer live with birds, we had to re-home four happy, healthy, loving pets, our amazing talking parrots. I still miss them but their new owners keep in touch with notes and pictures and videos. Not having them anymore didn't make me any less knowledgeable about parrots and I was happy to share what I knew with anyone who would listen so we continued our membership in the exotic bird club to which we belonged for many years. A year after transplant I ran for and was elected President of the bird club, Baltimore Bird Fanciers, (the oldest in the United States) and served for two years and am still the membership chair person. I also served on the reunion committee for Western High School class of 1961, chaired the nurturing committee of the Cedar Grove, United Methodist Women, flew to Phoenix, Arizona and drove to the Grand Canyon and visited many places in between. The elevation of the canyon slowed me down somewhat but I tried to do all I could while there and loved every minute of it. Breath taking is not an especially comforting word for people with lung problems but there really is no better description of the Grand Canyon. Since transplant, six years ago, I have attended parties and danced at several weddings of friends and family including a granddaughter. I've rekindled old friendships and kept relationships alive and well. These and many more things too numerous to list were all made possible to me through the miracle of lung transplant.

I couldn't possibly write any of this without also mentioning that I feel my transplant was first and foremost all to the Glory of GOD. I was not afraid of not surviving the transplant surgery because for me it was a win/win situation. If I made it, I was a winner and if I didn't I was still going to be a winner because I knew I would be with my Heavenly Father.

Thank you for giving me the opportunity to give you a little glimpse of what life has been like for me since transplant. I only wish my words were worthy of the honor bestowed on me by my God and my organ donor.

Carol Joyce, 66
Upperco, Maryland
Idiopathic Pulmonary Fibrosis
Single Lung Transplant, September 18, 2004
Johns Hopkins Hospital, Baltimore, Maryland

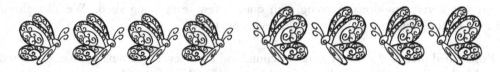

The 2008 U.S. Transplant Games and a Miracle Moment
By Mary Juneau

My husband, Robert, was born December 23, 1969. At age two he was diagnosed with Cystic Fibrosis; his parents were told he would not live to age 12. At age 10 his problems began, he had his first hospitalization for nasal polyps. At age 26, when lung bleeding episodes started occurring at a rate of three or four times a year he underwent a lung embolization.

At age 35, his lungs began to give out and they gave out fast. His health rapidly declined and he was forced to stop working. His doctor told him that only a double lung transplant could save his life.

After 11 months the call that a pair of lungs was available finally came. We took a medical jet to Massachusetts General Hospital, Boston, Massachusetts, where Robert had a very successful double lung transplant on March 14, 2007. Robert responded so well to his transplant that he was released from the hospital only 24 days later.

Robert's recovery was rapid from that point on. One of the things that he loved to do, which provided exercise for his new lungs, was play the game of table tennis. Robert had loved the game since he was a small boy. Before his health began to fail he competed in amateur tournaments. He was a good player and was often in the medals. The transplant helped him resume his love of the game. It is funny to note that on the day of the call for the transplant Robert had decided that he wanted to play table tennis one last time. We went to our local club, oxygen pack and all. I stood behind him to catch him if he started to fall and to retrieve the balls for him while he played. On the way home that night he decided that if he ever got his transplant, he was going to start playing competitively again. The call came in 10 minutes after we walked in the door that night.

During a check-up one day his nurse mentioned something called the United States Transplant Games. After Robert did a little research, he discovered that table tennis was one of the available sports for competition. He also was interested in the badminton competition.

Even though Robert had been playing table tennis for about six months after his transplant, he began more serious training to participate in the Transplant Games. He also began practicing badminton, which he had played years before. When the first day of the games arrived Robert was ready.

We traveled by bus to where the Transplant Games were being held in Pittsburgh, Pennsylvania. We were traveling with the rest of the Team Central New York competitors and their families. Also traveling with us were some of the families of deceased donors as well as a few living donors.

Opening Ceremonies were sad, happy and emotional. We realized at that time the games were more about honoring the donors and their families than, although important, about the competitions alone. It was a very emotional evening with quite a few tears being shed. We all realized how grateful we are to the donors that allowed the recipients to live.

Since Robert had practiced so hard at table tennis, and after several elimination games, he won the gold medal. It was an exciting and emotional moment as Robert stood on the top stand and was awarded the gold medal medallion.

Then the badminton competition began. The first game proved to be very exciting with the play very intense and physically taxing. The game was so exciting that people in the arena were beginning to gather around the court and the crowd that was watching grew. Robert lost the first game. Each player, the opponent having had a kidney transplant and Robert with his lung transplant, needed a rest between games. Badminton can be a very taxing and fast paced game. The second game began. The score teetered back and forth during the entire game, first Robert and then his opponent taking the lead. Finally, the game and possibly match point arrived with Robert's opponent in the lead by one point. Robert, by this time, had become very, very exhausted. The physical exertion required for this second game was taking a large toll on his stamina and lungs. What followed was a long and exciting volley. Robert's opponent won the second game and the gold medal. Robert, extremely pleased with his silver medal, was so exhausted from the two games that he was barely able to leave the court. When he finally got the strength and while breathing heavily and sweating profusely, Robert raised his arms in the air and said to the crowd, "Look how good my new lungs held up." The crowd cheered and most burst into tears.

Robert was so happy with his gold and silver medals that we left the arena both excited and teary eyed that Robert's health was now so good that he could participate in this type of competition. We thought, at the time, that things couldn't get any better than at that moment, we were wrong.

On the day of the Closing Ceremonies, Robert and I met two friends for dinner that evening. At the end of dinner, Robert wanted dessert but we were running a little late for the Ceremonies. One of our friends suggested that we meet after and have dessert then. Everyone agreed.

During the seating process we got separated from our friends that were supposed to have dessert with us. The Closing Ceremonies, like the Opening Ceremonies were extremely emotional. There were many, many tears of joy and sadness - joy for the transplant recipients who lived and sadness for those families who had lost someone so this could happen. We left the ceremonies with red eyes and a sense of wonder that the entire experience had been so very good.

Since we had gotten separated from our friends we decided not to stop for dessert afterwards. We boarded the bus for our hotel and went back. As we entered the lobby, Robert decided that he was in fact hungry and we should go next door to the convenience store and get something to eat. It was 11:30 p.m. by that time and the store had already closed. While heading back to the hotel lobby, we noticed a man and his daughter sitting on the steps in front of the hotel and the man was wearing a New England Team tee shirt and a Red Sox cap. We started back into the lobby. However, maybe because the man was wearing a Red Sox cap and Robert is a huge Red Sox fan or, as we believe, divine intervention, Robert turned around to talk to the man and the beginning of our miracle began.

Since Robert was originally from Maine but was now living in Syracuse, New York, he asked the man where he was from. He told us Warwick, Rhode Island. We asked if he was a participant of the games or a member of a donor family. He informed us that he was the father of a donor and his son had died the year before. Both of us hugged the man and thanked him for being so generous. He told us his son's heart and gone to a 16-year old girl, his liver went to a female school teacher, his kidneys had gone to two men who were exact matches and his lungs had gone to a man who was in his fifties and had Cystic Fibrosis. We were quite moved that so many people had benefited from this one tragedy. He then asked us if we were participants or a donor family and Robert told him about his lung transplant in 2007.

The conversation continued and it came to light that the man's son had died in March of 2007. Robert's transplant had been in March, too. The man said his son died on March 13 and Robert told him he got his call on March 13. At this time we started to get a little excited because on the day of Robert's transplant, a rare second transplant was performed at the same hospital for a man in his fifties. We knew, though, that this man did not have Cystic Fibrosis and Robert was 37 at the time.

Then the man's wife joined the group. She had been off calling a cab. She told us that there was no bus from the ceremonies to the hotel they were staying at because the hotel was not on the bus route. The family had gotten a late reservation and was not able to get a hotel associated with the games. The Kidney Foundation in New England sponsored one family to attend the games and her family was not picked. However, due to unknown circumstances, the family that had been picked could not make it and her family had been picked instead. Since cabs were hard to find when leaving the Ceremonies, the family decided to take the first bus they could and get off at the first hotel on the route and then call a cab from there. That was our hotel.

The man told his wife about us and she said that the family had received a letter from wife of the recipient of the boy's lungs. I had gotten to know the wife of the man who received the transplant after Robert and I asked if it was from her. The wife had an unusual name that would have been easy to remember. She said no and that the names from the letter were plain. She also corrected her husband and said that the organ bank had sent them information stating that the lung recipient was in his thirties and not in his fifties. She looked at our tags that were hanging around our necks and said that she thought that the letter might have been from Mary, about Robert, our names! Our hearts were pounding.

Then the wife started telling us about what was in the letter. She began repeating one particular sentence that was very specific and I finished the sentence for her. We had just met our donor family! The donor was the family's son and his name was Tim (Timbo) Packhem. He died on March 13, 2007 in a freak skateboarding accident.

The family we were with was Tim Packhem, Timbo's dad, Cari Packhem, Timbo's stepmother and Hannah, Timbo's half-sister. We started hugging and laughing and crying all at the same time. We simply could not believe that out of the thousands of people attending the Transplant Games that we could randomly bump into our donor's family on the street. It was an indescribable feeling.

After a few minutes, we all went into the lobby of the hotel. Timbo's mother, Paula Packhem, who was also attending the Games, was called and asked to come over immediately. She brought with her a representative from the organ bank. The representative called her office and gave us official confirmation of what we already knew: We had found our donor's family!

Word was getting out about what had happened and people started coming down from their rooms and joining the celebration. Also, there were still people coming in from the Closing Ceremonies and they were also joining in the celebration. Robert called his mother and father who live in Maine and told them the incredible news.

Since Robert had worn his gold and silver medals to the closing ceremonies he had them with him at the time. After meeting the Packhem's, Robert insisted that Timbo's father take the gold medal and Timbo's mother take the silver medal. After all, Robert would never have had the opportunity to win the medals if it weren't for Timbo and the thoughtful and heart-wrenching decision that his parents made the day Timbo died. The two gratefully and graciously accepted the medals.

At 2:30 a.m. everyone finally said goodnight. Robert and I went back to our room but neither of us slept that night. The next weekend, Robert and I went to Warwick, Rhode Island and spent a weekend with Timbo's family. We had quite a celebration. I think it was comforting for Timbo's family to see some of the good that has come out of their son's death. It also gave some closure to Robert to finally meet his donor's family and to be able to say, in person, "THANK YOU for giving me back my life."

I write this with a grateful and loving heart to the Packhem family.

Mary Juneau, Wife of Robert Juneau
Robert Juneau, 40
Marietta, New York
Robert, Cystic Fibrosis
Robert, Double Lung Transplant, March 17, 2007
Massachusetts General Hospital, Boston, Massachusetts
Read Jessica Water's Story, Robert's Donor's Sister, in this Edition of Taking Flight

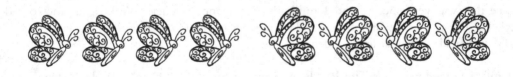

Promises
By Elizabeth Kellner

I was talking to a friend the other day about the decisions I have had to make in my life. Basic decisions such as, what to cook for dinner, or what to wear. Of course there are other decisions that I had to make where thinking about it, was not an option. It was a decision that was a matter of life or death.

The last thing I wanted to do at 25-years-old was decide if I wanted to have a lung transplant or not. I mean I always had an idea that the day would come. But never thought it would be at 25. I wasn't ready to face that reality yet. I was getting ready to graduate, planning a wedding and enjoying my life. But transplant was indeed a reality that I had to face whether I was ready for it or not. Three years later, I look back and do not regret the decision. If it weren't for my new lungs, I wouldn't have lived to see my wedding day, be writing this insert or go back to nursing school to become a nurse one day. I wouldn't have had the life I always longed for. I won't lie to you. There are days when I wish I didn't have my transplant or have to face the fact that I now need a new kidney. I no longer know who I am when I see myself in the mirror. I can no longer do the things I used to, and can't still adapt to my new life of kidney failure. However, it's on these days that I remind myself of the promises I made to keep myself from ever giving up.

I promise to always smile. To never give up. To always have hope. To never lose my faith. To be the best I can be. To be the loving wife I should be. To be a better friend. To always put others first. To bite my tongue as often as I can. To stay forever young. To always be inspired by music. To reach my goals. Always be happy. Always stay strong. To take care of myself. To do things for me. To never look back. To always go forward. Never let others bring me down. To cry when the pain is too hard. Look for the sun on a rainy day. To be a shoulder to cry on. To laugh at myself. Enjoy every breath. Enjoy moments with good friends. Learn from my mistakes. Stay true to myself. Remember my donor family. Hug my parents. Forgive others. To always be grateful. To show gratitude. To never take things for granted. To always learn something new. To be an advocate. To never doubt myself. To never give up. To ALWAYS fight CF.

Mrs. Brightside
I want to say that the hardest moment of my Cystic Fibrosis (CF) life was that month I was on the waiting list. I am very, very blessed that I received my lungs in a month after being listed, which is not very common.

That night, for the first time since I had been listed, I felt fear. But I had peace. I prayed to God that if it was meant to be for me to get lungs to please have them arrive quickly. And that if it wasn't for me then to let me go. I asked Him to give me peace and that I was not afraid to leave this Earth; that I wanted His will to be done. I slept peacefully which I hadn't done in a long time. But there I was just letting go, and saying to myself it's okay to stop fighting if I have to. I didn't want to stop, but if I needed to, it was okay, and I knew things were out of my control.

Today and for the rest of my life, I think I will always remember this day as well as tomorrow. I will always remember the struggle I had to go through to get to where I am today. I will always remember

[176]

that I did it with pride and a smile on my face. The days that were difficult were the days that kept me going. I had many days where I could not sit through my full class because I didn't have enough oxygen.

It Was All a Dream

In July of 2007, I never thought that my dream of breathing would become a reality. I mean growing up you know what the outcome of living with CF is. You hope you don't become a death statistic. You hope that a cure will be found, and you can pursue your dreams.

Everyday that passed, and every year that passed, my dreams seemed to fade more and more. I honestly thought there was no hope at times and my dream was fading fast. I thought, what if my dreams never happen? What if one day I can no longer dream? What if...my dream becomes a nightmare I would never bare?

On July 9, I had new dreams once I got my call for lungs. I had a dream that I would come out of surgery perfect. I had a dream that I was breathing for the first time. I had a dream that for the first time in my life CF was going to be a small part of me, and I was no longer going to be a part of CF. I was able to dream that I can for once take in a deep breath and not cough or feel the tightness in my chest. For the first time, I felt the way I should have felt 25 years before that day.

In the last three years my dreams have shifted, changed, or have been accomplished. My dream of marriage can get checked off the list, along with my dream of finishing my Associates of Arts Degree in Fashion Merchandising. I have a new list of dreams. I can spend hours thinking about them because honestly, three years ago I didn't think it was possible to sit here today and write this story.

I now dream of, becoming a Nurse Practitioner. I dream of being a great wife. I dream of living a longer life than expected. I dream of taking long walks in the afternoon with James when we are old. I dream of seeing the world. I dream of enjoying every single breath I can take until the day I can no longer dream. I dream of one day their will be a cure for Cystic Fibrosis. I dream of running next to my friends Mike, Joy, Sandy, and Cindy in the "ING Miami Marathon" a half marathon one day (ING Direct, the bank group). I dream of touching the lives of my patients. I dream of being an example to other CF patients who feel they can no longer dream and have lost hope. I dream where I can leave this Earth, one day knowing that I touched one life. At present, I now dream of the day, when I will get a new kidney from my husband James.

I am a true believer that no one can take our dreams away from us. I believe that we are the only cause of our dreams not being fulfilled. I don't know about you, but every time I dream, it gives me more reasons to pursue my dreams. My whole life before transplant I dreamed of breathing. Now that I finally have my lungs, I am living that dream and don't want to wake up from it.

Elizabeth Kellner, 29
Coral Gables, Florida
Cystic Fibrosis
Double Lung Transplant, July 9, 2007
Jackson Memorial Hospital University of Miami School of Medicine, Miami, Florida

The Mind is a Powerful Tool
By Kristina Kelso

On a dreary and bleak January night in 2006, as I was sitting on my stiff and uncomfortable hospital bed, I was given some seemingly devastating news. I was told that I was dying because my lungs were failing and I needed a double lung transplant in order to survive.

I have Cystic Fibrosis (CF), a genetic disease that can damage the respiratory system, digestive tract and reproductive system. I was a very healthy child and never had any illnesses to speak of, but I mysteriously started getting chronic lung infections in high school. The doctors had a hard time diagnosing me because I mainly displayed problems with my respiratory system. After years of testing different medications and visiting new doctors, my illness was eventually labeled as a variant of CF.

Being sick frequently as a teenager made it pretty hard to accept and deal with. I became rebellious and didn't want anyone to know that I had the illness. I just wanted to be treated like a normal kid. Relying on my parents, I counted on them to get me the treatments and care I needed. I tried to hide my illness as much as possible.

After I married, I depended on my husband for help. Being an amazing caregiver, he became my 'parent' in many ways while helping me deal with countless infections and hospitalizations. We struggled together through many rough days; yet, I always seemed to bounce back.

I was 37-years-old when I was told the news that I needed a lung transplant. My doctors came into my hospital room and were not exactly gentle in their approach. It was cut and dry, and laced with despair. After they left, I felt as though I was just given a death sentence. I went through all the stages of dealing with death. I couldn't believe this was happening to me. Would I actually get a transplant? I loved my lungs; they were, after all, mine. For a few days after I was discharged from the hospital I couldn't think straight. I thought that maybe I would be okay and that I didn't really need a transplant. Yet, I was very sick and needed to accept the reality of it all. I knew that this time in the hospital was different because I was put on oxygen and had to go home with an oxygen tank. I was told that, with only 15% lung function, I would need to use it for the rest of my life, or until after transplant, *if* I decided to have surgery.

Being on oxygen was a very hard thing to get used to. I knew that I didn't want to be on it forever. I was very self-conscious in public and had to get use to stares and even questions from strangers about why I needed to be on it. The time had come to decide... life or death?

The answer was obvious. I was going to 'Fight like Hell' to live. Looking at my two beautiful children and loving husband, I thought about the wonderful future I could look forward to with them. I hated the idea of me missing out on so much. I was already missing a lot from being so sick. The next eleven months were spent going through series after series of tests and preparations in order to be put on the lung transplant list. The ironic thing about being placed on the transplant list is that you have to be sick enough to need the lungs but healthy enough to survive the surgery. Being sick enough was easy. Getting in shape for the surgery was a different story.

Physically preparing for such an intensive and invasive procedure was at times, excruciating but also unbelievably empowering. My body and mind were tested in ways I never thought were possible. I had to be strong emotionally and physically. Despite the doctor's grim outlook and the fact that they gave me only a few weeks to live before I was activated in December of 2006, I knew that I had to believe in myself. I knew that my mind played a huge part in my survival… as much as my body. In order to survive and heal, my spirituality, my positive attitude, my will and my desire to live had to be very strong. Eventually I made peace with the idea of getting new lungs and was actually excited for surgery. My husband and kids were too. My husband could get his wife back and my children could get their mommy back.

Many remarkable things happened during the eleven months waiting to be activated. I grew more in those eleven months than I had in my lifetime. I took nothing for granted, began to see so much more beauty around me…in nature and in simple things. During a month long stay in the hospital just before transplant; my husband wheeled me outside for some fresh air. Almost four weeks had passed since I had seen the sun or been outside. My hospital room faced a wall!!! This new awareness may only come to those who experience a life-changing event. It was October and the leaves were gently falling to the ground and the sun was filtering through the trees. The breathtaking scene reminded me of a Monet painting. I experienced the most amazing feeling as the sun hit my face. It was as though a miracle was happening right then. Tears rolled down my face and I smiled at my husband. We both knew how significant that moment was. I wondered how all the other people around seemed to miss it. Were they too busy to notice the splendor of the scene? I wondered why I didn't see it until now… the beauty all around. This was an eye-opener.

Before transplant, I was in the hospital for over a month and lost 20 precious pounds. I *almost* felt defeated. It was a struggle just to sit up, but I really wanted to live, thrive and prove to the doctors that I could do it… just like I did when I delivered two beautiful, healthy babies years before. I knew in my heart that I could live, survive surgery and live a full life.

I imagined myself on a beach without an oxygen (O2) tank… running, playing, laughing and breathing… with my new, healthy lungs. I couldn't wait to start my second life with them. I did find myself worrying about the donor though. They would have to die for me to live. That fact was hard to accept. I came to realize though, that they would not die because of me, they would die even without me. Yet, I would live because of them. They were caring enough to think of someone else by becoming an organ donor. I felt that it was my responsibility to try to live my life to its fullest in appreciation of them.

On December 23rd 2006, I finally got THE CALL!! Only nine days after I was activated! All I could think about was the donor and their family. I cried, said a prayer and tried to re-gain composure as we headed to the hospital. I called my brother, my parents, and a few close friends after the nurse told me that the lungs were a perfect fit for me. I remember looking at my husband and thinking what a miracle this all was. My kids joined me in my bed as I was wheeled down to surgery. It was a ride of a lifetime. I was so happy and proud of myself for being able to get to that point.

The very next morning I was walking the hospital intensive care unit (ICU) halls with chest tubes, catheters, and IV's… but NO oxygen!! I was ecstatic! Nine days later I was out of the hospital and back to rehab where I was to spend several weeks gaining strength to start my new life. I surprised everyone except my husband and kids with my swift recovery. I was so excited to start living again that I could barely contain myself. I feel so fortunate that things went so smoothly. Preparation and patience was key to my recovery. Before and after surgery, I tried to stay out of bed, walk as much as possible on the clinic treadmill, eat healthy and follow doctor's orders. Planning fun and exciting things to do in the future also had a huge impact on how I handled the transplant experience.

It has been three and a half years now since my transplant and I feel so blessed. LIFE is amazing. I look at it as an opportunity to experience new things, spend time with those I love and also share my story...with those who are sick and those who are well. I hope my story inspires people to see the good in LIFE and not focus on the bad. The mind is a powerful tool. Believing in yourself can change your life! I see every day as a gift and I am forever thankful to my donor for giving me a second chance. What a miracle it is!

The best gift one can give is the gift of life.

Kristina Kelso, 43
Boca Raton, Louisiana
Cystic Fibrosis
Double Lung Transplant, December 23, 2006
Duke University Hospital, Durham, North Carolina

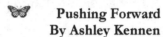

Pushing Forward
By Ashley Kennen

Growing up with Cystic Fibrosis was not necessarily what a person would want, but in my journey I've been blessed to go through it with tremendous support and have been able to live a fairly normal life. At 26-years-old, I can say I've accomplished a lot; I've earned a college degree, have an amazing husband and family, and I'm a homeowner. But the thing I'm most proud of is surviving a double lung transplant.

It took six months for my insurance to kick in, delaying my being listed. The hospital needed to know they would be paid, but we didn't have it. We had several fundraisers to raise the deposit on the transplant, family and friends donated, everyone dug deep. Prayers were said, money was raised, but oxygen was rapidly disappearing. My fear of not getting listed in time was growing stronger every day. Two days after our first fundraiser, I got the call that I qualified to be listed, but I was told it may take up to a year to get new lungs. I didn't know if I had it in me, but I was going to fight.

The day before Father's Day and only five weeks and six days after being listed, I got the call that my new lungs were waiting on me. When I got to the hospital and through all the pre-op, I did not know if these lungs were a match, so I tried to remain calm. Waiting the three hours for the signal the transplant was a 'go", seemed longer than the months I had to wait to get listed. I was not ready to be let down, I felt this was my chance to breathe - it was now or never. The lungs were perfect!

Waking up two days later with tubes connected to me everywhere, sore, and a little confused, I saw my husband and father standing over me. Smiling. I remember telling my Father that I was sorry I

[180]

slept through Father's Day. And apologizing to my Mother that I hadn't gotten her a birthday gift yet, since her birthday was the next week. Both told me I was their gift, and to watch me breathe was better than anything that could be bought in a store.

They encouraged me to get up and get moving, since exercise has been known to speed recovery. So I did. I was pedaling the first day I was awake, and walking halls the second day. I had my entire family with me the whole time, like a private cheerleading squad. Those moments that I wanted to give in, I just had to look at them and know they are why I needed to keep going. I learned how special breathing was for my family, my donor's family, and me. I had to keep setting goals and beating them.

Today, four months post transplant I have already done more than I could have even thought of. I've overcome some fears, blew up an inner tube, jogged, rode my bike for miles, and even signed up for a 5K. The life that I always wished I could have has now become a reality thanks to my donor. Every day I wake up pushing forward because of them. Besides, if it wasn't for them who knows if I'd get the chance to see tomorrow?

Ashley Kennen, 26
Lessburg, Florida
Cystic Fibrosis
Double Lung Transplant, June 16, 2010
Tampa General Hospital, Tampa, Florida

Breathe Me
By Stephanie Keustermans

I was born healthy, but soon something went amiss. At age three I got an adenovirus that began to eradicate my alveoli (air-sac) in my lungs one-for-one. Since that time, I was in a wheelchair and was on permanent oxygen. The sickness evolved so quickly that at seven years old; I could be compared with someone in the final stages of cystic fibrosis. We were told then that I urgently needed a double lung transplant. Unfortunately, Belgium had just started to perform lung transplants and nobody would risk the operation on a child. At that time, we decided against a lung transplant. At the age of 18 I was ready. Seven months on the waiting list, my phone call came.

No less than thirteen hours later, the transplantation became a reality and I was brought to intensive care. A month later I went home and could begin my new life. I could finally live instead of survive, dreams came true. I got my Art degree and could further study to become a teacher. A big dream comes true. Everything went fine. I could walk independently again and enjoyed a life where breathing finally became ordinary.

A year-and-a-half after my double lung transplant something happened. I was always tired and lethargic. Diagnosed with chronic rejection, the doctors only solution was re-transplantation. Within two minutes I accepted the proposal without a moment's doubt. All I wanted was to breathe. Unfortunately, the forecast wasn't that sunny, there were but three re-transplants in Belgium performed, and none had successfully survived.

Finally, on a Sunday morning, when everyone thought that the time had come too late, a donor was found. The doctors said I'd already lost since I was so weak and that there was only one thing I could do, WIN!

I have to say it was difficult to give up my first donor lungs; they were the greatest gift ever. Once at home the heavy rehabilitation began anew; learn to walk and use my hands, learn to sit. In a short time I had to learn everything all over again.

As of 2010, it's seven years later and I'm enjoying the fullest life with the air from my donors. Since my second transplant, I've been doing sports at the top level. I play badminton, table tennis and tennis. Annually, I take part in the "Transplant Games" and from six entries; I've earned twenty-five medals, all dedicated to my beautiful donors. Without them, I would never have been inspired to make it. I am so thankful. With each major step in my life, I think of those who have saved my life, those who were so brave to have made this decision.

Stephanie Keustermans, 28
Leuven Vlaams Brabant, Belgium
Bronchiolitis Obliterans – Caused by Adenovirus
Double Lung Transplant, October 21, 2001
Re-Transplant, Double Lung Transplant, October 19, 2003
University Hospital Gasthuisberg, Leuven, Belgium

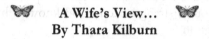

A Wife's View...
By Thara Kilburn

We met when we were kids. Our mother's were best friends. My husband Jason and I were married in 1998. I always knew he had Cystic Fibrosis (CF) and that once a year he went into the hospital for a "cleaning". Besides physiotherapy and inhalation meds four times a day, CF did not have a big impact on our lives.

Jason went in for a "cleaning", and this time his oxygen dropped and did not come back up. Oxygen tubes then became the norm in our home along with a Bi-level Positive Airway Pressure Machine (BiPAP). We use to call it the "Hannibal Lector Mask". Over the next several months the oxygen (O2) went up and his condition worsened. We were then told that his only option for survival was a double lung transplant. He was currently on eight liters of oxygen at rest. I was dumbfounded. A year earlier he was playing ball, golfing, and bowling. How could he have declined so fast? We did all the cleanings and meds and physiotherapy he was supposed to do. In the past few years prior we had bought a house and adopted a beautiful little girl. Life was going great.

Jason was listed 2008. We found out he was listed on the way to the hall, as it was our tenth wedding anniversary and we were renewing our vows. The term, "For better or for worse, in sickness and in health", took a very different meaning for us that day. We could barely say it through tears.

The wait was only nine months but seemed like forever. It was a long time to ponder whether lungs would become available in time for my husband. I had to think positively for him and our daughter but also figure out what I was going to do if it did not work out. It was a dark time for us.

My husband was in St. Michael's Hospital on 15 liters of oxygen at rest by mask now because the nasal prongs were no longer enough. The doctor came in and told us that he was being put on the critical list that day. Jason and I knew that list was for end stage of life.

Thankfully three days later he got "the call". The day before "the call" our daughter Jesslyn and I had been with Jason the entire day before to have a get-well party in his room. We were trying to spend as much time as possible with him. Jase and I had been told that he would not be leaving the hospital if he did not get a transplant. It was so hard to watch my husband decline so fast and feel so helpless. He was transferred to Toronto General Hospital, Toronto, Canada.

Jason did all the medicine and blood work while getting ready for transplant. The doctor came in about noon and told us there was something wrong with the lungs. Months before we had signed up for a study. Toronto General was taking undonateable lungs and putting them in a dome on a ventilator and healing them. It was called the Perfusion Study. Our surgeon was going to try this before he deemed it a false alarm. After twenty long hours of waiting the surgeon came to us, (now a group of over twenty friends and family); the transplant was 'a go'. Jase was wheeled down to surgery April 5th.

His surgery lasted twenty-four hours. There were some complications the most serious being how weak he was. At this point I found strength from God knows where, to keep on and so did my husband. There was no other option.

Jason is now twenty months post transplant. Jason will turn 38 this year. I now help him with home dialysis. A kidney transplant is now needed.

We now live a better than normal life. We are thankful for every minute of every day, every memory, and every plan for our future. This past summer we celebrated our twelfth anniversary and our daughter's fifth adoption anniversary....together!!!

To Jason's donor and family, "Our life would not be possible without you. We hope your father/husband is looking down on us proud. Thank you."

To my husband, "I am so proud of how hard you fought and how far you have come. I love you very much."

Anything is possible when you NEVER GIVE UP.

Thara Kilburn, Wife of Jason Kilburn
Jason Kilburn, 38
Oshawa, Ontario, Canada
Jason, Cystic Fibrosis
Jason, Ex Vivo - Double Lung Transplant, April 5, 2009
Toronto General Hospital, Toronto, Canada

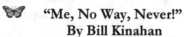

"Me, No Way, Never!"
By Bill Kinahan

I was transplanted on October 27, 2009 and my new life began.

Prior to transplant I was on 24 hours a day (24/7), oxygen for almost 12 years. Each year my pulmonary function tests continued to drop until my beautiful wife and partner Betty, along with my son Bill, investigated a lung transplant. My reaction was, **"ME, NO WAY, Never!"** But they continued the pursuit. Betty scheduled a lunch meeting with a post transplant patient and fittingly his name was, " Angel". This gentleman talked about quality of life, how mine was going downhill, and having a transplant my quality of life would rapidly improve.

I knew the risks involved and that there are no guarantees as to longevity, but I will tell you the quality of my life for the past six months has been truly amazing.

Here I will include a story that was written for a newsletter in February of this year: "Hello to all my new friends. I just want to pass along some good news for those of you who are waiting or contemplating a transplant. Also, those of you who had a transplant and know first hand the feelings of joy that we share in common. This week my son and his wife came from Connecticut to spend a week with my wife and me. This is the first time in a year that I have been well enough to have them here. It is also the first time that I have ever been able to lift either of my grandchildren, and give them big hugs. Today we spent the entire day at Busch Gardens in Tampa, Florida. We walked the entire park, climbed hills and stairs, went on some minor rides and in general I was able to not only enjoy them, but also join them in this special place. I never in my wildest dreams thought this day would ever come. So you can see why I wanted to share this special occasion with all of my new friends and to pray that you all may experience this pleasure in your new transplanted lives."

I recently completed a 5K walk in 45 minutes, when six months ago I couldn't walk to the end of my driveway. I may play golf next week the first time in a long, long, time. There are a lot of people to thank and the best way I can do that is to challenge myself to do the best I can in everything I do. I am very active on transplant web sites and some times, long-winded, but I attempt to be helpful and compassionate. I sent a note to all my friends and Facebook friends asking them to sign up to be a donor because the only person I cannot thank personally is my donor. She is in a better place and I pray for her every night.

Today May 26th, I played nine holes of golf and finished with a very good score. In addition to how well I played, I was pain free.

This being 'National Day of Prayer' I have every reason to Thank God for my new life.

Bill Kinahan, 69
Springhill, Florida
Emphysema
Double Lung Transplant, October 27, 2009
Tampa General Hospital, Tampa, Florida

🦋 New Lung Brings New Appreciations 🦋
By Stephen Knipstein

When I first considered contributing to the new edition of "Taking Flight", I pretty much thought that my submission would be a straightforward account of how great I have felt since my transplant, on January 19, 2010. It was wonderful to be free of the cannula feeding oxygen to me, which had been my constant companion for two years! How nice it was to be able to decide at the last minute to go away for the weekend, and not have to worry about arranging for oxygen at our destination. Or to just be able to not have to keep checking a watch to see how much time I had left on my oxygen tank whenever we went out somewhere.

But then, something happened which profoundly changed the way I looked at the blessings that my transplant brought to me. Appropriately, it was on Father's Day that my son called to tell me that I was going to become a grandfather, for the first time! He told me that the baby is due on Valentine's Day, 2011. I was thrilled, and I told him so. Later, after the news had sunk in, I realized that not only had the transplant given me a new lease on life, but also it had now given me the opportunity to see my first grandchild! This blessing was driven home recently, when I observed the third anniversary of my being diagnosed with Idiopathic Pulmonary Fibrosis (IPF). All of the literature I had read on IPF had stated that the average life expectancy, once diagnosed with IPF was 2-3 years. So, without having received my transplant, the odds are I might not have had the opportunity to live to see my grandchild.

Of course that blessing, while the most important, was by no means the only one. I have been truly blessed in so many ways throughout this whole process. Fortunately, I live close to Boston, Massachusetts, which has several of the most renowned hospitals in the world. The transplant clinic at Brigham and Women's Hospital, where I had my transplant, is an incredible place. Not only do they have a world class staff of doctors, but the nurses on the 11th floor, where the transplant patients are cared for, are also world class, especially when it comes to truly caring about their patients. Everyone worked together seamlessly to provide me with the best of care, and making for a quick recovery – I was able to go home just 12 days post-transplant.

Once a few minor glitches were addressed, my rehab has been very rewarding. Right from the beginning, I had a goal to work toward. Some people may have thought it was a bit aggressive, but ever since the day I became a candidate for lung transplant, I had set the goal of playing in my college's alumni soccer game again. I had played and coached soccer almost all of my life and the last time I had played in the alumni game was the very same week I was diagnosed with IPF. The game was scheduled for September 25th, 2010, so I had nine months to see if I could attain my goal. Thanks to my wonderful team at Brigham and Women's and the awesome folks at the Pulmonary Rehab Department at Concord Hospital, Concord, New Hampshire, as the "game day" approached; it actually looked like I could make it.

The day of the game was a gorgeous fall day; in fact it was a bit warmer than usual. Old memories came flooding back as I sat on the bench, lacing up my soccer shoes. This was the very same field that I have spent so many happy hours on, every fall from 1974-1980, either as a player or coach. It felt really great to take the field for the opening kickoff. I was by far the oldest alumnae playing in the game, but that didn't bother me – I may have been much older, and in a much poorer state of fitness than the others, but that didn't matter to me. I was once again a Plymouth State soccer player! So what if I only played a few minutes...the important thing is that I played at all! And for that I have to thank so many people – my all important lung donor, my transplant team, and all the nurses and rehab specialists.

As Thanksgiving Day, 2010, approached, I began developing increased shortness of breath again. After a checkup and vascular scan at Brigham and Women's, it was found that I had a blood clot in my upper right lung. This meant some intravenous blood thinners, and spending Thanksgiving with my "transplant family" – in the company of the people and at the place where I was given so much to be truly thankful for this year!

But just as importantly, perhaps even more so, I am most thankful for my wife MaryAnne, whose constant care and encouragement (not to mention the nights spent sleeping in my hospital room) were even more important to my recovery than any of the many medications I have to take. The entire transplant experience has reinforced my belief that family should be treasured above all else!

Stephen Knipstein, 59
Plymouth, New Hampshire
Idiopathic Pulmonary Fibrosis
Single Lung Transplant, January 19, 2010
Brigham and Women's Hospital, Boston, Massachusetts

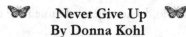

Never Give Up
By Donna Kohl

My name is Donna Kohl. I had a heart/lung transplant on September 26, 2000, at Barnes-Jewish Hospital in St. Louis, Missouri. I was diagnosed with Ventricular Septal Defect (VSD)/ with Eisenmenger Syndrome. My disease was diagnosed at six months of age at Children's Hospital in St. Louis, Missouri.

When being listed I chose to double list; at Barnes-Jewish and at University Medical Center, University of Arizona, Tucson, Arizona. During the wait, I continued to work and tried to maintain a so-called normal life.

I received a call from my transplant coordinator in St. Louis wanting to know if I was ready for my transplant. It was a long 40-minute drive to the hospital. I had contacted my husband and he left work and went to the hospital, where we all met. By the end of the night my whole family had made it to the hospital, along with some friends. Not really knowing what was going to happen, lots of emotions going through everyone's head and many emotions were going through everyone's head and lots of prayers were being said during this time.

When I awoke on September 26th, my body was ravished with lots of issues from the surgery, which happens with some surgeries, so nothing was abnormal. I was on my feet the next day walking behind a wheel chair, not fast but moving nonetheless.

Well, I never thought it would happen but I was eventually put into a step down room out of ICU. What a great day that was. My girlfriend came by and colored my hair, yes, right in the hospital room. I went back to work five months to the day after my transplant and I have never looked back.

My life with my new heart and lungs has been a great experience; I speak on organ donation and what it has done for my life. My husband and I also go on vacation each year to Cabo San Lucas, Mexico to celebrate the gift of life that I have been given. This year we were also fortunate to travel to Italy, which is something that I have always want to do, and because of my donor family, I was able to achieve this goal.

I thank my donor family each and every day for the gift that they have given to me, and very thankful that there are families that can go above their feelings and loss, and see that their loved one can help someone else, that would not have life without their gifts.

Donna Kohl, 49
DeSoto, Missouri
Ventricular Septal Defect (VSD)/with Eisenmenger Syndrome
Heart/Double Lung Transplant, September 26, 2000
Barnes-Jewish Hospital, St. Louis, Missouri

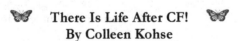

There Is Life After CF!
By Colleen Kohse

On October 22nd 1988, at 29-years-old, I had a heart-double lung transplant in Middlesex, England. There is life after Cystic Fibrosis!

Lung transplants were so rare then; we knew absolutely nothing and had just recently heard they were even possible. A few years before, I asked my brother, a doctor, if he thought lungs could ever be transplanted, he said, "No, they are just too fragile." When my doctor, in Vancouver, Canada said, "You need a transplant." I thought he was mad! I was assessed and sent to England, the centre with the best survival rate. Toronto had recently started performing double-lung transplants, but was not having as much success. My Cystic Fibrosis (CF) team knew I would not survive until a surgeon was trained in British Columbia (B.C.). I also didn't really want to be the very 1st candidate for practice!

I was totally terrified, but had great support from family, medical staff and friends. I was given a heart-double lung transplant because, at the time, they felt it was the best technique to preserve the lungs. My strong heart went to a 29-year-old man (we got to know him after transplant), who did really well too and went home to Greece, where he lived for 17 more years. Our surgeon, Professor Sir Magdi Yacoub, said he was glad I didn't know anything about the procedure, or I probably would have wanted to assist! My tendency to control everything must be really noticeable! Is that too a CF genetic trait?

Wow, what a feeling! To require 24-hour oxygen, suffer horrendous high-carbon dioxide (CO2) headaches, extreme shortness of breath, constant infections, coughing, reflux, etc. etc. (i.e.: end stage CF), then in a relatively short time, to feel better then I had ever known. I gradually got stronger and stronger, maybe not as energetic as the average healthy person, but incredibly good compared to life with CF lungs. I did very well post transplant and spent my recuperation period roaming London and the English countryside. Not too shabby indeed! Then I returned home to my old life, what a letdown! Just kidding. But just because you have a new lease, it doesn't instantly give you a new life!

After my transplant, I said, "I'm never going to die, I'll just keep replacing parts, ha ha!" Seven years later I developed kidney failure and didn't think it was so funny. I spent four years on dialysis, which was not a picnic, but at least there is life-preserving treatment for end stage kidney disease. I had a kidney transplant in 2000. It's a breeze compared to the heart-lung transplant.

So now my health remains good, and most importantly, my lung function is really good. Considering I don't do any regular exercise (this will get me in trouble!), it's rather amazing. I do keep active and usually get out and about daily. I also love traveling and try to get away (from my family), as much as possible! I've been very fortunate with my new organs, but I also try to maintain a healthy lifestyle. It's essential to have good relations with transplant clinic staff, take meds as prescribed, don't alter doses without permission, have monthly blood work, get all necessary tests done and attend clinic as directed (currently only every six months!). I try to get as much sleep as possible, don't drink too much alcohol or indulge in other vices that may adversely impact my health. In other words: I am a responsible adult. I'm not insinuating anything, but you know who you are, CF people, because I am one of you too! This doesn't guarantee success, but it certainly lessens the risk of failure.

I am not on any special diet and eat whatever I enjoy, but, oh, it is so much easier to gain weight! I have gained about 15 kg since my kidney transplant and I am getting fatter. How strange for a person with CF. I'm thinking, what is this? How do I get rid of it? Diet, you say, what does that mean!? On a recent trip, my friend noticed I was eating bacon most mornings, she commented that it's not very good for my heart. I just shrugged. Then she said, "Oh, why should I care it's not my heart." I quipped, "Yeah, well it's not my heart either!"

It has now been 22 years since my heart-lung and 10 years since my kidney transplant. There were many small hurdles along the way, but how amazing to still breathe deeply after all these years, although sometimes it feels like just yesterday. When I had my 50th birthday it was great; all my girlfriends were complaining about their age, but I was just smiling. I like the saying, "In life, as in cards, there are no winning hands or losing hands, it's how you play the hand you're dealt. Of course, a little luck is good too!"

Colleen Kohse, 51
Vancouver, British Columbia, Canada
Cystic Fibrosis
Heart/Double Lung Transplant, October 22, 1988
Harefield Hospital, Middlesex, England
Kidney Transplant, November 5, 2000
Vancouver General Hospital, Vancouver, British Columbia, Canada

Justin Masters - A Purposeful Life
By Noreen Labelle

"Your son has cystic fibrosis," the doctor said to me.

I had never heard of this disease before, and had no idea what a life-changing ordeal was about to face us. I say us, because it effected our whole family. So began the daily medications, chest physiotherapy, making sure he ate well and took his enzymes, and clinic visits. Justin was a healthy baby, toddler and youngster. It was just his digestive system that cystic fibrosis seemed to be taking a hold of; his lungs would get worse with age.

Justin was very active as a child. He loved to skateboard, right up into his late teens. He joined karate and kung fu. The gym became a very big part of his life, especially when he saw the benefits to his body and health. Justin graduated high school, and went to college, but by this time in his life, cystic fibrosis had begun to show its terrible ugly side. Justin worked various jobs, but would have to quit due to his health. Hospitalizations became more frequent and he wasn't able to maintain his health as before. This would really discourage Justin, but he was a fighter and would bounce back and try again.

At the age of 22, Justin started to use drugs. This became his downfall, not only to him as a person, but also as a person with cystic fibrosis. "I'm so sick of being sick" he said, "I need something to keep me going, so I'm not tired all the time, and so I can function as a normal person". He was addicted to many types of drugs. We tried as a family to help him with his addictions, but to no avail...he wasn't ready. By this time and many years before, I had been praying for Justin to make a change in his life. After so many hospitalizations and getting sicker from both drugs and his cystic fibrosis, Justin had to make a decision...drugs and dying or life and living...he chose life.

Justin is truly an amazing son, brother and friend. No re-habilitation would take Justin because he was so sick with his cystic fibrosis, so he got clean and sober with God's help. He had many cravings, but he fought hard. Justin knew that the Lord had given him a second chance in life, and he wanted to live his life for the Lord and for all to see.

Justin was on oxygen 24 hours a day (24/7) for the last year and half. He could not walk very far and became wheel chair bound. That didn't stop him from going out and doing activities. Justin did a feature newspaper article about his life with cystic fibrosis and also made a DVD for the cystic fibrosis gala in Ottawa. This DVD is also a teaching tool to help other cystic fibrosis people who also have battle with addictions.

The doctors told Justin, if you ever want a lung transplant, you have to make changes in your life, he did. We were now waiting for testing in Toronto for getting listed for lung transplant. These tests would determine if he was a candidate for transplant. It was a long and grueling week for him physically. At the end of each day, he would high-five me, and say, "We did it mom, one day done and four more to go". By the end of the week Justin was completely exhausted physically and mentally, but he was determined to finish the week of testing.

Three days after we returned home from Toronto, Justin collapsed. He was air lifted to Ottawa and put on a respirator. He was in critical condition, and it was an hour-by-hour wait to see his outcome. A Novalung (a treatment for lung failure with innovative artificial lungs that "breathe" outside the patients body) was inserted because his carbon dioxide levels were dangerously high. Toronto Hospital called and accepted him immediately on the transplant list. He was listed top priority in the Toronto area. Justin was then air lifted to Toronto by their excellent transplant team.

In Toronto, his condition worsened as the days went by. We waited and waited for lungs to appear...for three and half weeks we waited and prayed, and prayed. I have never seen time go by so slowly as your loved one is laying there, waiting for basically someone to die, so he can live. My husband and I tried to find the humor in this hard and difficult situation. We were looking at people and saying, "What's your blood type" or "Oh, you look about the right size. Come here for a minute", or even watching the news and seeing accidents and thinking, maybe these might be his lungs. Lungs arrived three times that we know of, but not good matches for Justin. Justin was put on an ECMO (Extracorporeal Membrane Oxygenation) machine, which is the last resort the doctors said, and each day brought complications.

Finally, on June 17, 2010...his lungs arrived. We were thankful to the donor family. All went well with his transplant, no complications during surgery at all. But, now his organs were shutting down, and the possibility of brain damage. The three and half weeks Justin was in the hospital before he got his new lungs, he was heavily sedated, and had pain medications, but we knew he could hear us. We were constantly by his side from morning until night to talk to him, sing, pray, cry and just to let him know how loved he was by family and friends. Justin was very big on family. In his eyes, we were his whole world, but he was the world to us. He loved to make people laugh with his jokes and stories. Justin liked to look at the bright side of things in life and to love each day, and not to take one day for granted.

In the end, the Lord took Justin home on June 21, 2010. Justin has the perfect lungs now, and can do all the things he has dreamed of doing. No cystic fibrosis in his way now.

"Justin you are missed so much and loved so dearly by your sisters: Justine, Cayla, Michelle, Rachel and brother Daniel, Mom and Dad." Thanks so much for the best of care that Justin received at the

Ottawa and Toronto General Hospitals. Please sign your donor cards today...you never know what tomorrow will hold!

Noreen Labelle Mother of, Justin Masters
Hawkesbury, Ontario, Canada
Justin, Cystic Fibrosis
Justin, Double Lung Transplant, June 17, 2010
Date of Passing: June 21, 2010
Toronto General Hospital, Toronto, Canada
"Forever 26"

 Part 2: Thanksgiving Miracle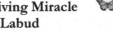
By Debbie Labud

I wrote my story for the 1st Taking Flight in 2002. Since then, my name has changed from Debbie Deloach to Debbie Labud; I was married in 2005, so life has ended up good! As I said in the previous book, I have Alpha-1 Antitrypsin Deficiency (Alpha-1); I was diagnosed in 1991.

My mother died when I was 15, after having suffered 13 years with Hodgkin's disease; she had to be a carrier of the trait Alpha-1. My father was tested and he was a carrier; that means he was an MZ. I inherited a bad gene from each parent; which made me a ZZ. I have two brothers, one was a carrier; he had the MZ gene. My oldest brother however, got a good gene from each parent; he is an MM. My daughter Amber is also a carrier. My father lived a very active life (he taught dancing; and had many awards in it). He passed away at the age of 91 in 2009.

In June of 1997, I started an Alpha-1 Support Group in the Gainesville, Florida area. My group was small, but being able to share has been a great support for me. Soon after forming this group, I was evaluated for a lung transplant. I went to Charlie's Corner at Shands Hospital at The University Of Florida, Gainesville, Florida where there was a support group "Second Wind" which I got involved with. They are a great group of people and have helped me feel comfortable about receiving a transplant. My caregivers were my boyfriend, and my grown children.

THE CALL:
Coming home from Thanksgiving dinner 2001, in Cedar Key, Florida I was beeped, after four years, four months, 22 days and three dry runs.

LIFE AFTER TRANSPLANT:
When I first came home from the hospital, it excited me just to walk to the mailbox or to take a walk down the street (what some people take for granted). I could now chase my two-year-old grandson. I had six grandsons at that time and a 14-year-old son at home; I could start enjoying my family. Less than two months after my transplant, I was riding my bike a mile a day. I was getting ready for the United States Transplant Games in Orlando, Florida June 2002. While I was waiting for my transplant my goals were to ride a bike in the Transplant Games and to walk with my kids and grandkids around Disney World without using an oxygen tank or a wheelchair. I did just that, I rode my bike in a 12-mile race seven months after my transplant in the 2002 Transplant Games in

Orlando. I came in last but I did finish the race. I also walked with my family for 12 hours around Disney World. Wow, what a new lease on life!

I have gone on a few bike rides with my husband and grandson in Florida; they were to benefit, American Lung Association. We did this ride with other Alphas (part of Team Alpha). My husband and I have gone to Massachusetts six times to join in with more of Team Alphas to do a three-day bike ride around Cape Cod, Massachusetts for the American Lung Association, yes, life has been amazing.

In 2004 my son and I flew to Minneapolis, Minnesota, for the United States Transplant Games. Again I did the bike race; I couldn't handle the hills, as a Floridian I am used to more flat land. I can say that thanks to my donor, I am able to attempt those hills!

2005 was a big year for me, due to my illness I hadn't worked in 10 years. I was hired as a Donor Service Technician with LifeSouth Community Blood Centers; now I am a Donor Recruiter. March 12th I married my boyfriend of 13 years; two days later my first granddaughter was born; she came a little early; so we had to hurry home from our honeymoon; but it was worth it. Again in 2005 my first great-grandson was born. Thank God for my new lung and my donor for being such a good match or I wouldn't be here to enjoy my family and my new additions!

2006 I was getting ready to leave for the Transplant Games in Louisville, Kentucky with my friend Karen Rodgers; she is a liver transplant recipient; when I received a call from Tampa. A woman from the organ procurement called and said that my donor's mom wanted to meet me. I have been writing letters for as long as they started letting me; it was such a rush to finally get this call. Off to the games we went, this time I did the 5K, singles in bowling and doubles in bowling with Karen as my partner. At the games I bought stuff to give to my donor's mom when we met!

Home from the games I had an e-mail from my donor's mom. We E-mailed each other and sent pictures; I now had a face and a name for my new lung. Christina was 29 and had an eight-year-old son. She also was an only child. That really made it hard; she lived in Crystal River, Florida and I lived in Gainesville; so in 2006 we met at Olive Garden for lunch in Ocala, Florida. My daughter Amber and a co-worker, Christine went with me. We enjoyed our meal and I brought gifts; we shared pictures. It just amazes me how much Christina reminded me of myself when I was that age. We still e-mail and keep in touch. I will always be thankful to Christina for having on her driver's license that she was an organ donor; or her mom wouldn't have donated her organs; she was too devastated by the loss of her daughter.

In 2008 I did my first half marathon. It was put on through my work and called 'Five Points of Life'; which are ways to share life through donation; such as blood, apheresis, bone marrow, and cord blood, organ and tissue donation. I walked it with my oldest daughter Michele; it was 13.5 miles. It was my birthday, so I carried a sign, on one side it said, "It is my birthday and I can walk if I want to", on the other side it read "Lung Transplant Recipient and Blood Donor"; the important thing is we finished 13.5 miles!

2008 off to the transplant games again. This time we were driving to Pittsburgh, Pennsylvania, with Karen Rodgers and her granddaughter Summer, and my grandson Jordan. Summer did the 5K with me and again I did singles bowling and doubles with my partner Karen. I recommend that everyone from donor families to recipients go for the experience of the Transplant Games; it is the best medicine!

2009, again I did the 'Five Points of Life' 1/2 Marathon; this time I did it with my husband Tony, my daughter Amber and my son-in-law Jared; again we finished (God is Good)!!!!

2010 I am going to Madison, Wisconsin for the United States Transplant Games; this time my husband Tony is flying with me. Tony will do the 5K with me; and again I am doing singles bowling and bowling doubles with Karen.

November 22, 2010 will be nine years for my transplant! I live to enjoy my husband Tony, my two daughters Michele, and Amber and Amber's husband Jared, my son Corry and his wife Stacey. I have six grandsons David, Steven, Joey, Kenny, Jordan and Caleb; and my granddaughter Kyrsten and great-grandson Gavin. I can say I am blessed!

Debbie Labud, 55
Micanopy, Florida
Alpha-1 Antitrypsin Deficiency
Single Lung Transplant, November 22, 2001
Shands Hospital at the University of Florida, Gainesville, Florida
Read Debbie's Lung Transplant Story in the 1st Edition of Taking Flight

 Whole New Life with New Lungs
By Gayle Lentz

I came into this world in early August. My first few years were tough, filled with tummy aches. The doctors tested me for various causes, and my first sweat test came up negative. I had frequent upper respiratory infections and was listed as "failure to thrive." When the next test came back positive for Cystic Fibrosis, (it was found that my original test was switched) they told my mom I wouldn't live past 16-years-old. They quickly rectified the situation with the other patient, but I fell through the cracks. I had a normal happy childhood; though always hungry.

As I got older I tried several new mechanisms to help loosen and strengthen my lungs. I got the usual amount of bullying and found a "protector" friend of sorts. Her name was Cathy. At 14, Cathy died in a car accident, but God must have known, because there was a new girl, Laura, at school right after Christmas break that I decided to take under my wing. She in return became my new "protector". She and I are best friends even today, though we are far apart in distance, I would do anything I could for her; and she the same for me.

At 18, the real trouble started. I planned to attend college but was late in starting due to an incident of hemoptysis (coughing up blood). In 1997 I was in a premarital seminar with my boyfriend Larry (now my husband), when I began coughing up blood. I was rushed to the emergency room. My dear doctor decided to put me the double lung transplant list in Buffalo, New York. Six months later, the lung transplant center closed, and my case was transferred to University of Pittsburgh Medical Center, Pittsburgh, Pennsylvania.

I seemed to stabilize for a while. I enrolled in a college in Rochester, New York and acquired a job in Rochester. Then I met Dr. Rob Horowitz and things stayed pretty much the same. During the summer of 2003 my husband Larry and I went to my 10-year high school reunion. I ended up coughing up blood once again. After that I continued to cough up various amounts of blood from a tablespoon to a liter. Landing back in the hospital for another episode, Dr. Horowitz came flying into intensive care unit (ICU) dressed in a black trench coat and said, "I've never been directive in your care, but you need a lung transplant!!" I then was activated at Pittsburgh for new lungs.

Two years to the day of transplant, I had no rejection. My lungs were doing well. I was happy with that, but still missing something…we found out on Valentine's Day what that something was. I took a pregnancy test and it came out very light, but positive. Larry and I were both shocked and ecstatic and a little scared, I think. The whole pregnancy I felt great. My lungs capacity actually went up.

Our little girl came into the world six weeks early at four pounds, 11 ounces. The first few months she sounded like a bleating lamb. I remember snuggling and cuddling her. I even nursed her for three months. Three and a half years later I have a precocious little girl who loves to learn, loves her veggies and is sometimes three going on 13. I have started going through chronic rejection, but hope to one day conquer it and have a sibling for my dear girl.

Gayle Lentz, 36
Spencerport, New York
Cystic Fibrosis
Double Lung Transplant, February 7, 2004
University of Pittsburgh Medical Center, Pittsburgh, Pennsylvania
Gayle had a Daughter, September 2006

 A Life Bigger Than My Own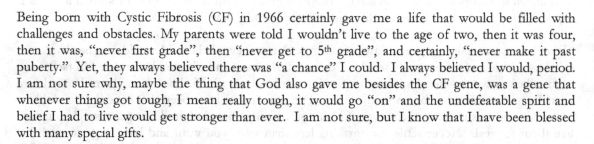
By Dottie Lessard

Being born with Cystic Fibrosis (CF) in 1966 certainly gave me a life that would be filled with challenges and obstacles. My parents were told I wouldn't live to the age of two, then it was four, then it was, "never first grade", then "never get to 5th grade", and certainly, "never make it past puberty." Yet, they always believed there was "a chance" I could. I always believed I would, period. I am not sure why, maybe the thing that God also gave me besides the CF gene, was a gene that whenever things got tough, I mean really tough, it would go "on" and the undefeatable spirit and belief I had to live would get stronger than ever. I am not sure, but I know that I have been blessed with many special gifts.

The gift of knowing what it is like to hurt so bad that you are not sure you can make it – but then you do. What a feeling of joy and pride that is. To see firsthand how precious life is and then get another day to live to appreciate the gift of deep breaths because you couldn't breathe deep at all. To know how important every piece of your body is for when a piece breaks down, the rest suffers. That makes you want to keep yourself healthy in a very real way - I feel lucky to understand that.

My disease and challenges have given me strength and knowledge I could never get anywhere else but from the experiences I have faced and lived through. It has all been worth it. I am a very blessed girl.

So when people ask me, so many times-especially in interviews, "Why have you never given up?" I simply tell them the truth, "I didn't know how" - because I don't. I cannot comprehend how to let my heart stop beating or to give the "okay" to stop breathing; it's not going to happen, ever. LIFE is too precious to treat that way and if you are still breathing, you are still living and that means you have the power to do all that is inside you to change how you will look at things and how you will fight for what you want. We must believe within ourselves first and foremost.

I'm human, and I have been scared, angry, and sad sometimes, but I never let it take control. I know I am not allowed that privilege. I always "turn that switch on" to the positive, the one thing that has a ray of HOPE that will keep me going to fight. Look for the positive in every situation because there is one and hold on tight to it for dear life, it will bring you through.

I learned to be the only Athlete I could be when I was little, play with the limitations I had - I found a way. I found a way to not give up hope when my CF started to control me - I fought back with exercise even if it was two minutes on a treadmill - I did it and it gave "me" the control. And when I saw there was a chance I could trade in these broken lungs that were too tired to work anymore I fought like heck to get my chance. And I did and have lived without restraints across my chest for 16 full years since my double lung transplant.

One thing I have learned and try to teach others in my career as a Life Coach is, "Life will not move over for you, you must move through it." Move. Move through life whatever way you can because you have to. You just do it because you are a fighter and because you want to live. It's kind of simple when you think about it like that. Take each day that comes, giving it your best, your absolute best, all you can, each and every day that arrives in whatever circumstance you are in.

You are all survivors and you all deserve a chance to thrive with deep breaths for a lifetime - this is my wish for you, and me. Live your life with Gratitude and you will always be fulfilled.

Never let anyone take your dreams away from you. No one ever believed I would ever be able to run or be an athlete and never mind me what I dreamed of most - an official Nike Athlete. In fact, some even talked over me when I spoke about it or even laughed. But I didn't hear them; I only heard what I was determined to be no matter what. For four years I have been that official Nike Athlete. Make your dreams real; live them even if it can only be in your mind until you get strong enough to live them for real. Never settle for anything less than what you want and little steps toward that create footprints to build upon. Never let anyone tell you, "you can't or you won't", because, "YOU CAN". And "You Must." If I have, you can.

As I celebrate my 44th birthday at the end of this year I am proud to live my life as if everything was new each day. My "numbers" may be considered old to some but my life truly, is not. I am young and determined to live a full life as a mother of the most beautiful six year old boy ever, as a proud athlete who will continue to remind the world to "never count anyone out", as a life coach and mentor to kids, young adults, and adults - anyone who wants to make their life better and do the work it takes to overcome. I will hold the hand of anyone who wants more for themselves and are willing to work for it. It is my honor to give back to others because the "gift" is mine.

I know I will always have obstacles to overcome in my life and that is why I do all I can do continue to create a strong foundation with my body through exercise, quality nutrition and a strong and healthy mindset. I am so proud to have been in the 1st edition of Taking Flight and now the 2nd. I am determined to break every statistic and barrier Cystic Fibrosis and Transplantation has put forth - for me, and those who walk beside me and also come after me. I want the same for each of you. May you all LIVE LIFE FULLY.

I have given myself a title: Mom, Athlete, Life Coach, and Very Lucky Girl.

I also have authored a book, <u>Seven Letters That Saved My Life.</u>

Dottie Lessard, 44
Haverhill, Massachusetts
Cystic Fibrosis
Double Lung Transplant, October 27, 1994
Massachusetts General Hospital, Boston, Massachusetts
Kidney Transplant, October 6, 2002
New England Medical Center, Boston, Massachusetts
Dottie Adopted a Son, Post Lung Transplant
Read Dottie's Lung Transplant Story in the 1st Edition of Taking Flight

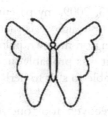

Breathtaking and Giving
By Angela Lewis

After enduring a frightening battle with my lawnmower in which it won, I decided it was time to see an allergist. That appointment in August of 2008 quickly escalated to a chest x-ray, then an immediate consultation with a pulmonologist. I just knew this had to be a lupus complication, because it always has been. After another couple scans and x-rays, the venerate Dr. Jim Curlee in Georgetown, Texas, took me back to his office where we spent two hours looking at results, doing online research, and drawing pictures of what "it looks like" and what "it should look like". He didn't normally deal with patients like me, but my condition – which was later diagnosed as Bronchiolitis Obliterans - caught his attention. The mention of lung transplant made me think he had lost his marbles. The insistence of wearing oxygen 24 hours a day (24/7) made me drive home in tears. Today, I can't thank him enough.

When I first went into the University Hospital San Antonio, San Antonio, Texas transplant clinic waiting room, I wanted to crawl inside myself and refused to admit I was like those other people. Little did I know I'd be the lady singing the praises of the angels behind the door. I met with those doctors and nurses who would later become my lifelines, listened to all kinds of frightening possibilities and freeing probabilities, and made the decision to begin the process not a moment too soon.

During my wait, I also rejoiced in marriage to a man who has the patience and understanding of a saint, and the work ethic of an army of one. I repeatedly gave Scott the opportunity to run away – leave with no guilt on his conscience – and I can honestly say that this was one time in my life I enjoyed hearing the word "NO". It has affirmed my faith that God does indeed have a hand here on earth, and that I am constantly surrounded by the priceless generosity and selfless capabilities of my dear family and friends.

The real call came on August 13, 2009, my parents' 47th anniversary. I was home in ten days and sleeping in my own bed. That first night was memorably peaceful – no concentrator rattling made me cry, waking up in the morning on my own pillow made me cry, swallowing pills without choking made me cry... then I realized it was probably the prednisone making me cry. Mom's 73rd birthday was fifteen days later and I was able to sing to her! Yes, that made me cry too.

The process from discovery to recovery took one year. I am still amazed by the blessed luck and skill involved in my transformation. Every time I sneeze or yawn, it makes me smile. When I complain about having to "get up" or "go do", I rejoice in not having to unwind myself from the oxygen tubing. Funny story: Upon returning home after transplant, my husband said, "Where are you? I can't find you anymore!"

I am not yet back to teaching, and am certainly not ready to even consider anything that may remotely jeopardize my new life. The risk of infection in a classroom is very great and may eventually become less of an issue as I move forward post-transplant. I am now six months out and still feeling like new.

My extended family that works at the University Hospital is made up of an incredibly diverse and talented bunch of loving people who tirelessly lend their lives to their transplant patients on a daily basis. There is no greater confidence than knowing your life-saving team is also a life-support system. I have also met and enjoyed the company of several pre- and post-transplant patients while spending my mornings there, and the stories are always the same: IT'S A MIRACLE. And that it is.

I have not had any contact with my donor family, but I hope that chance will come for me. Of the very little information I was given about her, I know she was 17 and quite possibly could have been one of my own classroom children. I have begun volunteering when I can, to promote organ donation registration, and will take on public speaking next. But it will always be difficult to fully describe the feeling of carrying a "Gift of Life", because it is the gift that is carrying me.

Angela Lewis, 38
Llano, Texas
Bronchiolitis Obliterans
Double Lung Transplant, August 13, 2009
University Hospital San Antonio, San Antonio, Texas

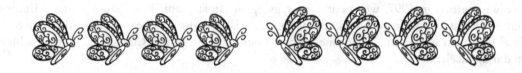

It Can Always Get Better
By Scot Longstaff

I'm 42-years-old, diagnosed with Cystic Fibrosis (CF) when I was three-years-old in 1971. At the same time, they tested my two-year-old sister, who was also diagnosed with CF. We had what I would consider the most common mutation of CF, that being the kind that affects both lungs and digestion. While at CF camp in Ontario, Canada when we were younger, we picked up the Cepacia bacteria.

Shortly before my sisters 16th birthday, she passed away from a serious exacerbation. As it happens, I was in the hospital room next to her when she died, as I was being treated for an exacerbation of my own. Needless to say, that was quite a traumatizing time for me. I listened to my sister suffer for days before the gasping finally stopped forever.

Unfortunately my health went progressively downhill as I went through puberty. By the time I was in my early 20's, I spent almost all day in bed and barely left the house anymore. It was then that I was placed on the lung transplant waiting list in early 1991.

On November 8th, 1991, I received a double lung transplant. I had approximately 32 chest tubes during this time and at one point the doctors told my parents that I would never be leaving the hospital. My prognosis was very poor.

Eventually I was able to overcome my complications. Almost a year later, I was on a solid path to recovery. I was actually healthy enough to take a part time job and join a sailing club in Toronto, Canada. It was at the sailing club that I met my future wife.

Before we married in 1997, we spent a year living in Amsterdam. Fortunately I am a European citizen as well as Canadian so I was able to get a social security number in Holland and access to medical treatment if needed. I had one exacerbation while there, but Ciprofloxacin Hydrochloride cleared it up nicely.

When we returned to Canada, we got married and bought a condominium. I obtained a full time job as a personal computer (PC) technician since my years spent in the house and in a body that wouldn't do what I wanted, had provided me with excellent PC skills; the computer was a way for me to escape my reality. We then went to an 'In-Vetro' clinic and were lucky enough to conceive a son.

Life has been wonderful since my transplant. I am now a senior systems administrator for a large insurance company. We built a cottage in 2004, and we've just bought our 3rd house this past summer. My son is nine-years-old now and the light of my life. I'm almost 19 years post transplant and my lungs are doing great. My kidneys are starting to show signs of extensive use of anti-rejection medication, but there is no immediate danger.

If you are looking for stories of inspiration or advice, I can honestly say that no matter how bad things seem, it can always get better. I was on my way out at one point, but was lucky enough to have been given a second chance. What I have done with that second chance is to try to live the life I was denied before the transplant. I couldn't be happier with the way things have worked out for me and hope there are others out there that can experience the same joy I feel on a daily basis.

Scot Longstaff, 42
Toronto, Ontario, Canada
Cystic Fibrosis
Double Lung Transplant, November 8, 1991
Toronto General Hospital, Toronto, Canada

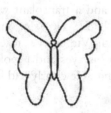

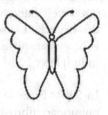

We All Won the Race
By Doris Lowenthal

My name is Doris Lowenthal from Severn, Maryland. I am married to the most wonderful man on the planet, Barry. We have two highly devoted, beautiful four legged children, Indy and Speedway. I stand before you today after receiving the most precious gift of all, the "Gift of Life", a lung transplant from an unknown donor. As a transplant recipient, we have walked a path with our illness behind us, and the hope of a long life due to transplantation in front of us. This path has been paved by those transplanted ahead of us and all the knowledge gained from their successes and failures.

A little bit about my journey. In 2003 it all started with a severe cough that would not stop. After much frustration and several misdiagnoses, I was finally led to a pulmonologist that properly diagnosed my condition. I clearly recall the day I sat before him with big eyes of hope when he delivered the bad news that I had Pulmonary Fibrosis and a transplant would be the most likely course of action. Otherwise death from the disease was likely. He went on to say that he would be willing to refer me to Inova Fairfax Hospital, Falls Church, Virginia because transplantation was out of his league. My husband looked at him with terror in his eyes and I looked at him as though he had two heads. You see I was 38, and a pretty young thing. He clearly had been smoking something and had it all wrong. But he was right.

We left his office and met with the Fairfax team. I was told I possibly could be listed and given a list of pre-transplant tests to be done prior to being listed. Three months later, I had done nothing. Denial and even more so, resentment set in. "This could not be happening to me." Again I felt I was too young and I focused solely on the mortality rate statistics that was shared on one of our visits. I concluded why go through all the surgery if I were only going to live possibly for five years. Then on one lovely Sunday afternoon, we decided to have brunch with a friend that was a dietician. During the brunch, I discovered she was not just a regular dietician, but also a dietician for one of the Boston transplant centers. It was truly divine. In two hours she changed my whole attitude. One month later I had completed what I had refused to even start three months earlier.

In 2004, I was listed. I had a wide variety of emotions. Some were good, some were awful. The pulmonary fibrosis really started to set in. April of 2005 during a breast examination, I found a lump. After having a sonogram, I was told it was benign. Although happy for the positive results, I still chose to have the lump removed and tested, after listening to my intuition in which I just wanted to double check. After getting a lumpectomy, it turned out that my intuition was correct. It was early stage breast cancer. My husband was devastated and I showed no emotions. At this point I couldn't feel any pain. I was so absorbed with getting back on the list, that I was numb to the breast cancer diagnosis. Within sixty days, I had another lumpectomy, a single mastectomy, and then was cancer free. Getting chemo or radiation was too much of a risk due to the lung disease. We were so delighted but it was short lived. Things changed for the worst. I was told that now I would need to be cancer free for two years before I could even be considered for a transplant, in that immunosuppressant drugs can cause cancer to spread if there is any cancer present.

With optimism, we said okay and moved forward. In January 2006, we decided to meet with the transplant team just to keep in touch and remind them that I was still holding on. During the visit, we discovered there was a discrepancy with what I thought we were told. I thought we were told two years to wait when the team insisted they told us five. We were devastated. I literally felt the walls closing in on me. The pulmonary fibrosis had really progressed. I now required six liters of oxygen. So we knew that a five-year wait surely meant death.

Then a ray of hope appeared. On the request of my transplant team, we met with their oncologist who felt I was young, vibrant, and worthy of the 20% risk that would be taken if I were transplanted. He felt the five-year wait, should not be a one size fits all and it should be evaluated on a case-by-case basis. Of course I agreed with him, so 2006, I was placed back on the list. Now my pulmonary fibrosis was in the final stages. My oxygen requirements had quadrupled and I required 100% oxygen, which had to be administered through a mask. May 8th 2006, I was transplanted with a single left lung at age 40. Seven days after being put back on the list.

The transplant was successful for about the first week. I then began experiencing what is known as primary graft failure. As the head of the transplant team, Dr. Nathan stated, "Everything that could go wrong, did." However things turned around for the better. After six more weeks at the transplant hospital, I was then moved to a rehab hospital. I began a daily routine of three hours per day of physical and occupational therapy to regain my muscles strength. I constantly felt depressed and my life was over. But with determination, and a persistent husband that never missed one day of being at my bedside by 8:30 a.m. before the doctors arrived, the entire five months I was hospitalized. I regained my ability to eat and talk after having the tracheotomy removed. As well as walk, and do all the things that used to seem small.

This whole experience has taught me that life is precious and we should treat each day as if it were our last. The fear of death, which initially kept me from pursuing a transplant, has now been replaced with a passion for life. I have the gift of gab and a strong desire to reach out to others. My dream is to start a Support Group Foundation that provides information and resources for individuals battling Pulmonary Fibrosis and/are pre or post transplant patients.

Finally, my quality of life has been restored. I pray for as many years, as possible. August 2010, I competed in my first United States Transplant Games in Madison, Wisconsin. I played on the volleyball team, and threw the shot put. I also ran the 100m dash and finished "dead" last, but in my mind, there was no first or last. We all won the race.

We have gotten back to traveling the World. In 2008 we took nine separate trips including a trip to Mallorca, Spain in what we labeled, "making up for lost time". Traveling without oxygen has been an amazing feeling after having done so for many years. We've also taken several trips to our timeshare in Grand Cayman Island. I was able to walk along the beach, swim and do all the things I did before getting ill. We had not been able to go there for many years.

Doris Lowenthal, 44
Severn, Maryland
Pulmonary Fibrosis
Single Lung Transplant, May 8, 2006
Inova Fairfax Hospital, Falls Church, Virginia

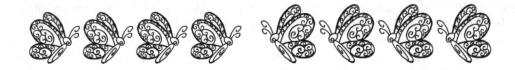

My Journey that Brought me to Where I am Today
By Scott Machowski

For as long as I can remember, my father told me never to do any thing half way. So as I grew up I did everything every other boy my age would do. As a child I played in the dirt and got my fair share of bumps and bruises. I never knew what was inside me was any different than anyone else. I would run and play all day, every day. I received decent grades in school, nothing spectacular. I was an average student and an average kid. I never felt different in my younger years.

My teens, I started coughing frequently. It was just one of "those" things in life you deal with. I also had several allergies that I was tested for, and they came back positive for just about everything they tested me for. So I had a runny nose and a cough, no big deal. Eventually my cough had become an everyday thing and I was coughing up this horribly tasting stuff. My best friend would joke and say I needed to bottle that stuff and sell it as glue. It was so thick and in such large amounts by now. It started to effect my every day life.

I was playing sports and having fun just like everyone else. I was on the track team, swim team, weight lifting team, and I even played football for a while. I was also in chorus from 5th grade until my second year in high school. It was right before my 16th birthday, when I was sent to Shands Hospital at The University of Florida to be seen by the pulmonary specialist. There I was tested for the genetic defect called Cystic Fibrosis. I still remember my moms face. Shear panic and sadness, followed by an abundance of tears. For me however, it was a different story. I knew absolutely nothing of the illness, so I wasn't upset or scared in the least. I was like, "okay, what now?" They explained all of the treatments and therapies I would need to do. I can remember thinking I wasn't going to let this thing kill me, because I had it in my head that I wasn't going to let it run my life.

We moved around a little. We moved to Louisiana and then back to Florida. My brother, who had already graduated from high school was already in the Air Force and wasn't around when I was diagnosed. Later on we found out my brother wasn't even a carrier of the CF gene. Which left us all very happy. I managed to graduate with a 3.0 Grade Point Average (GPA). I paid for college myself, when I enrolled at Bossier City Community College, Bossier City, Louisiana. There I received a certificate in Surgical Technologies in May of 1997. I started my first job as a surgical technician at Bossier Medical Center.

By the time I was 21-years-old I had been in and out of the hospital a few times but nothing serious. Due to aching joints almost every day, I enrolled in a nursing program hoping nursing would be a better career choice. I graduated from Shreveport/Bossier Vocational College as a Licensed Practical Nurse (LPN). I worked as a nurse until 2007, working in several different areas and I enjoyed my work. I was hospitalized numerous times over the course of those four years.

August of 2007 I had my first pneumothorax. I was left with a lung function of half of the volume I previously had and was faced with going on disability. Just weeks prior I was a thriving member of society and now I would lose everything.

So once again, I moved back to Louisiana to live with my father. I have to say that my father has always been there for me. Love you Dad. Don't get me wrong; my Mom was there for me too. Love you too Mom. By the beginning of 2009 I was in the hospital every other month for at least three weeks. I was now faced with a choice; did I want to die? Of course not. I am a lover and a fighter. I love life and I will fight to keep it. Do I want a lung transplant? I approached my CF doctor and asked the question, "Is it time for a lung transplant?" And she replied simply, "Yes". It was probably the toughest thing I have ever had to swallow. I know that it is just one more thing in life I will over come.

My name is Scott Machowski. I am 34-years-old and I am living with Cystic Fibrosis and my future is BRIGHT!

Update: Scott received his double lung transplant after writing this story.

Scott Machowski, 34
Galveston, Texas
Cystic Fibrosis
Double Lung Transplant, August 23, 2010
University of Texas Medical Branch at Galveston, Galveston, Texas

The Gift of Life, Love and Laughter
By Shelley MacLean

My name is Shelley MacLean and I am here today to share my story and journey through transplantation. I am 34-years-old and originally from Inverness, Nova Scotia, Canada. I have a beautiful 14-year-old son named Austin who means the world to me.

At the tender age of 25 I was diagnosed with a rare disease called Pulmonary Veno-occlusive Disease. This is a one in a million disease that causes the veins in your lungs to obstruct so the blood can't pump through to your heart, which then restricts your breathing.

Before my diagnosis I was very unsure of what was going on with my body. I was going to school for Police Foundations and I had to participate in physical activity. I would run the track and I would get an instant headache, and much too out of breath to continue running. At this time in my life I weighed 180 pounds so I was convinced that it had to be my weight limiting me, but the more I tried to exercise the worse I felt and there were many people heavier than me that had no problem exercising. I lived only across the street from work and embarrassingly enough, I would drive there because I couldn't bare the walk.

I went to Thunder Bay, Canada where the doctors thought I had a hole in my heart, and I was put on oxygen and sent home. I had regular visits to my cardiologist, and at times I wouldn't wear my oxygen. I think for me being so young I was in denial, and did not want to succumb to the fact that I was sick. On one of my visits to my cardiologist, I had my oxygen off, and he told me, "You are a very sick girl and you need to wear your oxygen or I can refuse to be your doctor." This was a shock, as well as a reality check that I was sick and that the oxygen was part of my medicine to get better. It was decided an air ambulance would take me to Toronto so they could better evaluate me. The Computerized Tomography (CT) scan was how they diagnosed that I had Pulmonary Veno-occlusive Disease (PVOD).

They had a specialist come from the United States who looked at my CT scan to ensure their diagnosis was right since, it is so rare and even at this they couldn't be 100 % sure. Six doctors told me; some of which were students, what the disease was and that I only had three to six months left to live, unless I chose to have a double lung transplant. Pre transplant patients must exercise and get as strong as possible before the operation, but my heart was too weak and fragile; so for me it was a waiting game.

We were very fortunate to get a lot of support from Inverness where I grew up and Marathon, Canada, where I was living at the time. My sister visited me at my hospital room in Toronto with money and cards from Inverness, where I had not lived since the age of 12; it was such a touching feeling. I felt so loved and grateful for the support from a lot of people that probably didn't even know or remember me anymore. At that moment I realized that no matter how appreciative and heartfelt I was, that no amount of money in the world could make my health better.

My family took turns taking care of me because I always had to have someone with me around the clock. I found it very depressing and frustrating with the realization that I was so dependent on everyone else now. I went to a lot of meetings about transplant to learn and meet new people going through the same thing as myself. My sister Natalie was pregnant with twins, and she told me she didn't think it was a good time to be pregnant, because she wanted to be there for me more. I told her I thought it was a good time because if I don't make it, she would have something to look forward too. She asked me to be present with her when the twins were born, and I hoped and prayed that I would live to see them.

I only waited a month and a half before I received my lungs. On February 27th, 2002, in the early morning a nurse came in my room and told me I would be getting my lungs. They said I was very lucky because three sets of lungs came in that night. All I remember is meeting the anesthesiologist and I was out for the count. The operation took nine hours with some complications, but I pulled through. I was in intensive care for 23 days after transplant. I remember being so thirsty I kept dreaming about fountains and water but when I would go to have a drink, there was none. When I finally went to 'step down', I was able to call my son and what an amazing feeling to be able to pick up the phone and hear his voice again. He was able to come see me but he wanted me to run and play with him.

The doctors would come in daily after my x-ray and check my lungs and I would pray that the leak I had, would close up, but everyday it was the same thing, I could see the bubbles in the Pleur-evac, which meant there was air, and the leak was still there. The doctors told me that most transplant patients that have trouble initially and stay in the hospital longer seem to do better when they leave so that kept me going. Spring came and when my son was visiting, we ventured outside. To have gone into the hospital in the Winter and come out seeing the grass again, I got so emotional just breathing in the fresh air, looking at the grass and feeling and seeing things like I never seen them before. What an overwhelming feeling of appreciation.

A doctor told me I was one of the most patient patients they had ever had and upon seeing my new pair of sneakers said, "Nice sneakers, I want to see a picture of you running in those one day." I needed to stay in Toronto for three months. My sister went into labor on May 29th but I was unable to be in the room with her, but happily she had twins and she named her daughter after me, which I thought was pretty special.

Once home, I went to my son's school and his teacher said, "All Austin's friends want to meet you, they want to help his mom get better." This was very heartwarming for me. I decided to start volunteering at my son's school but before I knew it I was asked to do lunchroom supervisor, then teacher's assistant. I pushed myself and continued working till I ended up with a full time position as a secretary in Human Resources. I do my best to focus on the positive and live a normal life. I ski, I have played hockey, I go to the gym, I started to square dance this summer and I have moved to the place I love, Cape Breton, Nova Scotia.

My son never lost his mother when he was six because someone took the time to sign their donor card, giving me another nine years of life so far…

On Christmas and my transplant anniversary, I anonymously write my donor family thanking them for the precious lungs they have given me. So please help promote organ donation, and sign your card today because you never know if it could be you, or a loved one, needing organs one day.

Shelley MacLean, 34
Inverness, Nova Scotia, Canada
Pulmonary Veno-Occlusive Disease
Double Lung Transplant, February 27, 2002
Toronto General Hospital, Toronto, Canada

❧ The Miracle of Transplantation ❧
By Nancy Matthews

I was born on October 7, 1974 in the shadow of the Grand Teton Mountain Range in Jackson Hole, Wyoming. I was a very healthy baby, who thrived; however, as I grew, my mother noticed some troublesome things about me. First, I had an insatiable appetite and at three was eating as much as a 200 lb man; second, I was spending hours in the bathroom each day. She raised her concerns to my doctor, but since I was thriving, he felt she was overreacting. She continued to push, and finally, at the age of six, the doctor conceded and sent us to Salt Lake City, Utah for further testing.

A sweat test came back positive for cystic fibrosis (CF). Normally there is relief when you get an answer to a nagging question; my parents found no relief in this diagnosis, only fear and disbelief. They were both teachers and had experienced children with CF; they knew the future was grim. CF was incurable and terminal; at that time the average life expectancy was only 18. They had received a death sentence for their little girl.

A CF specialist in Salt Lake City recommended that my parents send me to CF camp that following summer to allow me to meet other kids with my illness, my parents agreed and I attended my first CF camp. As the week progressed, I settled in and made some good friends.

The following year when it was time for camp, I was really excited to return and see my friends. The year before I had befriended a little boy named Josh, and looked forward to spending more time with him at camp. That first day I went in search of Josh, but couldn't find him. One of the nurses noticed that I seemed upset about something and approached me. When I told her who I was looking for, she sat me down and explained that Josh had passed away that year. He wasn't the only one who hadn't returned to camp. The reality of my illness came crashing down on me; CF was going to kill me. I never returned to CF camp and a few years later all of the CF camps across the country were closed down. Something awful had infected the CF community, two nasty bacteria: Pseudomonas and Burkholderia Cepacia (B.Cepacia).

I vowed to never let CF stop me. I set my goals high and didn't let my disease slow me down. I was active throughout my school years, participating in cheerleading, student government, volleyball, skiing, drama, speech and debate, track, tennis, and many other activities.

I attended St. Bonaventure University (SBU) in South Western New York. During my first semester at SBU, I was diagnosed with a non-malignant tumor on my pituitary gland and was put on medication to try to shrink it. The medication made my body extremely run down, and by the end of finals, illness had set in. I remained at home for the spring semester and, in August, underwent brain surgery to remove the tumor. I was back at SBU for the start of the semester, three weeks later.

Looking back, that probably wasn't the best decision, but I was determined to get back to school. A few weeks into that semester, I experienced my CF in a new and very frightening way. Walking home from the dining hall one afternoon I began coughing and my mouth filled with a warm liquid. I could not catch my breath and upon entering my room realized the liquid was blood. An ambulance was called; I was rushed to the hospital.

In the middle of all of this terror, something truly wonderful happened; my cousin introduced me to my future husband, Scott Matthews. Scott stood by me through each hospitalization. He chose to be with me despite my illness and we were married in 1996 between my junior and senior years of college. Three years later, after a difficult pregnancy, we were blessed with a beautiful daughter, Hannah Marie.

I graduated from SBU in 1997 with a Bachelor's Degree (BA) in Psychology. I began the Master's program in Counseling and was offered a wonderful assistantship at SBU's Learning Center. Upon completion of my Master of Education (MSEd), I was offered a position with the Learning Center as the Coordinator of Disability Services and served in that position for 7 ½ years. In 2006, I entered the end stages of CF and had to retire from SBU to pursue a life- saving transplant.

I spoke of the two types of bacteria that a CF patient can get, I have both of them, and the B. Cepacia made me a high-risk transplant candidate because the chances of success were less than 50% compared to a non-cepacia CF patient's 80+% success rate; despite these odds, the University of Pittsburgh Medical Center, Pittsburgh, Pennsylvania, accepted me for transplant. The wait was long and there were many times I almost gave up. I had to learn to depend on God and trust Him with everything.

On December 10, 2008 my cell phone rang. It was my doctor; they had found a donor for me! I don't know much about my donor, but do know that she was 34, the same age as me at the time, and that she was a hero. She made the decision to donate her organs in death, and by doing so she saved my life!

The transplant was, by far, the hardest thing I have ever been through, but those difficult days following the surgery were so worth it. 14 days later, on Christmas Eve, I was released from the hospital to spend Christmas in a Pittsburgh apartment with my family. We had been given the best Christmas gift of all, a second chance; all of our prayers had come true.

After transplant, I had to rebuild my muscles giving me the strength to become active again. I had become dependent on others during my illness, and had to re-learn how to be a strong and independent woman all over again. I was able to overcome those struggles and began to soar. I had been blessed with health again; better health than I could ever remember. I jumped into life and haven't stopped, celebrating each new day, opportunity, and small treasure. What an amazing second chance!

Not everyone is as lucky as I was. Across the country more than 108,000 people are waiting for organ transplants. One person dies every 80 minutes and 18 people die every day waiting for organs. I lost my closest CF friend, Emily, in 2007 because lungs did not become available in time. Emily and I had known each other for years, growing close through e-mail and phone conversations. Because of the ban on physical contact between patients with CF, we hadn't ever been able to meet.

Despite these things, I have never felt better. The entire journey helped me to grow as a person and gave me the strength to face any future adversity. It was all worth it and I praise the Lord each day for the miracle of transplantation!

I am the author of two books. "A Journey Toward Spiritual Peace" and "An Insider's Guide to Managing Your Chronic or Terminal Illness"

Nancy Matthews, 36
Westons Mills, New York
Cystic Fibrosis
Double Lung Transplant, December 10, 2008
University of Pittsburgh Medical Center, Pittsburgh, Pennsylvania

I Now See the Sky Bluer, than it Ever Was
By Chris May

My name is Chris and I have lived in the little town of Waterville, Ohio for over half my life. As a young boy, I grew up playing sports and living a very active life. When I turned 13-years-old I came down with pneumonia and contracted a disease called Sarcoidosis. The disease entered my spleen and enlarged it to the size of a basketball. My immune system was greatly affected and I became sensitive to illnesses. The disease did go dormant and my spleen did shrink down to close to normal size. So I found other avenues to explore instead of sports like singing in choirs, and theatre.

After close to 20 years of living a fairly normal life, at least in my mind, I started to get sick again with pneumonia. I was married and had a 4-year-old daughter and twin girls on the way. My oldest, barely remembers me being healthy enough to play and chase her around. My twins were born and I had to go to the hospital myself before they were a month old. I had seven pneumonias in a two and half year period. My lung capacity started to shrink with each illness. I went from 100% lung capacity to 36%. Instead of the 37-year-old man that I was, I felt as though I was in my 90's. Something was definitely wrong. The doctors didn't know quite what to do other than try to boost my immune system and keep me from getting any sicker.

I decided to go to The Cleveland Clinic Foundation, Cleveland, Ohio because my Father goes there for Multiple Sclerosis. I then found out how serious of a condition I was in. I was immediately put on oxygen 24 hours a day (24/7) and told I would be a perfect candidate for a double lung transplant. "A what!?!" I didn't know that was possible. I had heard of heart, kidney and liver transplant but I never knew they could do lungs. The news hit me harder then I've ever expected. I would have to go through all kinds of tests for every part of my body that I could imagine, to show that I'm healthy enough to go through a transplant, yet my lungs are sick enough for it also. The doctors needed to know that I would survive the operation.

I was placed on the waiting list and was told it would be very soon that I would get "the call" and would be breathing easier from then on. Well, three and half years later the phone rang. It was February 16th, 2009. I was so confused when the guy on the other end of the phone was telling me that my lungs are ready and do I want to accept this donation. So I told him to hold on and ran upstairs faster than I thought I could run to wake my wife and inform her that the time was now for my transplant. My wish had come true. I almost forgot about the guy on the phone but I remembered to accept it. Needless to say I didn't get a wink of sleep that night after that call. I kissed my girls goodbye and told them I loved them. I didn't know for sure if I'd ever see them again because surgeries always scared me. But I put up a brave front for my families sake.

During the wait, all I could think about was how I was going to be a better father and a better husband after this surgery is done and I'm healed. When they removed that breathing tube and I took my first regular breath, it felt like the greatest gift I could have ever received and I said a silent prayer for my donor and their family.

I was in the hospital for 10 days and stayed in the Cleveland area for two weeks; both a lot less time than what I expected. My recovery was moving fast. I had to have someone with me at all times whether it was my wife or my parents just in case I would need to get help or need assistance. But I was making leaps and bounds in my state of recovery that was amazing the doctors.

Once, I got home I rejoiced in the fact that I could spend time with my children, family and friends. It was a true miracle that I felt like I was 20 years younger than my true age. My kids where excited about the fact that their dad was for the most part healthy again. I've been able to help my oldest daughter train for softball. Also, my twins have been excited that I can now help them with their soccer skills and being an assistant coach for their softball team. I've been truly blessed.

I did have one unfortunate thing happen and that was my wife and I divorced. My children are with me and they surround me with the love that I need to keep up and I return the favor. After all, I'm back thanks to a donor whom I do not know. The gift he/she gave me and their family has allowed me to be the best father I can be.

I also competed in the 2010 United States Transplant Games. These are Olympic style events that transplant recipients compete in from all over the country. I didn't win any medals for my first games but I sure had a lot of fun playing sports again. This time my girls, Mom and a family friend got to see me compete. I loved the hugs I got before and after each event. My family has been a true inspiration to me.

I now see the sky bluer than it ever was. The rain doesn't bother me. I see shapes in the clouds again like when I was a kid. The world has become a more positive place for me. All this is due to my hero.... my donor...Thank you so much for giving me my life back!

Chris May, 41
Waterville, Ohio
Sarcoidosis
Double Lung Transplant, February 16, 2009
The Cleveland Clinic Foundation, Cleveland, Ohio

 Christine Victoria Come – "We Never Give Up" – 2009
By Harmony McCall

A spunky young six-year-old walked into her kitchen after attending kindergarten for only a little longer than two months. "How was your day?" asked her mother, "The same as yesterday… easy". The beautiful girl with long brown curls, and beautiful, deep brown eyes, replied with a sigh. Her mom just smiled and shook her head. The doctor's had warned her mother, Robin, that her daughter, Christine, might fall behind in school. They had warned Robin that she ought to be prepared for Christine to miss time due to the two-week-average-stays that a lot of Cystic Fibrosis patients become accustomed to, coping with, as a yearly addition to their illness. It would be hard for Christine to maintain her grades with such a disadvantage, they had said. Christine's birthday fell in November and the cut-off date to enroll in kindergarten was September so Christine remained one of the eldest in her class for the remainder of her school years. Fall behind she did not.

Christine never shared the true nature of her illness with most of her friends while growing up. She didn't want other people to feel bad for her, or look at her differently, and she never wanted to feel badly for herself. She played softball position as a catcher and also played third base. She got tossed high into the air as a cheerleader during the basketball season. She treated her life as a true gift and she fully embraced every opportunity she had to live it to the fullest.

After graduating in 2001, Christine attended hair styling school and went on to become a gifted hairstylist. Her happiness surmounted when she traveled to California and spent a year living with her brother, Brent. She then returned home to fall in love and become engaged to the man whom she felt was her true soul mate and eternal love. She traveled to the Bahamas, and is the only person that I have ever known to have adopted a 'vacation cat', which she nicknamed 'Scratches'. Her love for animals was inspiring. I have never seen somebody so pleasantly giggling while filming her cat being bathed, or somebody as concerned as Christine became when she was bed-bound and could spot a stray wandering around outside her bedroom window. Her own cat, Oscar, was her baby, and one of the greatest joys in her life.

Christine learned that she was to become listed to receive a double lung transplant in November of 2007. She became engaged around this same time, and as in the past, she never let the threat of this illness overlook her future. She shared in some of my happiest memories in the following two years while she waited to receive her transplant. Her alluring spunk and sassy sense of humor made every day a really good day...even when I knew that pain-wise, some of them had to have been her worst.

Christine liked to giggle during her hospital stays. One time she took the entire box of sterile gloves that was in her room and blew them all up like balloons. Then she had her friend proceeded to tack them all up to the ceiling so she could take pictures. She created a photo album on her MySpace titled, "Glove Love." Christine liked to laugh. She did not take much time to feel sorry for herself.

When it became clear that Christine did not have a lot of time left without receiving her new lungs, there was a quietness and calm sadness in the air. It took time for her to accept this and it became difficult for those who loved her. I remember just holding her and crying, not much else. After acceptance, it became a realization. Christine did not want to die. Yet Christine was not at all afraid of death. As scary of a concept as it can be for others, Christine had her own take on her own mortality.

In September 2009, Christine sat with her father, Ben, and had a serious conversation. "I know that I am never going to see my 27th birthday, Dad", she said. "But I am not afraid. I know where I'm going. And I am not afraid to die."

On October 21st 2009, Christine was admitted into Lebanon Hospital, Lebanon, New Hampshire and put on a ventilator. She was told that this would now place her at the absolute top of the list, but because of her rare blood type and small frame, a match was not imminent. After ten days on the ventilator, Christine was released freely and quietly into the arms of the Lord while those of us that loved and adored her gathered around and held onto her. On October 31, 2009, "We never give up," were Christine Come's last words.

Christine Come will forever remain a hero to many. Through every obstacle and every challenge that she faced with her illness, she never lost courage or hope. She remained strong and insistent that this disease will be cured very soon. A cure is so close, and medical advances become so much more refined every single day. Christine became such an inspiration to me, and many others who work very hard to continue to spread the importance of organ donation and help collect funds to benefit the Cystic Fibrosis Foundation.

Little annoyances in life often have a way of distracting us all from what is truly important. Christine taught me that we cannot let our difficulties lie in the way of our dreams and that we can never give up.

Harmony McCall, Friend of, Christine Victoria Come
Pittsfield, New Hampshire
Christine, Cystic Fibrosis
Passed Away, Pre-Double Lung Transplant
"Forever 26"

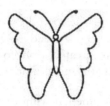

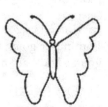

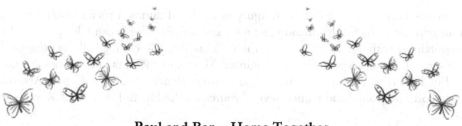

Paul and Ben – Home Together
By Shelby McDaniel

Paul Andrew McDaniel, 22, was a senior at Christian Brothers University (CBU) in Memphis, Tennessee who loved life and loved his University. His grass roots while attending Christian Brothers High School (CBHS) gave him such a disciplined way of life he wanted to continue at CBU and then attend law school. Paul was our youngest son, passing away on September 14, 2008 due to a stroke. He was majoring in finance. Paul was certified brain dead at 2:00 a.m. on a Sunday morning giving the "Gift of Life" to four people through vital organ donations as well as helping eighty people live a better life with his tissue donation.

When Paul was declared brain dead we had to make a decision concerning his organs so we signed the necessary papers with Mid-South Transplant Foundation. Paul had expressed his desire to be an organ donor. He was on a ventilator for two days while they matched his organs up with his recipients. Even in death Paul continued his life of service to others as he had while he was alive. When the word 'service' is included in your life you always wonder how far the journey will take you. For Paul, 'service' was a large part throughout his twenty-two years.

At an early age he started spending time daily with his grandfather who lived about two minutes from our backyard. When Ben Baker (Paul's Grandfather) who was called Paw Paw developed Parkinson's disease Paul was right there to help. It was a joy to see how he provided his grandfather with transportation, spent time with him and ministered to his needs. Paul had a natural drive to serve and care for others! His friends described him as loyal and supportive and always there to help and listen to anyone who needed a friend. He had a gift with young children, as he was the lifeguard at our day camp. The young kids loved being around Paul. They enjoyed their swim times in the pool.

As Paul started CBHS his service expanded to tutoring elementary school students. For his efforts he was given the De LaSalle award. Paul was also the recipient of three honor student awards. At the 2004 CBHS graduation he received, "THE BROTHER ANDRIAN POWERS ACADEMIC IMPROVEMENT AWARD" given to the senior who over a period of four years at Christian Brothers High School, has shown the greatest academic improvement.

Paul loved to work for the local law offices and run their errands for them, and became fascinated with law and decided that he wanted to be a lawyer as this was another way he could help others. He was very good and thorough in his researches to gain knowledge about everything he could get his hands on, especially involving legal issues. He was an "Apple" fanatic and thought Apple Computers was the only way to survive. He could do anything with his computer.

Paul early on was very good in golf but an injury to his hand during a rock climbing trip would not allow him to grip the clubs firmly anymore, so rock and ice climbing became his passion. He became an avid mountaineer with a deep passion for the rock and ice. He climbed all over the United States including his most recent expeditions to Engineer Mountain in Durango, Colorado and Boulder, Colorado. But his favorite spot was Horseshoe Canyon Ranch (HCR) in Jasper, Arkansas. Paul's brothers Ben and Tim bolted and named several routes on the North Forty at HCR in his honor and memory.

Ben and Tim started the Paul Andrew McDaniel Foundation in his memory. The foundation strives to raise awareness of strokes in young people and to promote organ and tissue donation. Paul has left an undying fire in his brother's hearts to make him proud. Every day the foundation makes a difference in the lives of people touched by a stroke. Community involvement and donations go a long way toward helping the foundation achieve its mission. By getting involved today you could be helping a family member or friend tomorrow.

The foundation's mission is to raise awareness, promote education and support for people to be an organ donor. On any given day there are over 100,000 needing a transplant! We were chosen as Paul's parents, by The Mid-South Transplant Foundation to attend Washington D.C. for the National Donor Recognition Ceremony July 2009, as donor families were honored. We attended workshops in brain death, sudden death and musculoskeletal transplantation, allowing us to better comfort and share how loved ones live on as Paul is living on.

Even in death Paul continues to give life to others through organ donation. We have heard from three recipients and the heart recipient and his family will be coming to meet us for Paul's annual "Fall Farm Festival" fundraiser on October 23, 2010. We will be able to put our hands on Paul's heart and feel it beating!

The foundation website can be found by going to Google, and entering: Paul McDaniel Foundation. It is a 501 (c) (3) nonprofit. The night before his stroke Paul posted his climbing photos for all to see at: http://web.me.com/paulandrewmcdaniel/Site/Welcome.html

At a young age Paul accepted Christ as his personal savior. He just went to sleep and woke up in Heaven. Paul was a very loving and special young man. He was a well-rounded individual. We will miss him dearly.

Late August 2010, Shelby and his family experienced another tragedy. Their son Ben McDaniel went scuba diving into a cave, and never returned.

Ben McDaniel
Somehow we believe God will use Ben's life to enhance the glory of Jesus, his Savior. His Facebook page is a testimony to his relationship with the Lord. His daily devotion time writing his prayer requests and thoughts reflected just how far he had grown as a believer. For some reason as with Paul, God decided that it was Ben's time to leave this earth and enjoy what we all desire, to live in Heaven.

We are so thankful God let us borrow Ben and Paul for these few years. Both lived a full life! It is such a comfort knowing they are together again! We must go on with our lives though and the real meaning and purpose set before us----to share the " Good News " and sow the seeds expected of us to those who are blinded or to those who are down in the valley and encourage them to return to the joy of their salvation.

Every family has challenges, some more than others but as believers we know the Lord never puts more on us than what we are able to endure. As a matter-of-fact, we should grow in His grace and allow the Holy Spirit to lead us and be there for those less fortunate who need a shoulder to cry on.

Deuteronomy 4:29 says, "When you search for God, you will find Him when you search for Him with all your heart and soul." Ben did this, and found the peace that the Father promised.

Shelby McDaniel
Donor Father of Son: Paul Andrew McDaniel
Collierville, Texas
Paul Passed Away, September 14, 2008
Paul Andrew McDaniel – "Forever 22"
Father of Son: Ben McDaniel
Ben Passed Away, August 18, 2011
Ben McDaniel, "Forever 30"

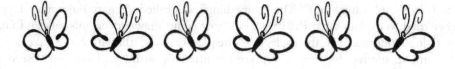

Christmas Miracle
By BreAnn McFarland

When you hear of someone suffering from a terrible illness, you offer your prayers and support, and yet, you never think that something like that could happen to you...especially when you are only fourteen-years-old. At that age, we all think that we're invincible, that we can take on the world.

I was fourteen when, the summer before starting high school, my whole world came crashing down around me. I started having trouble breathing along with chest pain and dizziness while walking home from the bus stop at the end of my 8th grade year. When it got to the point that I would have to sit down in the middle of the street to keep from passing out, I knew something was very wrong. I tried to hide it until one day when I came home, my mom was vacuuming the foyer, and I barely made it inside the door before I had to sit down. I was too worried about the room spinning around me to hide what was happening anymore.

My pediatrician could not find anything wrong, but my symptoms worried him enough to refer me to a cardiologist. The cardiologist, in turn, diagnosed me with a hole in my heart. Surgery to repair the hole was scheduled to be done during my summer vacation. Before they could do surgery, a heart catheterization had to be done to learn more about the hole. So, what did they learn? There was no hole! Great news, right?

I went home, ecstatic to know that I would not need surgery. The following day my parents came home from what I thought had been work but was actually a meeting with some doctors. They sat me down to talk about "something." The "something" was called Primary Pulmonary Hypertension (PPH). They tried to explain what PPH was, but how could they explain this rare and fatal disease when they didn't understand it themselves? The doctors said that it would take a heart/lung transplant for me to survive, for me to even see my fifteenth birthday. I had never seen my father cry, but his cheeks were wet as he hugged me close, sharing in my fear and despair. At that moment, I knew my life would never be the same again.

And it wasn't. I was sent to Emory University Hospital in Atlanta, Georgia to Dr. E. Clinton Lawrence, who was not only the pulmonary transplant doctor, but who also specialized in pulmonary hypertension. I spent a week in the hospital doing the testing that was required to be placed on the waiting list for a bilateral lung transplant; and, yes, I said a lung transplant. Dr. Lawrence explained that once I had new lungs, my heart would go back to normal. Before I made the decision to have a transplant, however, Dr. Lawrence wanted to exhaust every other option available to me. We learned a lot about PPH at that point, mainly that the "primary" meant that they could not find what was causing the pulmonary hypertension.

My sophomore year of high school, I was started on Flolan, a drug that had to be continuously infused intravenously through a catheter implanted in my chest. I had to carry a pump around with me at all times because the medicine could not be stopped for more than a few seconds, and I had to mix my own medicine every twenty-four hours. When the Flolan did not lower my pressures like it was supposed to, the doctors got more aggressive with it, increasing my dose very quickly; however, my body was not responding to the treatment. I finally had to accept that it was time to go on the list for transplant. So, on my eighteenth birthday, I was put on the waiting list for a bilateral lung transplant.

My family, friends, school, and community were absolutely amazing; they showed more support than I ever could have hoped for. My school held a blood drive and collected donations to help pay for my surgery. The support I got was what helped me get through each day--what gave me the courage to fight for my life.

After I graduated, I was not able to start to college as I had planned. Instead, I waited day after day for the next four-and-a-half years for one telephone call. Each day I got weaker and had more trouble breathing. In October 2008, I had seizures due to a medication interaction, and I ended up on a ventilator in the Intensive Care Unit (ICU). I was struggling to breathe, and my family was told that it was time to say their goodbyes. Dr. Lawrence had to go out of town while I was in ICU; my mother later told me that before he left, Dr. Lawrence stood by my bedside telling me that he had to leave, but that, I *WOULD* be there when he got back…and I was.

I was sent home with an oxygen tank. December 7, 2002, I lay in bed knowing that I was out of time; we all knew that without new lungs, I would not make it through the weekend. That's when it happened. The phone rang with *THE* call we had waited so long for.

As we waited for Dr. David Vega to arrive with my new lungs, I felt very peaceful. I knew this was my last chance, but I wasn't scared—it was in God's hands. A nurse later told me that as they wheeled me down to surgery, I had one request; I asked her to take care of my parents if I didn't make it out of surgery. My parents had fought just as hard for my life as I had, and I knew that they would have been devastated if something had gone wrong. There were some complications, and I spent more time in ICU than expected. It was not the ideal place to spend Christmas, but I had no complaints that year.

I have had some problems over the past eight years, but I celebrated my thirty-first birthday two weeks ago, proving to all those who said I would not see fifteen that there is always hope—like the hope that Dr. Lawrence always kept alive in me. I fought hard for my life, but I could not have done it without the love and support of my family and friends. More importantly, I could not have done it without my faith in God. That faith brought me a miracle. I have a pillow that is embroidered with, "Miracles Happen to Those Who Believe." I know I believe, do you?

I want to thank my family and friends for being there for me during the most difficult time of my life. I want to thank Dr. Lawrence and Dr. Vega for all that they have done to make it possible for me to see my thirty-first birthday, and hopefully many more. I love you all! I want to say thank you to my donor's family, you will always have a special place in my heart.

Finally, to an unknown hero—thank you for the precious gift you have given me. We may have never met, but you will always be a part of me.

BreAnn McFarland, 31
Acworth, Georgia
Primary Pulmonary Hypertension
Double Lung Transplant, December 8, 2002
Emory University Hospital, Atlanta, Georgia

 Oodles of Smiles
Cathy McGill

As a long time recipient of a heart/double lung transplant, Cathy has seen many changes in the 'world of transplants', a nice statement to add to anyone's "transplant resume".

Because of my long time friendship with Cathy, my life has been brighter, more energized with the determination and kindness she radiates! Anyone who meets this 26-year recipient cannot help but delight in her smile. I feel like leapfrogging or yelling a cheer when I am in her presence.

Everyone needs a sense of cheerfulness, every day of his or her life. Cathy is that sunny soul who has inspired many around the world. She draws people to her, and they listen to her tales of travel, adventure and her continued bouncy outlook on life.

Cathy and I met in person about six years ago in Iowa with several other lung recipients. What is the thrill of meeting others who are wearing the same shoes as you? Shared happiness, similar fears and concerns are the start of the list of reasons. I believe that all lung recipients are truly kindred spirits; we share the uniqueness and the very special gift of life – the gift of breathing. I knew immediately when I met Cathy; I truly met a kindred spirit.

Summer 2010, Cathy and her parents, Don and Jackie met a large group of "kindred spirits" at the 2010 Transplant Games in Madison, Wisconsin. The anticipation of having Cathy at the "Lung Gathering" was pure excitement for everyone. I was asked, "Is Cathy here yet?" I cannot count the number of times...oodles of times!

Cathy also had a kidney transplant in September 2005 after a year on dialysis and shared that she was glad a kidney donor was available at the time of her need.

Cathy is an inspiration to us all…and while it is not "official", we believe that Cathy is the World's present longest surviving heart/double lung recipient!

Cathy McGill, 57
Moline, Illinois
Eisenmenger Syndrome
Heart/Double Lung Transplant, July 13, 1985
University of Pittsburgh Medical Center, Pittsburgh, Pennsylvania
Kidney Transplant, September 28, 2005
University of Iowa Hospitals and Clinics and Iowa City VA Medical, Iowa City, Iowa
(Story Written by Joanne Schum)
Read Cathy's Lung Transplant Story in the 1st Edition of Taking Flight

 My Journey Towards "Breathin' Easy"
By John McHale

My journey towards lung transplantation, and eventually towards "Breathin' Easy" (which I'll explain further later on) began in November 2000 at age 38 when I developed a dry cough that wouldn't go away. I went to my local physician who referred me to a local pulmonologist who diagnosed it as, "cough variant asthma". I thought this diagnosis was rather strange since I was otherwise a healthy man, never had asthma as a child and never smoked, but I accepted the diagnosis as the cough was merely an annoyance at that point and wasn't affecting my quality of life in any way.

Things all changed while on a vacation trip to the Grand Canyon in August 2005. That is, one day while hiking in the canyon suddenly I couldn't walk 50 feet without becoming extremely short of breath. I had that "gut feeling" right then that this was something more serious than cough variant asthma, but I never dreamed what was to come.

My pulmonologist sent me for an X-ray Computed Tomography (CT or CAT) scan. The scan revealed pulmonary fibrosis (scarring) in both lungs. The doctor referred me to a surgeon to do a surgical lung biopsy to confirm or refute what the CT scan said. My lung biopsy surgeon called me at work and told me that I had "UIP - usual interstitial pneumonia".

Curiosity got the best of me and I looked up UIP on the Internet. I stared at the screen in disbelief as I read a *New England Journal of Medicine* article which explained that UIP was another term for IPF – Idiopathic Pulmonary Fibrosis, a disease of unknown origin resulting in the progressive scarring (fibrosis) of the lungs for which there currently is no cure. The average expected survival period is 2-5 years from diagnosis unless the patient receives a lung transplant.

As I read this information and then went on to read additional articles, I couldn't believe it. "This must be a mistake"; "I'm only 43-years-old"; "I have a 12-year-old son"; "The holidays are coming up"; "How am I going to tell my wife and son?"…"How can it be that I'm dying?" were some of the thoughts that flew through my mind.

My local pulmonologist candidly told me that he was only a "country doc" when it came to IPF so he referred me to the Hospital of the University of Pennsylvania, Philadelphia, Pennsylvania (HUP) to investigate the transplant process. From the moment I met the staff there I felt at ease and never doubted that they would do their best to help me.

I tried to stay as active as possible. I even continued to go to work with a portable oxygen tank when commuting and a concentrator under my desk at work. I found maintaining my "normal" daily routine to be helpful as it made me think about things other than my disease.

Three months to the day of being listed, I received "the call". However, it turned out that the donor lungs were not viable and I was sent home. I received a second call a month later, but again the lungs were not viable and I was sent home. Finally, on May 25, 2008 I received the third call and the "third time was the charm" and I received my new lungs on May 26 – Memorial Day.

I had some post-op complications, but I continued to progress towards the goal of getting my "normal" life back and the journey was marked by "milestones" – being able to walk to the end of the driveway with a walker; walking to the end of the street without a walker; being able to drive again; having my feeding tube removed and being able to eat "real" food again; and returning to work on a limited basis in January, 2010.

I consider my biggest milestone to date to be the fact that I was able to walk 3K (2 miles) on April 18, 2010 as part of the Gift of Life's 15th Annual Donor Dash in Philadelphia with my wife, son and 18 other members of our "Breathin' Easy" team. The Dash is held to honor organ donors and their families and to raise awareness of the importance of organ donation. It was very emotional for me to participate in that event as it was a great day for me to celebrate my second chance at life with my family and friends while at the same time thinking about my donor and their family. I plan to participate in the Dash every year to honor them.

Throughout my entire ordeal I have had the overwhelming love and support of my wife and son, brother and sisters, in-laws and other relatives, friends, neighbors, and colleagues. Having such a great support system was critical to my recovery as there were many days when I wondered if I could make it through another day and their unwavering support helped to pull me through. I will be eternally grateful to them for that.

In closing, I thank God, my donor and their family, all of the doctors, nurses and other medical professionals who treated me and all those who were there to lend their support. I would not be here today was it not for you and I have no words to thank you enough for that.

John McHale, 48
Bridgewater, New Jersey
Idiopathic Pulmonary Fibrosis
Double Lung Transplant, May 26, 2008
Hospital of the University of Pennsylvania, Philadelphia, Pennsylvania

If God Brings You to it, He Will Bring You Through It
By Sandy Metheany

My life has been an exciting journey. To say it has had its ups and downs would be an understatement. As the fifth child of ten, I was destined for an exciting life. I experienced polio at age two, two broken arms at eight and a diagnosis of Cystic Fibrosis at nine. A brother and sister also had Cystic Fibrosis, and life expectancy for all of us was grim.

When I was just sixteen, my older sister died. She did not have a desire to live with such a devastating illness, but I did. I followed every bit of advice I got from the medical community and knew I would fight until the last moment. But I couldn't have imagined all that my life would turn out to be.

For years I faithfully took all breathing treatments, did my postural drainage, thumping, took medicines and even slept in a mist tent, as prescribed by my doctors. One of my legs had been severely compromised from the polio and this further limited what I could possibly accomplish in life. I assumed I would never find someone to love me with all of my problems, yet the day after Jon came home from the service we met and were married in seven months. Our joy was complete when, five years later, our daughter Jodi was born.

My faith, which has dominated my life and given me strength, grew and grew during these years. With each hardship, God sent all the graces I needed to overcome as many health problems until finally in 2001 I was told I needed a double lung transplant. My physical strength was completely depleted yet somehow I was able to see my only child through her wedding preparations. By this time I was on prayer chains literally around the world.

In 2003 my beloved mother-in-law died and my daughter announced that she was pregnant. My emotions were twirling in so many directions!

Only five weeks after achieving the waiting list the first call came in. But eight hours later we were told that the donated lungs were infected and could not be used. So the wait began again. Three months later, the second call came.

So by God's goodness, and against all odds, I have lived to see three of my grandchildren born. I will be forever grateful and so will my wonderful family, to the family, which was generous enough in their own grief to give me the gift of life.

Now I am able to experience life pretty much to the fullest. I no longer need oxygen 24 hours a day (24/7), any breathing treatments, or help with my home and garden. I love camping with my family. It was awesome to be fishing with my grandson, Braeden when he caught his first fish at age three, then again with his sister, Serena when she was four and caught her first fish. I now look forward in the future to teaching Annika how to fish.

We all love riding 4-wheelers, especially to go rock hunting. On one trip with my hubby and sister and brother, we rode 56 miles in one day just enjoying the beauty God created, among which were wild horses, antelope, badgers and bald eagles. While hunting rocks in eastern Oregon I found a 68-pound thunder egg (the Oregon State rock).

My koi and goldfish are a great source of joy for me. When I was extremely ill my oxygen hose would just allow me to go out as far as my pond and sit and meditate and watch the fish. Now I enjoy planting flowers and bulbs and caring for the pond mostly by myself. I do wear a mask and gloves to keep from contact with the fungus and life threatening organisms. This is a very important part of maintaining health post transplant along with taking many pills every day.

It now seems there are not enough hours in the day to accomplish all I want to do. Besides all the outdoor activities I like to bake and do many crafts. I can now care for all our household needs, as well as preserve the many fruits and vegetables from our garden. But my most favorite thing is to spend time with my grandchildren. Being a "Grammy" is about the most important and most enjoyable job I have ever had.

These days I have a passion for talking to school kids and others about organ and tissue donation. I also participate in two bible studies each week, one of which I frequently lead. These wonderful new lungs also allow me to sing in the choir at church. Words cannot express how thankful I am for this gift of new life I received from God and from a stranger.

When you die, don't take your organs to heaven, please. Heaven knows we need them here.

Sandy Metheany, 58
Molalla, Oregon
Cystic Fibrosis
Double Lung Transplant, June 24, 2003
University of Washington Medical Center, Seattle, Washington

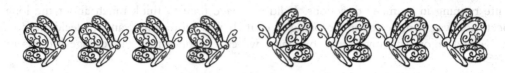

Breathing with Joy
By Piali Mukherjee

"God, can I ever again have the luxury of taking in deep, lungful breaths, one after the other?" I cry out in agony! Woken up all of a sudden by a coughing fit, in the middle of the night, I frantically search for my nebulizer mask. As the machine starts its gentle humming lullaby and a steam of mist makes its way towards my scarred lungs, I know that God has once more held me in His loving embrace, and I can hear Him whispering of a better day waiting ahead-a day of easy, unlabored breaths…

Breathing is an activity that most people take for granted, paying little attention to it unless there is a hindrance. And there are a group of people, who have to be thankful for the few moments, when they do not have to be consciously aware of the act of breathing. In the 31 springs that I have seen till now, I have the experience of both and that is why to me every breath is a blessing, no matter whether it is easy or labored…

Diagnosed with bronchiectasis, asthma, osteoporosis, atrial fibrillation and retinal degeneration of both eyes, medical management is a normal way of my life. Living most of the time with the feeling of breathing through a large-bore coffee straw isn't very pleasant always. Add to it the fact that I stay alone in a city as a paying guest and handle a job in the media and Public Relations department in a leading international-standard hospital. Life just can't get more interesting!!

Childhood charms and salad days…
But it wasn't like this always. I had a relatively healthy childhood, with occasional chest infections, measles and a diagnosis of retinal degeneration in both eyes. An avid biker, I crisscrossed our town many times a day and by the age of 18 years, toured most of India with my parents. I had my first serious bout of a chest infection and hospitalization at the age of 16, when the severe respiratory distress made me turn dirty blue and cold. Before I could recover from the hospitalization, with oxygen and intravenous (IV) antibiotics, our family received the terrible blow of losing my only elder sister, aged 32, due to sudden cardiac arrest in her sleep.

During my college years, I developed some heart issues (alas, not the romantic ones!!). Known as atrial fibrillation. I was diagnosed with uncontrolled asthma with severe chest infection. We were so concerned with the cardiac issue that the 'asthma' bit did not sink in at all. We were more eager to get the curative therapy for heart trouble. But with my problem area lying very close to my natural pacemaker, the ablation therapy (frying of the short-circuiting wire) was not possible. While prescribing medicines to slow down my heart rate, my Cardiologist told my father 'her heart will be fine but you need to closely watch for her lungs. They need good care'.

With life running in so many directions, I did not have time to think much about the long-term prospect, nor was I interested in brooding over it. It was more important to decide as to which movie I could enjoy with my friends or where we can fix up a picnic!! Teenage life has its own charms☺

After my graduation, I took the tough decision of leaving the loving nest of my parents and come to Kolkata, the Metro city in search of a career. Tough for me but more so, for my parents. After the tragic loss of one daughter, their heart wrenched to let me go. Still they let me fly. Parents can only make a sacrifice like this!!

Out in the city…
In Kolkata, I maintained two jobs; one in an informational technology (IT) company as Centre Manager and Chief Trainer and the other; in a heart hospital as a writer, working seven days a week. By this time I had mastered (or so I thought!) the art of asthma management. Chest infection, shortness of breath and weakness increased gradually making movement difficult. It went to an extent when my doctors advised me to use wheelchairs to conserve energy. It was a tough decision for an active and independent individual. But staying miles away, my parents somehow convinced me to carry on with the treatments and inspired me to make the best of each day.

It was in 2006 that a computerized Tomography (CT) scan detected bronchiectasis and emphysema. A port-a-cath was implanted for easy antibiotic injections. I had countless hospital admissions and visits to the emergency room but with the support from the hospital and my doctors, I managed to maintain an active life. At that point I came in contact with Pranic Healing, a no-drug, no-touch complementary energy therapy, developed by the Chinese Filipino Energy Master Choa Kok Sui. It helped improve my condition physically, emotionally, mentally and spiritually.

Getting a firm ground and steady support…
For any chronic patient, it is very important to build up a strong bond of trust with the doctor, who can and will do anything to help his/her patients. When we were utterly frustrated at my decline, thankfully I found that doctor. Dr. Raja Dhar, an accomplished pulmonologist, joined our hospital and I was immediately placed under his care; the best medical decision taken about me to date. The first thing he did was to put me at ease with my health. We started working as a team where my family and I always play an important role. Today he is not just my doctor but also a brother, someone whom I can look up on for support anytime for anything. Through him, I came to know Chandrima De, his friend who immediately became a very sweet sister of mine. After my parents, they are the greatest support person I have got to date.

Bacteria and fungus…in love with my lungs…
Much to my dislike, lately my lungs have been pretty gracious host to different species of bacteria and fungus!! While I had to be admitted on some occasions for IV tune-ups, mostly I have been able to manage the treatment outside the hospital, carrying on with home IV therapies. During August 2009, I had a severe bout of hemoptysis. In 2009, after two months of oral and nebulized antibiotic therapies, the bugs started getting smarter, which in medical jargon means multi-drug

resistant!! So in went another port-a-cath for IV therapies. (Thanks again Sandi, Med-Comp, USA for the free Port a Cath).

What lies next?...

Dr. Dhar explained me that bronchiectasis is an irreversible condition. Since all the lobes of both my lungs are affected to an extent, surgery to remove the diseased portion will not help me. But they are not bad enough to be thrown off for a new set☺. With my symptoms, he strongly suspects that I have a variant form of cystic fibrosis. While the risk of infection and further deterioration always looms large, we are totally focusing on maintaining stability. With God's blessings, I look forward to that day when I can walk and talk without getting breathless, enjoy a full meal without coughing fits, wake up in the morning and not spend hours clearing my lungs but draw in the first breath with ease...

Life gets better every moment ...

I am involved with Pranic Healing and Astara (a spiritual school) where I am learning to focus on the positive aspects of life. It is not about denying the occasional lows but expressing it in a constructive way and replacing it with hope. It's about making best of each opportunity that I get. Prayers, feeling of gratitude, letting go of the old hurts and pains and meditation help me a lot.

Staying alone in a city involves a lot of responsibility, which at times get overwhelming. But my parents are there with me, guiding me all along and supporting me through thick and thin. My relatives pitch in whenever needed. My colleagues are understanding and helpful. In lonely nights, when I wake up coughing and choking on blood and I am afraid, I know that I can call my doctor just to listen to his reassuring voice "you will be fine darling, just rest" or a cheerful message from Chandrima De to brighten my day. They do everything possible to make me happy; planning out a movie night, surprise gifts, celebrating my birthday in a grand way...the list continues!! A steady shoulder to rest on, they help me add the extra bounce to my steps. With so much of love and support, life becomes worth every moment!

My dream ...

I have a love affair with pen and paper since my early days and poetry gives me maximum creative freedom. Getting my poetry book 'Reach Out' published is a dream I nurture closest to my heart. I have written more than 60 poems on different subjects. Some of them have been published in international magazines and received awards. But I dream to reach out and touch many more hearts with my writings. With God's blessings in so many forms, I try making the best of every day. I believe that for anyone living with a chronic condition, it is important to learn from the Past, dream about the Future but focus more on the Present. That is something I learnt from my parents.

I strongly believe that my condition is meant to bring out some positive experience and that is what I strive each moment. I am involved with a number of support groups on bronchiectasis and cystic fibrosis and have recently hosted my website. Spreading awareness about bronchiectasis treatment and prevention is a mission I peruse enthusiastically. Working for underprivileged children, taking part in charitable service, speaking and writing projects motivate me to march ahead. I also have a dream of penning down a book on living a full life with different chronic lung conditions. My doctor has agreed to edit the book, which I have fondly named, 'When every breath is a Challenge, when every breath is a Blessing'.

I feel that Life is much more than medicines, hospitals, breathing treatments, injections and cough-punctuated nights. To me, it's the energy of basking in the first sunshine, the joy of watching a dazzling rainbow, the thrill of a joyride, whispering of a sweet nothing in ears, the assurance of always being there and the hope of a brighter day. No wonder, each breath of mine turns to Blessings Unlimited…

Update: Sadly, Piali passed away October 12, 2010. Her family, friends in India, and her "family of friends" around the world miss her very much. My good fortune has allowed me the pleasure of being friends with Piali for the past 10 years. ~~ Joanne Schum

~~~~

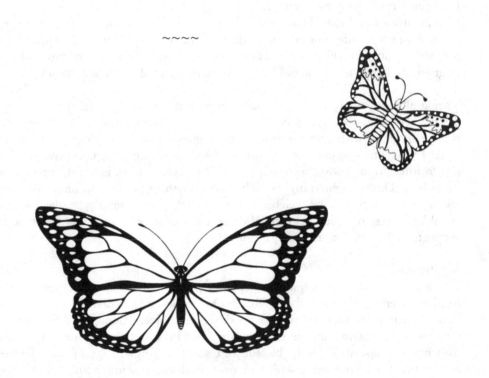

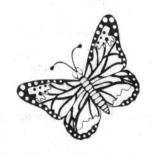

Looking for a Rainbow

As the scorching rays of blazing sun
Torch the heart of the globe,
I know rain clouds are on their way
To drizzle the Earth with showers of hope.

When relentless rain halt the life
And dark clouds rule all the while –
I search for a rainbow in the horizon
Waiting to dazzle with colorful smile!

As blanket of snow covers the forest
And lulls the entire nature to sleep,
Eyes wide open, I wait eagerly
For the tiny flowers of spring to peep.

When Life becomes a battle of breath
And seems to slip out like a handful of sand
I fight with both my body and mind
And look forward to hear God's command.

Till date He has made me the winner
On me His blessings do pour-
I celebrate the victory of each of my breath
And go on to love my Life even more!

~~Piali Mukherjee

Piali Mukherjee, 31
Kolkata, West Bengal, India
Bronchiectasis, Cystic Fibrosis
Pre-Double Lung Transplant
Apollo Gleneagles Hospitals, Kokata, India
Piali Passed Away, October 12, 2010
"Forever 31"

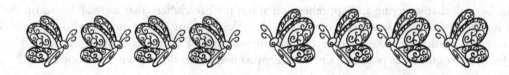

[228]

Nothing Short of a Miracle
By Mandy Murawski

Sitting here contemplating where to begin and how to go about explaining the progression of my life since my double lung transplant is more complicated than I could ever imagine. I have accomplished more than I ever dreamed I could, and I, also, feel compelled to inform other transplanted friends some very important tidbits I wish I had known after transplant. Plus, I have a very dear story to my heart I want to share with all of you about a very strong friend of mine. Adding to the complication of writing this story is I recently broke my very first bone, which happens to my pinky finger. Ha-ha, I don't even mean a little broke, I have wires and a pin sticking out of my little finger!

In the first edition of "*Taking Flight*", I talked about starting college and taking gym class for the first time in my entire life, after transplant. In gym, I learned who Billy Blanks is (Tae Bo) and that running is not my forte! My college days were the best of times (partying) and yet one of most stressful periods I tackled. I put a lot of pressure on myself to get good grades because I had missed so much school when I was young because of Cystic Fibrosis; I somehow felt I needed to prove something.

Fast forward a bunch, I graduated with a Bachelor degree in Accounting and a Master's in Management. I currently work for a small business owner doing accounting and administrative duties, which I enjoy very much. This month I flew my little sissy to see me for a quick visit, and it is awesome to have a relationship with my sister as a young adult. She is so beautiful and a fantastic artist. She is just starting college herself and plans to move to California soon. I am so excited for her and love being able to watch her grow and laugh (snort). In the first edition book I didn't mention my boyfriend because, hey, they sometimes just come and go. However, I am excited to brag we met soon after my transplant and he is still by my side.

If it weren't for my donor families' most unselfish gift of life, I wouldn't be here to keep experiencing life and all its wonderful moments. A second chance at life means more than just breathing; it means I am still growing and changing. I look back at my struggles and realize they have made me who I am. However, if I could go back to the first day I was transplanted, I wish I could tell myself so many things. I have talked to other transplant patients about the biggest regrets we have made or things (tidbits) we wish we had known. For some of us, we felt like our new lungs were like a ticking time bomb and we needed to live for today because tomorrow we might get rejection and "BOOM", second chance over (game over). We are told statistics on life expectancy, but we shouldn't really count on that "long" because of added risk factors. So this day has yet to come for me, and I want to take back all that worrying and apprehension about my life choices that were all based on the fear that I had limited time. I want to be more care free like so many others my age who don't dwell on mortality. I would also like to take back some mistakes I made in thinking I needed to live everything up as quickly as possible, when I really just needed to slow down and enjoy life!

I would, also, tell myself to stay concentrated on my health even though I felt good. It is easy to focus solely on your health when you're dying because that consumes your psyche. However, it is another story when you're feeling great and you're busy with friends, family, college, work, etc. I got a little too passive with my healthcare and want to warn others not to make the same oversights I have made. To all transplant patients, you need to understand your pulmonary function test (PFT's) and lab numbers; be sure to have them checked often. They should also recognize normal ranges on all tests/labs and watch any trends. I know this seems like common sense but never assume anything when it comes to your healthcare. Stay aggressive!

I have been thinking a lot about my donor family. I plan on writing them again; I never heard anything from the first letter, but maybe it was too soon. I want to meet them and tell them they have given me more than just "lungs"; they have given me a "life"! Another reason I have been thinking so much about them is because of a dear friend of mine's gift. I was on the receiving end of the "gift", which felt nothing short of a miracle, but never allowed myself to fully comprehend it came from someone else's tragedy. I guess it was my mind's way of minimizing the guilt of living because someone else died. I have now witnessed the strength it takes to donate the most unselfish gift of life, and that is "nothing short of a miracle"!

Let me tell you about my dear friend, Nick. I met him and his mother at my campaign fundraiser for my transplant over 13 years ago. They both helped with my campaign and continued to stay in touch with me throughout the years. Nick was always a good friend to me, so I was happy to hear he was blessed with a healthy baby boy. His little baby boy was named Andrew, which everyone called him "Roo". Nick was a wonderful father to little Roo, and you could see Roo was his everything! I felt like I knew little "Roo" through all Nick's Facebook updates. I remember Nick was so excited about Roo's upcoming birthday party when he would be turning three-years-old. However, little Roo never made it to his third birthday. He had a rare, unfortunate condition called Acute Hyponatremia, which causes cerebral edema. Nick's mother called me from the Children's Hospital and told me that Nick's little Roo had passed away and Nick was filling out the organ donor papers. Tears ran down my face because they were suffering through the most heartbreaking circumstances imaginable and somehow they still wanted me to know of their generous gift of life. Later at the funeral, Nick came up to me and said, "Mandy, did you hear? Roo and I got to save a little Mandy. Roo's lungs went to a little five-year-old girl with Cystic Fibrosis." The strength my friend possessed said it came from his love for his son. I believe his strength was nothing short of a miracle!

As you can see, I had a lot to share and was worried it wouldn't come out adequately. If you didn't like my story, I am blaming it on my broken pinky (ha-ha). It has been over 10 years since my transplant and I hope for many more years. My breathing numbers are still super high and I feel great. My future goals include one day becoming a homeowner and hopefully, adopting a child. I would, also, hope to be in the next edition of "Taking Flight" if the fragile Joanne Schum is up to it (bubble wrap)! I hope she knows we really appreciate all the work (patience) she does compiling these stories; they mean so much to us, the transplant/donor community! Again, like in the first edition, "my future has endless possibilities," this in itself is nothing short of a miracle!

Mandy Murawski, 30
Dickson, Tennessee
Cystic Fibrosis
Double Lung Transplant, February 10, 2000
University of North Carolina Hospitals, Chapel Hill, North Carolina
Read Mandy's Lung Transplant Story in the 1st Edition of Taking Flight

A Little More Time on This Earth
By Katie Murray

While I do not have Cystic Fibrosis (CF) myself, my journey with the disease began before I was even born, and is something that I will carry with me all my life. My dad, Roger, has CF. He was diagnosed at age 10, and made it through 37 years of life before he was truly 'sick'. Technology in the 1980's did not allow men with CF to have children, and as such, my parents made the extraordinary decision to have a baby using donor insemination. A donor, who I will never know anything about, is the reason that I am lucky enough to live in this world today. Throughout my life I have watched the trials and tribulations of this disease affect some of my closest relatives and loved ones. Working with the Canadian Cystic Fibrosis Foundation both as a staff member and volunteer has allowed me to meet countless CF and lung transplant patients, and seen first hand the amazing impact that organ donation can have. While I have many stories to tell, including the one of my own father who is now 17 years post-transplant, the story that will always resonate the loudest is of my aunt and uncle.

It was always their running joke that their eyes met across the treadmills. Where else but the hospital gym do you meet someone when you're a CF patient waiting a double-lung transplant? Despite their CF, both my Uncle Shawn and my 'soon to be' Aunt Annie always had an amazing zest for life. They shared the unique CF sense of humor and worldview – a world where things do not come easy, nothing is taken for granted, and yet life is an amazing blessing. We should all be so lucky as to see the world in this light.

Uncle Shawn was born twelve years after my dad, and diagnosed with CF at birth. Thanks to the mystery of modifier genes, Uncle Shawn was always a lot sicker than my dad, and faced more health struggles than anyone should have to. In the early 1990's, lung transplantation was still a fairly new technology, and when my dad, and then my uncle, was faced with the decision of being put on 'the list' for transplant, it was a challenge for even the strongest members of my family. I was very young at the time, but remember well the doctor office walls, the looks on people's faces, and the perceived urgency of the entire situation.

My dad and my uncle ended up on the waiting list for a double lung transplant at the same time – my dad was 37, my uncle 25. The wait would not be short for either of them, but while we all waited, the most extraordinary thing happened – our family expanded. The people that we met while attending support group meetings and other functions at the hospital (this, of course, was before the days of superbugs and other such scary things) became our family. We had things in common with these people that even my parent's closest friends could not understand – we shared a common bond where the threads of illness wound through our lives. And then, of course, there was my future Aunt, Annie.

Looking back 'soon to be' Aunt Annie and Uncle Shawn helped form my understanding of love, and perhaps even my unwavering belief in love and romanticism. They truly were like one soul in two bodies sometimes, and could have been mistaken for siblings, if not twins. They both had long brown hair, raspy CF voices, clubbed fingers, and a rebellious streak. They both had tattoos before it was 'cool', and they both shared an amazing sense of humor. Annie, almost instantly it seemed, became a part of our family – both our transplant family, and our 'real' family.

To look back on their love, I think of how difficult it must have been at times to allow themselves to fall for each other. It is because of them that I know that true love is a force stronger than any illness – capable of overcoming fear and filling lives with light. There is always a great unknown in the lives of those living on a transplant wait list. The thoughts of timing always exist in the back of one's mind – "Where will I be when the call comes? Will the call come on time? What if it's a false alarm?" We must force ourselves to not let these questions take over, and to go about with our 'normal' lives, even if beneath the surface there is always some anxiety, some fear mixed with excitement, and even if our hearts skip a beat whenever the phone rings. To not only fall in love while awaiting a lung transplant, but to fall in love with another transplant patient laughs in the face of fear, defies the odds and is proof that there is no mountain to high.

While we all waited, 'soon to be' Aunt Annie and Uncle Shawn's relationship grew. Finally, on October 3rd, 1993, after almost two years of waiting, our journey to becoming a post transplant family began. I somehow knew as soon as the phone rang – it was my Dad's time. My mom drove while my dad sat in the back, writing down notes, instructions, and other things that he needed to share before going into surgery. Much of the hospital trip is a blur, aside from watching the elevator doors close behind my dad when they took him to the operating room – while I was not yet even a teenager, I knew enough to know that I might not see him again. The gut-wrenching night we spent waiting in the lounge outside of the intensive care unit mostly blurs together for me, though I do remember 'soon to be' Aunt Annie and Uncle Shawn bringing me a chocolate chip muffin. It's funny the things that stand out in a young mind.

My dad's transplant was an amazing success, though it was difficult to understand seeing him attached to tubes in the intensive care unit. Within days he was moving, and within two weeks he was in 'step-down'. His first trip out of the hospital was to take in the Blue Jay's Championship parade after they won the World Series of Baseball! In the years that followed his transplant, my dad has been able to spend time with me and watch me grow up, return to work, and take up an active lifestyle again. Amazing!

Only a few short weeks after my dad's transplant, Shawn received his call, and came though his transplant, and after two heart-breaking 'false alarms', Annie also received her transplant – the following May.

Finally 'soon to be' Aunt Annie and Uncle Shawn could live their life together as a (mostly) 'normal couple'. They were married in November 1994, in a beautiful ceremony in Sarnia, Ontario, Canada. They moved into a cute ground-floor apartment in Toronto, where I visited them. Aunt Annie was the first to allow me to wear make-up – applying natural colors to my face before a family event. She gave me a sweater, perfume and lip-gloss for Christmas. I looked up to her, and admired both her and Uncle Shawn. It was nothing short of beautiful having both of them around, breathing like 'normal' people.

Our family gathered together for Easter 1995 at my grandparent's house. I remember distinctly remarking, once we got in the car to head home, how skinny Uncle Shawn was – hugging him goodbye I could touch my arms together, elbow-to-elbow. Uncle Shawn was sick. That Easter dinner would be the last time I saw Shawn alive – he passed away the next month. The summer that followed was chaotic and sad. While Uncle Shawn's death was not entirely unexpected, the emotions that came with it were difficult for everyone. This was compounded by the knowledge that Aunt Annie's life was coming to an end, too.

One of the last times I saw Aunt Annie was when she gave me a small diamond ring that had been given to her by her older sister. The card, which has a simple teddy bear on the front, housed the words, "I hope one day you will wear this, and remember how much Shawn and I love you." I wear your ring often Aunt Annie, usually suspended from a chain on my neck, and I do remember, not only how much you both love me, but also how you taught me to believe in love, and in life. Annie left this world in the first days of September 1995, her bed surrounded by family, her sense of humor intact.

I carry Aunt Annie and Uncle Shawn's spirits with me – I think of them daily, sometimes simply cherishing their memory, sometimes selfishly frustrated that they are not here anymore. I take comfort in thinking that wherever they are, they can finally breathe. I carry their memory with me forever – both metaphorically and literally in the form of a tattoo in my left ankle that reads, 'Forever Young'. They both lived to be 28.

The gift of organ transplantation gave Aunt Annie and Uncle Shawn the chance for a little more time on this earth. They got to enjoy building the start of a home together, and we got to enjoy knowing them and watching their love grow. Aunt Annie and Uncle Shawn were inspirational in every way – teaching me both directly and indirectly how important it is to appreciate what we have, live life to its fullest, and that love is capable of helping us overcome life's biggest obstacles. I am honored to not only be related to Aunt Annie and Uncle Shawn, but to have been able to call them my friends.

All our donor families are heroes, to whom I owe not only the opportunity to grow up with a father, but the lessons of love and strength that my aunt and uncle showed me.

Katie Murray, Daughter of Roger Murray
Roger Murray, Cystic Fibrosis, Age 56
Ontario/Alberta, Canada
Roger, Double Lung Transplant, October 4th, 1993
Toronto General Hospital, Toronto, Ontario Canada

Katie Murray, Niece of Shawn Murray and Annie Riley Murray
Shawn and Annie Murray, Cystic Fibrosis
Shawn Murray, Double Lung Transplant, Late October 1993
Toronto General Hospital, Toronto Ontario, Canada
Annie Murray-Riley, Double Lung Transplant, Spring, 1994
Toronto General Hospital, Toronto, Ontario, Canada
Shawn Murray passed away: May 19, 1995 – "Forever 28"
Annie Murray-Riley passed away: September 3, 1995 – "Forever 28"

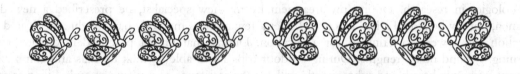

My Spirit Keeps Me Strong
By Ramesh Nankissoor

My spirit kept me strong, even when, at age 60, I faced the most difficult challenge – a double-lung transplant. Today my faith still keeps me strong.

Over 15 years ago I had a cough that wouldn't go away, even after several treatments. Eventually I was sent for a chest X-ray. I was diagnosed with pneumonia. This was not possible because my temperature was normal and I was not sick.

I was a very active person and was the type who would normally run up and down stairs rather than walk. One day I was completely out of breath and had to stop running halfway up the stairs. I knew something was wrong. This time my family doctor referred me to a respirologist who requested a lung biopsy. The biopsy revealed a condition called 'Sarcoidosis'. I was devastated. Little was known about Sarcoidosis, (an Internet search resulted in four lines total) but it was treated aggressively with steroids. This treatment seemed to stabilize the "raging fires" in my lungs.

Many years later, having lived a reasonable life, my lungs started showing signs of declining function. At this time I was referred to another respirologist, one involved in more up to date treatments and technologies in research. During my treatment by my new specialist, he prescribed a new drug regimen, but my body had a bad reaction. After a few months my body had fought and cleared the infection and I went to Trinidad for a vacation. During that time I practiced meditation every morning. I found new strengths. During outdoor trips I was able to walk up hills and climb stairs without losing my breath and subsequently without the assistance of my oxygen tank. Life was great once more and I was full of hope. Then I contracted another infection.

Life was becoming very difficult. I was losing weight and was coughing incessantly. My doctor recommended the option of a lung transplant. At that moment I was overcome by so many emotions: shock, fear, and disbelief to name a few. I was aware that lung transplants were done in Toronto, Canada, but now it was my reality.

During a meeting with the transplant team in Toronto, I was told the life expectancy post transplant is five years. Despite the risks, my family and I agreed that five years was a decent amount of time and I was ready to take my chances with the transplant. The potential benefits of a successful surgery would be better than the life I was living now.

I am involved with an organization that teaches meditation, and offers support to families that are faced with life crises. We are also taught about dealing with death and dying. I believe that my body is a vehicle to carry me through life, but it's not all that I am. I am not the body. My spirit and faith are what keep me strong.

While undergoing the transplant medical assessments, my body was too weak to commute so I stayed at the hospital. Due to another infection, I was there for a month. During that stay I developed acute anxieties. I had a real fear of running out of oxygen. I was afraid of running water; I thought I would drown in the shower, I was afraid of lying down and falling asleep forever.

While I was hospitalized my house had to be sold. My daughter and her husband had to move back to Toronto from Australia. My oldest son and his wife spent hours by my bedside. My youngest son prayed for me and visited every chance he got while studying at University.

Six months of agonizing waiting passed when the phone rang and the hospital told my wife, "WE HAVE LUNGS FOR HIM". We prayed all the way to the hospital. My nine-hour operation was a complete success.

Three weeks after the surgery I was home and on my way to living a full life. I was walking out in the park almost every day and fully enjoying nature. Breathing in the fresh air is a wonderful feeling. I can easily walk 5km and even organized a group to participate in a fundraising walk. My kids who walked with me joked that they were the ones keeping up with me!

My wife and I are finally able to travel freely. I've been back to Trinidad twice; to Orlando, Florida twice and look forward to many more trips. We plan to see as much of the world as we can. Our next trip includes Vancouver, the Rocky Mountains and an Alaskan cruise. I attend family gatherings regularly and it's a joy to see my family change and grow, especially my youngest son. A year after the surgery I was able to see him graduate from University. Only a few months later, we were in Orlando, Florida celebrating his wedding. It was a grand event that ended with all of us dancing the night away. It was the first time I danced post surgery and I was the only one on the dance floor with gray hair. I should have been embarrassed but I have too much to celebrate.

I can walk, I can talk without coughing, and I can breathe.

I thank God every day for inspiring the donor family who gave me a second chance at life and for keeping my spirit strong. I am forever grateful, and pledge to take good care of my precious new lungs. Special gratitude goes to my ever-supportive wife and children, and of course the transplant team at Toronto General Hospital, Toronto, Canada.

Above all it was made possible by God's grace.

Ramesh Nankissoor, 62
Toronto, Canada
Sarcoidosis
Double Lung Transplant, May 9, 2009
Toronto General Hospital, Toronto, Canada

Waiting for Lungs - September 23, 2007
By Andree Niefield

One day my life will be full again
My lungs will take big breaths out and in
My step will be lively; my laugh will be brilliant
My life will be filled with hope and resilience

But now I am waiting and wanting in my transitory life
Holding on to each moment that comes free of strife
Inhale, then exhale, no more can I take this for granted
As I wait for the day with new lungs transplanted

Every day is a struggle, who knows what my plight is
My chest tightens, my breathing is shallow, a continuous fight
It would be easy to shut down, to cry, to give up the struggle
But then where would that leave me, so in spiritual strength I nuzzle

I reach down so deep to bring out the strength buried inside
It's been in reserve building up, as I dig through vanity and pride
Cut through that ego, just do what needs to be done
There is no time for excuses; the game has begun

The game is to stay alive, the game that keeps this tired soul going
Breathing in - breathing out – please keep this process flowing
I anxiously wait for the call, for a miracle, day or night
To receive the gift of life and soar into flight

~~~~

My First Thanksgiving
In Honor of Dolly, My Organ Donor - November 20, 2009

It is hard to believe my good fortune that today I am still here

It is hard to believe that I've been given a second chance to live with no fear
One year ago my breathing were encumbered
One year ago my days were numbered

Today I am breathing freely by the grace of an angel who saved me as my time was just about to end
My time was running out; I could no longer pretend
That everything was still fine as I gasped for each breath that was so difficult to attain
I was preparing for the worst when finally the call that saved me came

And now it is Thanksgiving – a time to reflect and remember the year that has passed
How much more meaningful this has become when I thought that would have been my last
I am joyous, I am grateful; I am overwhelmed with the presence of life's existence
How fortunate I am to experience every day with persistence

So thank you my donor for the greatest gift I will ever know
You have given me a chance again and I promise you that although
You are no longer present yet your soul shines through my eyes
Forever I hold you in my heart, my soul and my cries

Thank you my dearest donor

Andree Niefield, 57
New York, New York
Idiopathic Pulmonary Fibrosis
Double Lung Transplant, March 19, 2009
New York Presbyterian Hospital/Columbia University, Medical Center, New York, New York

The Mountains that Surround our Home
By Steve Ollila

The first visit to the Louvre Museum, Paris, France is a revelation. The scope and size of the paintings is a shock, in a book the small reproductions give no hint that the originals cover entire walls two and sometimes three stories high. Another surprise is the diminutive size of its most famous treasure the Mona Lisa. It was in these magnificent galleries that I shared some of the last days of my mother Betty Lou's life.

Like so many who will be reading this book she was diagnosed with Pulmonary Fibrosis. A rural Minnesota housewife she had always loved art and actively painted on everything in sight, flower pots, light switch covers, cards, decorating them with squirrels, flowers, trees. Weeks after her diagnosis I struck upon the idea of a trip to Paris, so she could see the great art of the Western world. She bravely embraced the idea and a few months later we were checking into a small hotel near the Tuileries Gardens. It was a memorable week, with oxygen tanks on her lap; I would push the wheelchair to a new gallery each morning. The Parisians were gracious as they waved us to the front of each line.

As she slept each night her lungs would gasp for air with a terrible rattle. The sound was unsettling and left little doubt about the deterioration of her fragile body. Unknowingly I was also glimpsing my own destiny.

We returned safely home after our memorable week and resumed our routine. I would call each morning to check on her day ahead and the night before. She would report on the birds at the feeder or the Minnesota weather, never a complaint about her own struggles. Then one morning it was I who got the call, Betty Lou had passed away that morning.

[238]

Years later while skiing at our local area I abruptly pulled up to the side gasping for air. Normally I would have cruised non-stop to the bottom without a thought. After catching my breath I continued on, attributing the puzzling stop to a lack of my usual conditioning.

Ten months later during a routine physical, Dr. Frank Batcha reported that he could hear crackling in my lungs and recommended an appointment with a pulmonologist. A bout of pneumonia and a couple months later, Dr. William Bergquist diagnosed idiopathic pulmonary fibrosis. Shortly after the diagnosis I simultaneously contracted a bacterial, viral and fungal pneumonia, the impact severely compromised my pulmonary function and my physical deterioration seemed to be accelerating. With little hope available from traditional pharmaceutical protocols I was referred to renowned pulmonologist Dr. Ganesh Raghu at the University of Washington Medical Center, Seattle, Washington (UW), perhaps a clinical trial could offer a ray of hope.

Drug therapies failed to halt the advance of the tissue scarring, so Dr. Raghu suggested lung transplant as our last option, he described it as, "Not a big deal, but the biggest deal". Since we live ten hours by car from the UW Medical Center we arranged for a jet charter when the call came. Amazingly two days after listing the phone rang and we rushed to the airport. Just as we were ready to board, the transplant coordinator called to declare a dry run, the donor lung would not be viable for our transplant.

With winter approaching we moved temporarily to Seattle, renting an apartment with Transplant House to ensure easier access to the medical center. My resident angel and wife, Becky Ross diligently kept working in Idaho and would fly to Seattle on the weekends to prepare my meals for the week as well as doing the apartment housekeeping. The selfless support and love of caregivers like Becky is the parallel story to the experience of a transplant patient. During the week, transplant alums Kim and Julia Lebert and many close Seattle friends kept a watchful eye on my progress. Co-workers, family, friends and local businesses held a fundraiser at home while I was in Seattle; the emotional and financial support was invaluable.

I continued to work remotely on my laptop as we patiently waited. The pull of gravity was growing stronger with each passing day. Becky and I always joked that the call would come while she was en route to or from Idaho. I called her while she was driving across the high desert on her way home, that UW had called. She did an about face on the snowy highway as I headed to the hospital.

On December 14, 2009, Dr. Michael Mulligan transplanted a single lung for me and another recipient, a real life Santa Claus no less. A selfless loving family had saved our lives while struggling through their own personal tragedy.

For Becky and me, they not only saved my life, but they preserved our dreams. We had only been married a year when our personal tragedy struck. We were working hard so Becky could finish school and begin a teaching career. The recovery has been slow, but steady and once again we can dream of Becky in her own classroom. I hope to find ways to pay it back and forward, contributing to finding a cure for pulmonary fibrosis and improving the viability and availability of lung transplants.

Dr. Raghu continues to monitor my progress from all parts of the world and Becky continues to take care of me here at my side. The mountains that surround our home will soon be our destination.

Our gratitude to the donor family, the incredible doctors, family, neighbors, friends and our community is something we'll never forget. My gratitude and love for my personal angel and wife Becky is boundless.

Steve Ollila, 58
Hailey, Idaho
Idiopathic Pulmonary Fibrosis
Single Lung Transplant, December 14, 2009
University of Washington Medical Center, Seattle, Washington

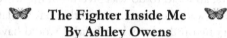 **The Fighter Inside Me**
By Ashley Owens

My story is one of love, faith, and a lot of luck. I have always thought of myself as a lucky person. Don't get me wrong, I have had a lot of bad luck, but I have had a whole lot of good luck as well.

It was Friday the 13th November 2009, a day that is notorious among superstitious believers to be a day of misfortune. For me, it was the day that set in motion the events that would ultimately save my life.

I knew I was dying, everyone knew I was dying. As much as I tried to cover up my cold blue fingers, purple lips, the oxygen I wore at night and should wear during the day, and my gasping for air, it was still no secret. It was also something all of us knew would happen one day. It was simply the nature of cystic fibrosis. For two years my doctors and family tried talking me into going on the list to get a double lung transplant. To be honest, it scared the hell out of me. I was determined to put it off for as long as possible.

Friday the 13th I drove myself to school and parked right by my class. It was pouring rain and I had trouble walking with a lung function of 20%. I tried to take a breath to prepare for what I knew would be an excruciatingly painful walk. My body began to shake and tears built in my eyes from the pain of my worn out lungs. I only had to cross a street, but to me it might as well been a hundred miles.

I collapsed on the other side of the street and let the rain pour down on me. I managed to get out my phone and dial Jesse's number. Jesse is my amazing boyfriend. This would be where my good luck comes in. Jesse and I met when we were both only seventeen in a study hall at our high school, and we have been madly in love ever since. He has stood by my side and helped me fight this disease outstandingly, passionately, and with love. Jesse had gotten a tattoo of "65 Roses," which is what little children call cystic fibrosis. He got the tattoo on his wrist and told me, "That way I will carry it with me too. We are in this together." He also sat with me while I did my treatments, spent time with me in the hospital, he would carry me around since I stopped being able to walk, and he even would wear oxygen out in public with me, so I was not alone in this war.

Jesse came to my rescue as soon as he could. We were both students at West Chester University, West Chester, Pennsylvania and his class just happened to be beside mine. He lifted my small, 69-pound body up effortlessly and whisked me away into the shelter of the school building.

"You cannot keep doing this!" he said frantically trying to dry me down and warm me up with his jacket. "I can't watch you suffer anymore… I can't lose you… Please… as much as I don't want to admit it - you need to go on the list… before it's too late." My whole body was so weak from no body fat and high levels of carbon dioxide. "Now I'm going to take you home, but you seriously need to consider going on the list." I then said, "Well I made it this far - I might as well go to class," I panted. It took some convincing but that's what I ended up doing.

Once home I called my doctor. "I'm ready," I breathed into the phone. I had already done the three-day evaluation, signed the papers, all I had to do was give them the word, and that is what I did. They told me I would probably have to wait six to twelve months. Hours later, my right lung collapsed. I was later told that if I had not gone on the list when I did, I would have been considered too sick to go on the list. I made it just in time.

Jesse and my parents rushed me to St. Christopher's Hospital for Children, Philadelphia, Pennsylvania. I spent the next week in critical care. My cousin Adrian left her job and drove all the way from Virginia to be with me. My family was told not to expect me to make it to Christmas. I was at the top of the list. In the next few days, I actually started to improve. Unfortunately, I started coughing up blood. The doctors informed us that the best chances of survival would be if I were transported to the Hospital of the University of Pennsylvania (HUP), Philadelphia, Pennsylvania, where my lung transplant would take place.

I called Jesse. Jesse, my dad, and brother Robert all left their job so they could be with me during my time of need. (My mom was already with me.) I then, shaking, set out to write my good-bye letters, and prepared myself to die. Jesse's embrace provided me with the comfort I so badly needed. His eyes were teary, but he remained positive. "We are going to get through this. You are going to get the surgery and everything will be okay. I will be right here beside you the whole time, and I promise to be there for you no matter what happens. We are going to get through this and grow old together. I want to spend the rest of my life with you," with that, Jesse dropped down on one knee. He pulled out the most beautiful ring I have ever seen, and my breath was officially gone.

Everything he said was so beautiful and I knew he meant every word. He honestly believed I would survive and that we would spend the rest of our lives together. I wanted so badly everything he said, to be true. His courage and faith gave me the courage I needed to keep fighting. I agreed to go to HUP. I would make it; I would survive! After all, I had a wedding to plan now.

Miraculously, just three days later, on November 23, 2009, I received new lungs. And so far everything Jesse said has come to be! I am now 23 and just celebrated my one-year survival! I will be graduating December 19, 2010 to be an elementary teacher. Jesse and I are still doing great and are planning our wedding, which we hope to celebrate June 2011. During our years together I had written letters to Jesse, highlighting my battle with cystic fibrosis, and how I would not have survived without Jesse's love. I hope to try to even publish these love letters into a book. This is a real life tragic love story with a wonderful, uplifting ending.

Also, another amazing thing that has happened is that I found out my lungs came from a professional athlete! His name was Paco Rodriguez, and he was a lightweight boxer. "Gift of Life" and ESPN even arranged it so I could meet his family and thank them! His wife Sonia, daughter Ginette, and the rest of his family welcomed me with open arms. We are all now a family and I am so happy to have gotten the chance to thank his wife for making the decision for her 25-year-old husband to donate his organs. That decision saved mine, and four other lives! Paco's story is being aired during April; organ donor awareness month, on E-60, channel ESPN.

A little over a year ago I was sure I was going to die. Now, I have a bright future where I will get to teach young children, get married to the most amazing man in the world, and have health I never dreamed of possessing. I can actually say that I have lungs of a fighter - in many ways that is what I am. I feel as though I truly am the luckiest girl in the world!

Ashley Owens, 23
Spring City, Pennsylvania
Cystic Fibrosis
Double Lung Transplant, November 23, 2009
Hospital of the University of Pennsylvania, Philadelphia, Pennsylvania

I Come to You Through the Courtesy of Love
By Alex Pangman

Since yesterday, I have spent six hours on stage singing. Singing, and clapping, snapping and laughing, smiling and breathing in and out beautifully through new lungs. I've held long notes, made soft breathy sounds, expressive, and belted it out—all things I couldn't do anymore in the time leading up to my double lung transplant in 2008.

You see I am a vocalist by profession. I was also born with Cystic Fibrosis (CF); something I kept a guarded trade secret, fearing it was not nearly as romantic as the blind blues musician in popular culture. No, indeed: a jazz singer doing her intravenous antibiotics backstage at a music festival, or coughing up blood on intermission, is not sexy. Nor beautiful. But it was who I was, and I dealt with it privately. Cruelly ironic to be a singer so afflicted, but that's just the way it was.

Most of my life I was healthy enough, managing to go to school, ride horses most days of the week, and make music. But as the hemoptysis got worse and the antibiotics stopped working, we started to see my lung function drop into scary territory.

You all know the story: your life gets whittled away until you are just a shadow of your former self. I still rode my horse several days a week; it was the only form of physiotherapy that would gently help to move the mucous that was clogging up my lungs and scarring them (every other form of physiotherapy made me choke up rivers of blood). I have an amazing old pony named Gypsy who has been my companion since 1989 and we've done it all together. She is always adaptable and always in tune with my health. And for the two years prior to my transplant she miraculously changed from a feisty beast to one who stood for me patiently as I fiddled with oxygen lines, and waited as I endlessly caught my breath. From her I borrowed legs, lungs... I borrowed freedom.

And apart from riding, the other thing that defines me is singing. Singing isn't something I do, it is WHO I AM! Even at 28% lung function I was still in the recording studio, although, even I had to admit that some days the slavish editing to remove all the phlegm and crackles was becoming excessive.

Blessedly it did, after I'd been half a year on the list. After one false alarm (we call those a "rehearsal" in show business!) the real call came on November 4, 2008. As they wheeled me into the operating room I looked around at everyone—and though I can hardly believe I said this to the crowd of folks assembled to SAVE MY LIFE—I nervously said, "Hi! I'm a singer, so please can you be careful passing those tubes past my vocal chords?!"

Well, it's been over a year now, and the vocal chords survived the ordeal, though the lungs not without some minor complications along the way. But would you believe I'm back to working again and singing all night and dancing and galloping around on horseback. I'm back to being MYSELF again! And can I say that singing is fantastic! To identify as an artist, a vocalist no less, it is so mind blowing to be given one's craft back. Yes, we all need lungs to breathe, to survive. Yet for some, like athletes and musicians, breath defines us. In tiny increments over many years I watched as my art was stolen from me by CF. Miraculously, in the space of an eight-hour surgery and through the most generous donation of my donor, it was given back to me; completely. In fact, I think my craft is better than ever, as I don't have to plot a verse around a coughing fit or phlegm. I open my mouth; my lungs flood with air to support my voice and music comes out – not disease or illness, but MUSIC! I've gone from singing through the equivalent of a straw to singing through a giant mega phone! I've gone from dreading walking up a flight of stairs, tangled in oxygen hose, to trotting up the stage steps.

Singing love-songs has always been a joy of mine. And now? Now when I sing a love song—think of a lyrical beauty from the 1930s—those love songs make all the more sense to me. Lyrics like "I know why I've waited," or "you came to me from out of nowhere" are all easy dedications to the donor of my new lungs and the second wind I've been given. There's one song I have recorded that particularly fits the bill here: it contains the line, "I come to you through the courtesy of love". And yes, yes I do!

So now, with this gift I've been given I hope to spread the word: to tell people just how it is that I come to sing for them! I am in fact singing with somebody else's lungs. Doesn't that blow your mind? Though they feel as one with me now, I can't ever know whom these lungs belonged to, (that information being kept anonymous in Canada) but they raise my voice in song and my heart to wonderful heights with every breath.

Thank you. Thank you, a million times over to my donor and their family who made this possible. Thank you to the great doctors who saw me through this and who continue to help me along the post-transplant journey, which is not without challenges, I admit. If "health is wealth", then I pray this good fortune continues. *Thank you!!!!*

Alex Pangman, 34
Toronto, Ontario, Canada
Cystic Fibrosis
Double Lung Transplant, November 4, 2008
Toronto General Hospital, Toronto, Canada

Life is "Breathtaking"
By Amber Payne

Breathtaking. It's a word in the English language that automatically seems to evoke emotion in all of us. Whether we are describing a view from the top of a mountain range, the water of a crystal blue ocean that seems to stretch out for miles, or even our first kiss, the word "breathtaking" seems to take on more meaning than most others.

For me, *breathtaking* means so much more.

At the age of nineteen, after battling cystic fibrosis since birth and seeing my lungs deteriorate beyond repair, I came home from college and my life was put on hold for ten months until I received a double lung transplant on September 25, 2005.

The road to transplant, though, was by no means easy. I was on oxygen therapy 24 hours a day (24/7) and was running on very low reserves. I also experienced two false alarms before my actual surgery, planned my own funeral with close friends and family, and honestly wondered if I would even live to see my earthly miracle occur.

I went from being an out-going, vibrant college freshman to a young woman who literally stayed in her room for the better half of a ten-month period. I used to be the one doing everything for everyone, but during that time, I needed my family and friends more than I ever could have imagined.

Once I received my lungs, I never looked back. It has been over five years since my surgery, and I am so humbled that not only can I *breathe;* I can breathe *well* – better than I have my entire life. I went from having less than 20% FEV1 (the amount of air one can breathe out in one second) to around 110% at this time.

I've had a fuller five years than I could have ever imagined. I have not only written a book, but traveled the country proclaiming His sovereignty and goodness, graduated with highest honors from college (the same one I had E-mailed to say, "I'd be back"), started my career, and married my best friend, John. The latter is my most important earthly accomplishment, if you ask me. I adore my life, especially now that I get to share it with my wonderful husband. I could never ask for more.

The book, *Breathtaking* - published under my maiden name - Metz, is a gut-wrenching account of my journey to transplant, written from a compilation of E-mails I wrote from March through Christmas of 2005. My desire was – and still is – to give my life back to *others,* as I have been given the ultimate gift of life here on earth through my transplant, a life that is *abundant* and *free.*

I also have become an advocate for organ donation awareness, speaking to nurses and students about the importance of making the crucial decision to become an organ donor and also respect the people involved if the difficult process of discussing organ donation, does need to be put into effect.

I can never say thank you enough to my donor family for giving the gift of life. I pray that I am able to one day meet them in person and thank them face-to-face for their decision, which has in effect allowed me to embrace life once again and ready to face the unknown.

Amber Payne, 25
Lima, Ohio
Cystic Fibrosis
Double Lung Transplant, September 25, 2005
Nationwide Children's Hospital, Columbus, Ohio

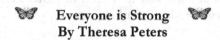

Everyone is Strong
By Theresa Peters

On December 15th of 2003 I received the "Gift of Life" in the form of two pink, perfect lungs at Duke University Medical Center in Durham, North Carolina. Now, nearly seven years later, I celebrated my 34th birthday.

I was born in 1976, the first child of two young parents. Growing up with Cystic Fibrosis at this time, it seemed unlikely that I would ever live to be 34. I often imagine what it was like for my parents to hear my diagnosis. In January 2003, I underwent a series of medical complications, and my lung capacity fell dramatically. It was time to begin the process of getting listed for transplant. I worked really hard at rehab so that my body would be in good shape despite my broken lungs. When I was transplanted, the organ allocation method was based on time on list, and I didn't have much time. I was accepted as a transplant candidate and officially listed.

On the day that I was listed I went into the hospital and stayed there until December 14th. In mid-November I went into respiratory failure and was told that I was too sick to receive a transplant. These were my darkest days. I didn't give up, but it seemed unlikely that I would recover enough to become eligible for transplant. With a lot of hard work and prayer, I did recover. I worked harder than ever walking and exercising, and was discharged. The next morning the call came that they had lungs for me.

Nearly eight hours later, my surgeon told my parents that the surgery went well, the lungs were perfect, but that I still had a long road ahead. I had a successful post-surgical experience. I moved to the step-down unit that evening, and insisted on walking there. I started walking up a storm around the nurses station and had very little pain issues. I was discharged in six days, and at that time it was a record.

My rehabilitation program was five days a week, four hours per day for six weeks. I made huge strides in rehab, and even jogged by the end of it, though my jogging at the time was comical while my body learned to get back in sync. Despite all of this success, there were hard times after transplant. Relationships can also take a toll, and I did go through a divorce in 2005. One thing has always been forefront in my mind is that I would do it all again for just one day where I didn't have to worry about breathing.

Since my transplant I've had so many special experiences. At the 2008 United States Transplant Games, I won three medals in swimming. I am so proud of that accomplishment. In 2009 I went with my sister on a cruise to the Bahamas. That was one of the best times of my life.

My day-to-day life is so normal. I live on my own with my two cats and one dog. I work full time as an accountant for the Medical University of South Carolina. I don't see myself as having any physical limitations. My biggest problem is working too much! I've dabbled in new hobbies such as gardening and photography. I've been involved with a local charitable organization and we held very successful fundraisers, volunteered at children's homes, retirement communities, and soup kitchens. This year I am so proud to say that I was able to witness my sister's lung transplant, and I hope that I am a good mentor and can provide guidance for her journey.

Before my transplant, I never imagined that it would be difficult to remember how hard it was when I couldn't breathe. I wonder how I managed for that year. I think about going around with a literal time limit, how long my tank would last, and I'm so grateful that is something I no longer worry about. I've learned to appreciate that things really do always work out the way that they are supposed to. I have so much less stress since I figured that out. It's pretty amazing, but, everything works out. If I see myself on the wrong path, I stop, figure out how to fix it, and start again. Things seem simpler now, and when I'm starting to feel things spinning into a direction I'm not happy with, rather than worry and stress, I assess the situation, make a plan, and start putting it into action. People often will say things such as, "Wow I'm sorry you've been through so much. You're so strong." Really, I think everyone is strong; they just may not have been tested the same way.

When I first went to back to work my interviewer asked me the age-old interview question, "Where do you see yourself in five years?" At that time, I thought it was hard to imagine being alive that far in the future. Now, five years from that question, I'm able to think long term. I'd like to be married again. I'm not afraid of love anymore. I can commit to having a pet and buying a house. To me, the future no longer has a pending end date.

I'm so thankful for donor families and living donors everywhere. I couldn't have done it at all without my family. Thanks of course to my transplant team at Duke, especially Dr. Michael Reidy.

Theresa Peters, 34
Mount Pleasant, South Carolina
Cystic Fibrosis
Double Lung Transplant, December 15, 2003
Duke University Medical Center, Durham, North Carolina

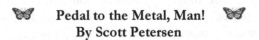

Pedal to the Metal, Man!
By Scott Petersen

My story? Hmm ... To be honest, to me it's a non-story. I suppose that any person who has endured a lifetime with chronic lung disease (Cystic Fibrosis in my case) has quite a tale; however I just feel I've been simply living my life. Understand that as time goes on, all the extraordinary experiences and struggles just become how you live and it's hard to realize that most folks "day to day" is far easier and simpler health wise. Plowing through my days with a component of dealing with health issues and being a Cystic Fibrosis (CF) and now Lung Transplant warrior is the only way I know how to live. Nevertheless, by age 54 a person has had to accumulate a history and I'm happy to share mine.

As an infant, the first problems indicative of CF were digestive and my parents went from one pediatrician to another before a diagnosis was finally made. "Enjoy that boy" was the recommendation along with a prognosis of a five to six year life expectancy. (Remember, this was the late 50's!). I can't imagine the shock and subsequent sleepless nights my folks must have experienced. Lucky for me, my real breathing issues were yet to develop. In those day's CF people slept in mist tents with giant nebulizers hanging from the frame spewing out whatever medication was in vogue at that time and man, it was hot and humid in those things! Plus the noise from the little air compressor. But hey, you get used to it. When my family moved in the early 1960's my Dad built a house next door to my Grandmother and he cleverly put a large compressor in the basement and ran tubing up to the bedrooms for my younger brother and I. Well that got rid of the noise at least!

By the time I graduated from high school I had had five sinus surgeries, if memory serves me correctly. (In fact, in the post transplant world my perennially infected polyp infested sinuses draining into the lungs are of great concern to the transplant team). I honestly don't know how many times we've removed these things and why should I? You just get it done and move on. I'm not worrying about the past, man!

Ah yes, most importantly my teen years were the time I really fell in love with music. I had always participated in athletics and played basketball and ran track as a high school freshman, but when I started listening to Jazz, my already large interest in music went 'tilt'! I had been playing clarinet since grade school and was good at it but I assure you, it was not from diligent practice! When I started playing Tenor Sax that was it! All interest in athletics (or almost anything else for that matter) faded, although I still am a sports fan. I practiced and practiced and started working 'gigs' before I was out of high school.

Playing the saxophone to a professional standard requires a lot of air and support of that air. I truly believe that all that blowing has significantly helped me get to this point in time. Playing also has been a good barometer of my pulmonary health. When I've had infections over the years they were noticed early, as I perceived compromises in my air for playing. Over time as my lungs deteriorated my skills to utilize what air I had to the fullest continued to develop and allowed me to continue pursuing my career. I have always been determined and found a way to take every gig; even rigging intravenous antibiotics drips in my car when needed to keep on my med schedule when I was sick. My famous cough (especially after a long held ending note) was a cue, but no one except my closest friends knew that I was dealing with CF.

Alas, the inevitable deterioration reached a point where the process began to be listed for lung transplant. I had known that this step was coming for quite a few years and prepared myself by viewing it as a bump in the road, and that I would cross it and continue and thrive in the new life. Still, it was rough mentally as I had to start curtailing my schedule. At first I still worked and traveled on oxygen, but later, first the travel and then even working at all was no longer possible. This dark time was exacerbated by my Dad's deterioration and passing from cancer. I was thousands of miles away and powerless to help. I wish he had lived to see my transplant but passed six weeks prior to "the call".

"THE CALL!" I bet every transplant person can remember the words spoken to them when the phone rang. Dr. Charles Hoopes and his staff at University of California San Francisco Medical Center, San Francisco, California, performed my surgery in January 2009. I am very fortunate to receive care here. Every visit, I have to resist the urge to give a big hug to every one of the fine doctors and staff who are responsible for me being alive today. My mate Susan did a heroic job of putting all our organizational plans into reality while still working her job! How she did it and stayed sane, I don't know. Hey all I had to do was recover. Seems like an easier gig to me!

And what a life it is! I got back on the horn after six weeks, and two weeks later played my first gig in a long time. After all the years of compromises, I don't take being able to blow like I can now for granted as well as striding up the hills of San Francisco lugging all my horns and equipment and barely breathing hard. The road post transplant has been a bit bumpy: two surgeries, three rejections, and some other problems but I consider myself to be the luckiest person alive and I feel that in my heart.

The true way to honor the incredible gift my donor gave me is to press on and live each day to its fullest. Nobody knows what the future holds, but through my donor's extreme kindness and the help and work of so many, I'm here ... and I'm living "Pedal to the Metal", man!

Scott Petersen, 54
Novato, California
Cystic Fibrosis
Double Lung Transplant, January 22, 2009
University of California San Francisco, San Francisco, California

 My Transplant Experience
By Cheryl Peterson

My journey began in June 1999 when my doctor told me I was going to have to be on oxygen because of my chronic obstructive pulmonary disease (COPD)/Emphysema. He then suggested a lung transplant but cautioned the life span was only about five years. I had a big decision to make.

My family and I talked about it in depth, and decided on the transplant. I was in the hospital twice with breathing problems prior to the transplant. At the time, my son Clinton, daughter-in-law Maggie, and grandkids Aubrey and Jeramiah and I all lived together in a two-story duplex. I spent most of my time in my room upstairs as I had a difficult time going up and down the stairs.

My pulmonologist got in touch with Oregon Health & Science University Hospital (OHSU), Portland, Oregon. "The call" came in on October 11, 2000. My sister Barb rushed me up to OHSU. From what I have been told, I was one of the last lung transplant patients they performed at Oregon Health & Science University.

I now have fun doing the things I couldn't do before transplant. This last summer we spent our vacation in Disneyland…what a fun experience for the whole family; it was a little hot for me, but I managed just fine. We put in a container garden last year and plan on having another one this year. A couple of other years we had a small ground garden.

I don't know what I would do without my family around me. We take life as it comes and always hope and pray for good health and happiness. My son Clinton and daughter-in-law Maggie keep me in check, regarding my health; making sure grandkids stay away from me during their colds and any other health issues. My beautiful granddaughter Aubrey is now 17-years-old and a junior in high school. My handsome grandson Jeramiah is 11-years-old and in 6th grade. They purchased a rose for me that was displayed on the "2010 Donate Life Rose Parade Float" which was very special to me.

During my grandson's elementary school days, I was able to help out at his school. I helped with making popcorn on Friday mornings; helped in his classroom(s); and corrected math papers at home. When my granddaughter was in middle school, her dance performances would be a blast for all of us to attend, even traveling to Portland, Oregon once a year for regional competitions. There have been numerous school projects and performances by both kids that I would have missed if not for my lung transplant. We didn't get to go camping this summer, but we're hoping to go next year. We attend many of the celebrations around town during different times of the year and sit out on the sidewalks downtown, with our hot cocoa, and watching the Christmas Parade.

I am back on oxygen now, but can still do so much more than I could before my transplant. My doctor tells me I'm doing well and to keep up the good work.

I would like to say a special 'Thank-You' to my sister Sandy and nephew Michael who stayed with me in Portland. They were sure I made it to all my appointments and returning to 'home' for visits.

Cheryl Peterson, 58
Springfield, Oregon
Chronic Obstructive Pulmonary Disease/Emphysema
Single Lung Transplant, October 12, 2000
Oregon Health & Science University Hospital, Portland, Oregon

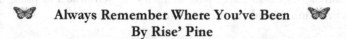

Always Remember Where You've Been
By Rise' Pine

As I blew out my birthday candles at my thirty-sixth birthday party, I made a special prayer that I could stay alive for one more year. It was not too long before that time that I'd been told that I had less than a year to live, because I was dying from Cystic Fibrosis.

In the event that I needed emergency assistance, I decided to leave my apartment door unlocked. This plan of action saved my life. On January 18, 1996, my respiratory therapist found me semi-coherent, on the bathroom floor, with my cannula detached from my face. Sandra had come to give me a breathing treatment. I was taken by ambulance to the nearest hospital. When I became conscious, I looked over at my parents in the intensive care unit (ICU) and felt a great appreciation that they were called to meet me at the hospital as I lived alone.

A few evenings later, I asked the ICU nurse to help me get out of bed. I wanted to walk in place for twenty minutes, because I knew how important it was for me to get some exercise. I wore my oxygen cannula in my nose as I proceeded to slowly march in place. While I held the nurses hand, I said aloud, "I will never give up! I want to live!" It made me feel so alive, unlike the way I looked. I felt a little shaky and my skin tone was a bluish color. After I said my famous marching words, I looked over my shoulder to see my parents' reaction. Their emotional reaction will remain indelibly ingrained in my memory. My determination was so alive. I was going to fight this battle!

Later that evening, after midnight the lights flicked on. I was being taken to Chicago for new lungs, at Loyola University Medical Center, Chicago, Illinois.

After I received my new lungs I was only on the ventilator for an additional eight hours. When I woke up from surgery, my first request was for ice, because my throat was very dry. I then asked if I could listen with a stethoscope to hear my clear sounding new lungs. Later, I asked for a mirror so I could see my lips and fingernails, which were pink. The entire transplant team was very impressed with my enthusiasm.

To write a letter of appreciation to my donor family was paramount to me. I have written four letters in the past six years. I wrote about the gratitude and respect that I have for the family. They had the foresight to see life for another human being. They gave me the chance to breathe freely for the first time in my life. I always pray for them. I had not received any replies so far. I had an intuitive feeling about his race and his birthday. I found this to be a true discovery by family services from the organ donor program.

After returning to Hollywood, Florida, I contacted several charitable organizations and civic groups to arrange speaking engagements on organ donation. This is my way of giving back to society for the precious gift that was given to me.

In 2000, I created the website TransplantBuddies, which you can Google. Currently, many patients, both pre and post transplant, enjoy helping one another on a daily basis. There are topics for almost all facets of transplantation. I also participate at Jackson Memorial Hospital, University of Miami School of Medicine in Miami, Florida in their mentoring program.

I enjoy fast walking, aerobics and weight training. Deep-breathing exercises are part of my routine during resting periods. I believe in holistic therapies and find a great benefit from them. I met a wonderful man named Cary shortly after my first transplant; he has been a big support to me throughout all of the years we have been together.

Facing a near-death experience has taught me a great deal of appreciation for life, for my family, friends and doctors who have stood by my side through good and bad times alike. Regardless of what I might experience in the future. I feel as though I can handle anything. However long I shall live, will be God's plan. As one can imagine, this life changing experience has enlightened my spirit in many ways.

I lived with a great lung capacity for eight years. In 2004, I was diagnosed with chronic rejection. I decided to go back to Loyola University Medical Center in Chicago for a treatment called, Photopheresis. After three months, I decided the treatment was not helping and decided to head back to my home in Florida.

My transplant team at Jackson Memorial Hospital, University of Miami School of Medicine re-transplanted me in July of 2006. Fortunately, my health improved day by day once I left the hospital! I had a difficult operation due to the fact that I had my lungs for almost ten years. I received Campath induction therapy with my second transplant and I believe that is a big help especially for re-transplantation, as I no longer have to take steroids.

I never dreamed that I would do as well as I did especially for a second transplant. I will be 51-years-old, October of 2011. Twelve days before my second transplant anniversary. Cary and I were married, and we are living life to the fullest. My lung function has been stable at 99 percent. I am extremely grateful. I believe that a healthy high fiber diet, exercise will keep your overall health in good condition. Since 1996, I have been able to maintain normal kidney function, which I claim to be a result of my healthy diet. Currently all of my labs are normal.

God Bless my Donor and his Family!

Rise' Pine, 50
Pembroke Pines, Florida
Cystic Fibrosis
Double Lung Transplant, January 21, 1996
Loyola University Medical Center, Maywood, Illinois
Re-Transplant, Double Lung Transplant, July 25, 2005
Jackson Memorial Hospital, University of Miami School of Medicine, Miami, Florida
Read Rise's Lung Transplant Story in the 1st Edition of Taking Flight

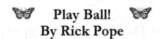

Play Ball!
By Rick Pope

On June 24, 1981, my wife, Cindy gave birth to Andrew Douglas Pope, our second child. During the birth, Dr. Jarrell recognized that I was getting weak-kneed, and sarcastically, ordered me to, "Sit down boy I don't want you passing out in my delivery room". Drew's birth at the Medical Center, in Columbus, Georgia, for all accounts and purposes was normal. The following morning, the doctor came into Cindy's hospital room and informed us that Drew was having some difficulties with breathing due to an abnormally low oxygen level. After an x-ray was taken, the doctors diagnosed our baby boy with a pneumothorax. A chest tube was inserted and relieved some of the immediate issues and his oxygen levels went up as well.

Over the next two and a half years we were in and out of many doctor's offices. After several years, our worst fears were confirmed; our son had all the classic symptoms of Cystic Fibrosis (CF). A "sweat test" was performed and the results were positive. His sister Melissa, who was five-years-old was also tested for CF. We were delighted when her negative test results were delivered to us.

In a "blink of an eye" our lives were changed forever. We immediately developed "a life plan." It consisted of many visits to the CF Center in Atlanta where Dr. Kaplan became Drew's CF doctor. Dr. Kaplan was a Godsend for Drew and many other CF patients. Like many children with cystic fibrosis, his "life plan" included several intravenous antibiotic infusions. Many of the symptoms of patients with CF are low weight gain, clubbed fingernails, and salt residue left on his brow after playing sports.

Drew faced his lot in life head on. I think this attitude, carried his family through even the most difficult times. Most of our time, between his 8th and 13th birthday, were spent at the baseball field. Drew loved playing baseball! Our family embraced baseball as part of our life plan. He did not want to be different or allow himself to "take it easy."

Drew went to University of Alabama Hospital, in Birmingham, Alabama for the evaluation of a lung transplant. Anyone who has gone through this ordeal knows this is a multi-step process. You also have to time the need for the transplant with the patient's ability to survive the operation, and their psychological stability, combined with their support system. Drew did well in all categories.

Less than three months had passed when we received THE CALL! We are about 150 miles from Birmingham and the drive to Birmingham was quiet, as we were going over in our minds our "life plan". Our family would pace the waiting room and cry. Cry for hope, cry for fear, and cry for all the uncertainty the day would bring. Many hours passed, when Dr. David McGiffin came out and delivered us the news we were all so anxious to hear, "The surgery was a success." We all wept even more, knowing that Drew's life was about to drastically change for the better.

Drew was trying to wake up in the intensive care unit shortly after the surgery was completed. He wanted the breathing tube out right away! He was tough. As a family, we were tough. But we knew who to give the real praise to, God.

When the team of doctors released Drew from the hospital, he proudly, "rang the bell". The "Ringing of the Bell", is a symbol to all on the transplant floor that Drew had completed a major victory and the start of a new life.

Drew fully took advantage of the next eight years of his life. He graduated from Columbus Technical College and worked full time as a pharmacy technician. Drew was an outdoorsman to say the least. He loved hunting and fishing with his best friend, Bill Woolf. Bill was Drew's backbone, always standing by his side at all times. I was so proud that my son had such a first rate friend like Bill.

Drew, like others, always tried to appreciate life, love others, and do the very best he could each day! Drew did all these things, and jumped out of a perfectly good airplane! He loved skydiving!

Unfortunately, after a long illness, Drew lost his fight with CF on Feb. 23rd, 2010. On what would have been Drew's 29th birthday, on June 24th this summer, Drew's niece, my granddaughter, Kayla and I went parasailing. In Drew's honor, she wore his mother's locket, which contained some of Drew's ashes. It was one of the greatest feelings in the world and a memory that her and I will share forever!

In our everyday lives since Drew's passing, we celebrate and honor his memory. We celebrate the wonderful gift of organ donation. Drew would not have had the privilege if it were not for the gift that we received from a perfect stranger. Drew touched all of our lives and he will be greatly missed until the day that we are all reunited with him in our Lord's house.

Rick Pope, Father of, Drew Douglas Pope
Columbus, Georgia
Drew, Cystic Fibrosis
Drew, Double Lung Transplant, January 21, 2002
University of Alabama Hospital, Birmingham, Alabama
Drew Passed Away, February 23, 2010
"Forever 28"

🦋 Perfect Match 🦋
By Addie Benton Poudrier

"Lung transplant!" Two words you never expect to hear in reference to someone you love, let alone your own father. My dad was diagnosed with Idiopathic Pulmonary Fibrosis (IPF) in October 2009. A condition I was unfamiliar with, however, I quickly understood very little was to be understood about this unique disease. He was 65 at the time and the thought of a man his age qualifying for a transplant blew my mind. Fortunately we all live in Jacksonville, Florida, one of the homes of Mayo Clinic.

My dad was deteriorating very fast. He required oxygen (O2) much of the time and began having trouble tying his shoes and taking a shower. After two dry runs and as a result of mild post-traumatic stress syndrome (PTSD) he was finally called in for a successful single lung transplant on June 26th 2010. His donor was a young man, very athletic and was a "perfect match". My dad spent only five days in Mayo Clinic Florida, Jacksonville, Florida, and was released and had zero rejection. He is roughly three months post transplant and is already back on the golf course (with a mask and mild swing) doing what he loves the most...LIVING!

The road to recovery is frightening. The delicate balance between healing and thriving, living and loving is thin, but it becomes so clearly defined once you are able to look back and realize you have survived the odds. With a positive outlook, faith in yourself, your doctors, your body, your loved ones and your higher power, nothing is impossible.

Addie Benton Poudrier, Daughter of, Robert Benton, 65
Jacksonville, Florida
Robert Benton, Idiopathic Pulmonary Fibrosis
Robert Benton, Single Lung Transplant, June 26, 2010
Mayo Clinic Florida, Jacksonville, Florida

Life After Bilateral Lung and Liver Transplant
By Patti Prince

I was born in June of 1981 and six months later, I was diagnosed with a hereditary disease, called Cystic Fibrosis (CF). When I was diagnosed, my Mom was told that she shouldn't expect me to live past the age of twelve-years-old. That was the median age at the time. I did fairly well in my childhood years, with few hospitalizations, and surpassed all the things the doctors said that I wouldn't be able to do.

When I entered high school, I started to have more frequent lung infections and I was diagnosed with Cirrhosis (liver disease), portal hypertension (high blood pressure in the liver), and an enlarged spleen. I had evaluations at two different hospitals, both of which said that it would be years before I would need a liver transplant. After many illnesses and hospitalizations throughout high school I was told that I would not graduate on time. I was out to prove my teachers wrong, and I graduated on time. I then went onto a community college and graduated. Two months later, I was married to the man I had been dating since I was 17 and his job moved us to a different area.

We bought a house, settled in, and were making a great life together. We were both working and enjoying life, until I started getting sicker. During one of the admissions I was told that I needed to look at transplant centers that would be willing to do a bilateral lung and liver transplant. Dr. Sexton called the doctors at The Cleveland Clinic Foundation, Cleveland, Ohio. They said they had never done one before, but they were willing to look at my case. It was determined, that with an FEV1 (lung function) of 40 percent, that I was likely too healthy to be listed at that time.

I found out in August 2005 that I was nine weeks pregnant. I was told by my CF specialist, the OB/GYN, and the transplant teams to terminate the pregnancy. After talking to my husband and family, I decided that I wanted to try to move forward with the pregnancy, being that it may be my only chance to have a biological child. I was hospitalized 28 weeks into the pregnancy and my son was born, seven weeks early, in January 2006. He was healthy and after a month in the hospital, he came home.

I was listed at the Cleveland Clinic for a bilateral lung and liver transplant in August 2006. I was air lifted to Cleveland due to a very large bleed from my lungs. Three days later, in the hospital, I was told that they found a donor. I was Cleveland Clinic's first bilateral lung and liver transplant on January 31, 2007. I recovered rather quickly and was home in New York only four and a half weeks after the transplant. I have had two episodes of rejection not too far out from the transplant. One of them was treated with Solumedrol and the other one went away on its own.

Since the transplant, I have been enjoying life with my husband, and now, four-year-old son. We have traveled a few places across the country (Washington, Virginia, Oklahoma, Texas, Tennessee, Ohio, and New Hampshire) to visit friends and family. Traveling was something that was very hard for me to do beforehand. I couldn't handle the air pressure up in a plane, car rides were too long and exhausting, and between having a child and having all of my medical equipment, it was just too much to carry. It's such a different experience now and I love it!

I also had a very hard time just taking care of myself. It was exhausting just to take three showers a week, change my clothes, or even comb my hair. Now, I can take a shower every single morning, get dressed, comb my hair, get my son dressed, make breakfast for both of us, and I still have more energy for the rest of the day; no more getting out of breath, no more sleeping all day, no more admissions to the hospital, and no more asking other people to watch my son because I just couldn't do it. I can read long books to Brady, play games with him, chase after him around the house and outside, and join him in activities at his preschool. We enjoy day trips to the local zoo and doing other things together that I never could have imagined before the transplant. My husband works 40 hours a week and can now come home to a clean house, clean laundry, groceries in the cupboard, and dinner on the table about an hour after he gets home. All of which, I couldn't do for about two years before the transplant.

Since the transplant, I have also joined online CF and transplant communities to share my story and help others who are facing the same obstacles that I faced. I have met a lot of people with Cystic Fibrosis, including two others who had a bilateral lung and liver transplant two years after I had mine. I am also currently talking to one other person who is waiting for a bilateral lung and liver transplant and a wife of someone who needs one. I like to help in any way that I can, and because of this, I was named a CF 'Hero of Hope' in July 2010.

Meeting and talking to so many people in the CF community is not always easy, though. I became very close to one girl and met her in person twice. She became very ill in 2009 and even after a bilateral lung transplant in September 2009, she passed in November 2009. I left home the day after Thanksgiving to fly to Texas for her funeral, where her family asked me to speak about her. I did so, and it was probably the hardest thing that I ever had to do. Other friends with CF have also passed on, and it never gets any easier to hear the news.

At this point, I am three and a half years post bilateral lung and liver transplant and I'm very healthy. I live my life to the fullest every day and I am very thankful to my donor, their family, and all of my doctors for giving me the gift of life and allowing me to be here for my husband, son, other family, and friends. I get to continue to be a granddaughter, daughter, sister, niece, aunt, cousin, wife, daughter-in-law, mother, and friend. I will turn thirty, next year. It's the major milestone that I was told I would never reach. There is no greater feeling in the world than this.

Patti Prince, 29
Yorkville, New York
Cystic Fibrosis
Double Lung & Liver Transplant, January 31, 2007
The Cleveland Clinic Foundation, Cleveland, Ohio

🦋 Pushing the Boundaries 🦋
By Anonymous Lung Recipient

The last time I attended my transplant support group meeting, I was asked if I could do things AFTER the transplant that I couldn't do BEFORE. I blurted out "I can garden!" and, the whole room burst out in laughter. You see, my transplant coordinator was sitting right there and gardening is a no-no for transplant recipients. She just laughed and said that I just "ousted myself." So, yes, I'll admit it, I sometimes break the transplant "rules."

It got me thinking of all the ways I have worked around the rules that I was given post-transplant in order to live the kind of life I wanted. The first rule I broke, concerned my cat, right before I was discharged. My transplant doctor told me that I needed to get rid of him. But, how was I to part with such an important member of my family? Apparently, he was concerned that I might catch cat scratch fever. So, I offered, "What if I had him declawed?" "Then, alright, you can keep him," my doctor muttered. So, the operation was scheduled and he had his front claws removed. After I saw how painful it was for him, I decided to forego having his back claws done.

At the same time, I had my cat tested for toxoplasmosis. Toxoplasmosis is a parasitic disease that can live in cat feces and can cause serious complications in transplant recipients. Transplant recipients are instructed NOT to clean cat litter boxes for fear of acquiring the disease. Fortunately, my cat was NEGATIVE for toxoplasmosis since he had spent the better part of his life inside my apartment. Apparently, cats can get the parasite from eating small animals while hunting outside. As another precaution, I purchased one of those automatic cat litter boxes, but it didn't work very well and I still had to clean it by hand. But, I always wore a pair of gloves and made sure to wash my hands afterwards with soap and water. My doctor never asked again about my cat and he lived with me for many years!

Gardening is a no-no for transplant recipients. But, it is one of my most enjoyable hobbies. No matter where I have lived, I've always had household plants, and, even if I didn't have a space of my own, I'd plant a garden. I just really enjoy connecting to nature and seeing things grow from seeds. So, after I was transplanted, I wore a mask and gloves whenever I was stirring up dirt. I started to collect orchids because they don't grow in soil like other plants. But, even with these precautions, I developed an *Aspergillus* infection only a few years after my transplant. I asked my transplant physician how I got it. He told me that *Aspergillus* is EVERYWHERE in the environment and it is almost impossible to avoid it. So, it may or may not have been caught when I was gardening. Unfortunately, as time has progressed, wearing a mask has become too difficult for me when I garden. I had lost too much lung function over the years due to chronic rejection. So, I had to ditch the mask, but I still wear my gloves and shower afterwards.

Another one of the rules I broke concerns sushi. After my transplant, I didn't eat sushi because it is another no-no for transplant recipients. But, one day a friend told me that there are some items of sushi on the menu that are COOKED. So, I tried eating the cooked salmon, crab, and shrimp rolls. It was delicious, and more importantly, it was safe for me to eat! Later on, I learned all seafood that is to be consumed RAW in the United States, by law, must be frozen for a period of time. This process kills any parasites that might be lurking in their flesh. So, I now order as much RAW sushi and sashimi as I desire and I don't worry about parasites, but I always go to a reputable restaurant. However, the one thing I won't do is eat RAW shellfish.

The next rule I broke was perhaps the worst one of all. It occurred when I began dating my husband. Up to that point, I did not drink alcohol. But, on our first date, I ordered a beer! You see, I wanted to fit in and appear "normal" and healthy since it was too early in the relationship to discuss my transplant. So, I continued drinking whenever we got together. I knew that my transplant team did NOT recommend it since alcohol may interact with my medications and damage my liver. But, drinking alcohol became a regular habit for me for a number of years. I justified that I had worked hard all day and having a drink was my just reward. Later on, as I saw my health decline due to chronic rejection, I gave up drinking all together; no need to add fuel to the fire, so to speak. This was one rule that I shouldn't break.

Now, it is true that keeping pets, gardening, eating sushi, and drinking alcohol are risky behaviors for a transplant recipient. But, so is everyday life. A bus tomorrow could hit me. So, I just weigh the amount of risk versus the amount of reward. I've concluded, in my case, that the rewards of having pets, gardening, and eating sushi are greater than the risks. It has been 13 years since my transplant, so I must be doing something right.

Now, I don't want you to think that I don't obey ANY rules. I haven't had any grapefruit since my transplant, even though it was one of my favorite breakfast foods. I wash my hands and take my medications religiously. I never take anything with ibuprofen or aspirin. I don't take any dietary supplements or herbal remedies. I don't own any reptiles and my husband takes care of the fish tank. I am leery of swimming in public pools, oceans, lakes, etc. and am careful not to swallow any water. I wear a mask when flying and I put it on whenever I hear someone coughing near me. And, I've never gotten a tattoo or body piercing; my operation scars are all the body adornment that I'll ever need!

Anonymous Lung Recipient

A House Can Be A Home
By Carol Riker

Married to a man who lives under clouds of uncertainty and fear is hard enough, but when the clouds also rain on you, well-----. For a year my husband Ray and I waffled back and forth about the risk of a double lung transplant or just waiting, severely handicapped by Chronic Obstructive Pulmonary Disease (COPD).

In June of 2007, Ray and I went to Pittsburgh to await a donor's lungs. We were sure the operation would afford us a better life. When we arrived at the Neville Family House, a Ronald McDonald type residence for adults, the sun was shining brightly, not a cloud in the sky.

We were given a tour of the beautiful house. When we got to the kitchen, Ray pointed at the gas stove, his oxygen tank, and then at me. He was laughing when he informed me that I would now be doing the cooking unless we wanted an explosive relationship. A week later, he chided me for letting him cook the last 30 years while I professed a culinary ineptitude. For the seven and a half months that we were in Pittsburgh I cooked, very well, if I may say so myself.

The camaraderie in the house was exceptional. The other residents and Ray and I became both speakers and listeners. We shared experiences and fears. The seven weeks waiting for the double lung transplant were eased by new and strong friendships.

The call came at three o'clock in the morning of September 11, 2007. My friend Betty had told me to wake her no matter the hour. I knocked at her door and she ran out into the hall to hug me. The door to her room slammed shut. Betty stood there in only in her nightgown with no key. We both looked at the locked door and started laughing. Ray and I rushed to the hospital. Betty spent the night on the family room's couch trying to keep warm by using throw pillows as a blanket. To this day we laugh about it, because laughter is what kept us sane.

At first, I was so scared and alone at the hospital waiting for the surgery to be over. Five of our friends from the Neville, including the thawed out Betty, came to be with me. I often wonder how I would have gotten through the ten hours of waiting without their support.

It's stressful and lonely in a city far from your friends and home. We were so lucky that a wonderful family adopted Neville House. Once a month the whole family, from grandfather to grandson, made a gourmet meal for all the residents. Christmas, the family held a party with games and prizes.

Many of the local college sororities and fraternities made treats for us. One such ambitious group made us a pancake breakfast. I looked around the kitchen and marveled at how many of the residents were from other countries, coming to the Pittsburgh hospitals and, thus Neville, because of a transplant doctor's excellent reputation. I announced for that day Neville House, in honor of the lovely breakfast, would be called The International House of Pancakes today. Laughter was a good thing.

When Ray and I left Pittsburgh in February of 2008, we felt like we were leaving family. Before getting into our car, I was stopped by a staff member. He thanked me for helping new residents adjust to the family house. I told him that I was thankful for their friendship. The staff and fellow residents were always there for us through tears and laughter. The friendships that we made through the hardships were strong and lasting. They are more than friends. They have a special place in our hearts.

Carol Riker, Wife of, Ray Riker, 65
Rochester, New York
Ray, Chronic Obstructive Pulmonary Disease
Ray, Double Lung Transplant, September 11, 2007
University of Pittsburgh Medical Center, Pittsburgh, Pennsylvania

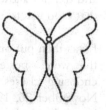

Never Give Up
By Jill Conner Roberts

When I was three-years-old, I was sick a lot and exhibiting odd symptoms so my pediatrician sent me to a neurologist whose clinic was in the same area of the hospital as the cystic fibrosis (CF) clinic. The CF doctor accidentally picked up my chart and looked over my symptoms. He assumed I was his patient and he entered the room and told my parents he wanted to do a sweat test. The doctor returned later with the results and told my parents that I had cystic fibrosis and that I would probably not survive to be five-years-old. What a devastating day for my family.

However, my parents did not give up on me. They taught me the art of goal setting and they encouraged me to set goals that would not be achievable for several years. For example, at a young age, they drove me around the University of Missouri and we talked about going to college there. At age five, they were told I would not live to be 10. At age 10, they were told I would probably not live to be 18. At 18, we were told my life expectancy would not exceed 25 years of age. My family never gave up on me and I never gave up on myself.

I spent most of my life in and out of the hospital. The nurses and doctors were like my family. In my early 20's I noticed it was getting harder and harder to walk to my college classes. I became very sick and was hospitalized for over four months. Towards the end of my hospital stay, my doctor told me that there was nothing else that they could do for me. I refused to believe that so I got a second opinion. It was then that another CF doctor suggested that I go to Barnes-Jewish Hospital in St. Louis, Missouri for a lung transplant evaluation. I went and was evaluated. On the final day of tests, I went into respiratory arrest and was not expected to live. I was immediately transported to intensive care unit (ICU). While there, every rule was broken. My nurse allowed my mom and sister to stay with me all night long. I should have died that night, but once again, my family was with me and did not allow me to give up. Miraculously, I pulled through. That was the first time I realized that God was taking me on this journey for a reason.

I was then put on the lung transplant waiting list. Now, all I had to do was wait my turn for lungs that were a perfect match for me. While I was waiting, I continued my college education, often choosing classes that were in buildings with no stairs and handicapped parking nearby. On November 26, 1997, I told my mother that I felt worse and needed to drive to St. Louis to be hospitalized. I called my coordinator and she said to come for an appointment and be prepared to stay for a tune-up.

That morning was a sunny day and as my mother and I got in the car and prepared for the two-hour drive to St. Louis I said to her, "Today is a great day for surgery." Little did I know that it really was a great day for surgery. I arrived at admissions and was kept waiting for several hours. A nurse finally came down and told me that they were keeping me waiting because lungs had become available. A good match for me had to be determined, so hence the wait. Depending on that decision, I would either be placed on the transplant floor or the CF floor. Guess where I went? I went to the transplant floor. I have never experienced such a peace about me. It was as if, I knew this was my time and I was ready for it. It took several hours for the Barnes doctors to fly to Louisiana to get my lungs and get back to Barnes, but they made it safely and my surgery was successful.

I was on a ventilator for 36 hours and after it was removed, I was up walking, with several tubes attached of course. The first thing my mother told me after I woke up was, "you are not blue!" When you are struggling to breathe, blue becomes the way you look and people get used to that. I was moved back to a regular room and stayed there for 10 days. After I was released, my family and I stayed in an apartment not far from the hospital. Our apartment was on the 21st floor. About a month after my transplant I would walk up one flight of stairs and take the elevator the rest of the way. Eventually, I gained strength and walked up more and more flights of stairs. Although I never made it to the 21st floor, I did great. Imagine going from using eight liters of oxygen to walk, to going up several flights of stairs, in just a few months. Amazing!

Three months after my transplant I moved back home and returned to college. In preparing me for life well into adulthood, my parents taught me to be responsible for my own health. As a result, I studied the effects of all the medications I took and would be taking after my transplant. I discovered how much the medications effect the muscles and bones. While I was waiting for my transplant, I changed my major to nutrition and fitness so I could understand better the ways to help myself be healthy and strong after my transplant. I graduated at the top of my class and went on to get my master's degree. I decided to attend the University of Florida, Gainesville, where cutting edge research was being done on the muscles and bones of heart and lung transplant recipients. A professor that was studying the effects of prednisone on lung transplant patients took me under his wing and I started my own research study. The title of my research study and thesis was "Glucocorticoid-Induced Osteoporosis in Lung Transplant Recipients." As part of the study, I had to become a personal trainer to several lung transplant patients. Like them, I had osteoporosis from being on prednisone for years. Our study showed that resistance training significantly reduced the amount of bone loss after transplant. I began a rigorous exercise program and my osteoporosis and diabetes were reversed. Still today, several years later, I do not have to check the osteoporosis or diabetes box on health care forms.

During graduate school I met my husband. We are the proud parents of one rescued cat and two rescued dogs. David was in the Navy so we moved around the first part of our marriage. We now live in the Tulsa, Oklahoma area. I work full-time as a Cardiac Rehab Exercise Physiologist and I volunteer at the Ronald McDonald House. My family loves to travel and since my transplant I have seen the world and all it has to offer. I decided to train for my first 5K and set a goal to run it in under 45 minutes. I ran my first official 5K in 36 minutes and 14 seconds and two weeks later I ran in the Tulsa Run with over 2,300 other runners. A week after the Tulsa Run, I participated in the Tulsa Cystic Fibrosis Foundation's Climb for Life, climbing to the top of a 36-story building. I made it to the top in just over 10 minutes. Remember when I could go up only one flight?

I went back to Barnes-Jewish Hospital recently for my 13th year anniversary of my transplant. My pulmonary function tests were amazing, 109%. I never imagined that I could run a 5K or climb 36 stories, but with hard work, a positive attitude, and help from God, I was able to do them both. My motto is to never give up, whether it is drug side effects or a mountain I need to climb, I will conquer it. I was given the gift of life and I love to use it. My donor family has not written back to me, so I do not know anything about my donor. I do know, though, that I live to honor the person who saved my life.

Jill Conner Roberts, 36
Sapulpa, Oklahoma
Cystic Fibrosis
Double Lung Transplant, November 26, 1997
Barnes-Jewish Hospital, St. Louis, Missouri

A Journey of Faith
By Barbara Roupe

My name is Barbara Roupe. I am a 69-year-old mother of four, grandmother to twelve and have been married to my husband Jim for forty-eight years. I am a retired Registered Nurse (R.N.) having worked for thirty-seven years as an obstetrics nurse at our local hospital in Washington, Pennsylvania. Loving my profession I often wondered if I would know when it was time to retire. Little did I know it would be decided for me.

An active woman I walked three miles every day and my husband Jim and I loved to hike and ride bicycles when we vacationed.

Fall of 1999 I noticed I was becoming more fatigued on exertion and was experiencing shortness of breath with many of my normal activities. It was a bike ride of that year that made me realize something was wrong. A twenty-two mile ride that we'd done before without difficulty, turned out to be very different. On the return side of the trip I became very short of breath and we found ourselves stopping at every mile marker. I just couldn't get my breath and was becoming exhausted.

After an appointment with my family doctor, Dr. Michael Falcione and months of diagnostic testing, I was referred to a cardiologist, Dr. John Wilson. A right heart catheterization verified pulmonary hypertension (PH). Even though I am a nurse I knew very little about the lungs. I told Dr. Wilson the only thing I know about my chest was breast-feeding.

I was referred to the PH Center at University of Pittsburgh Medical Center, Pittsburgh, Pennsylvania, (UPMC) and the first appointment was with Dr. Srinivas Murali. I owe my life to Dr. Murali. His words to me during that first visit were. "Barbara, you have a disease for which there is no cure, you can be treated, but there is no cure." Those were very profound words. My head seemed to be spinning with all the information. Forms had to be signed and papers filled out. I went on the transplant list and also registered with National Organization of Rare Diseases (NORD). We went home as a family bewildered and devastated. We cried, and we cried.

After a heart catheterization at UPMC was performed, I was immediately started on Flolan intravenously. I would remain on Flolan for the next six years. My world as I knew it was gone or so I thought.

My husband, family and friends were very supportive and caring. Two of our children are nurses and my son's wife is a Nurse Practitioner, their knowledge and encouragement was very helpful.

After the initial shock and confusion I realized I could and would go on. I had tremendous support from Dr. Murali and two of his nurses, Michele and Carrie. With their support and encouragement I met each day with hope. I also new my faith in God was sustaining me and that He did have a plan for my life. "Great is Thy Faithfulness" had always been a favorite hymn and I was prepared to trust that promise.

January of 2001 I was diagnosed with breast cancer, resulting in a partial segmental mastectomy followed by radiation. Life went on, although I would have to be free of cancer for five years before I could go back on the transplant list. During those five years my faith grew and I knew in my heart I would get a transplant. My sister Sandy always reminded me that God had a set of lungs out there for me, but that person still needed them.

May of 2006 I was placed on the transplant list again. Prior to the "real deal" I was called three times all of which were "no go". I received my lungs on June 8th, 2006. As I went into the operating room I could feel the prayers of the people and God's presence. I would be all right. My entire family was in the waiting room. It was a long night for them but with joyous results. My surgery was performed by, Dr. Yoshiya Toyoda and his team. I was told the lungs I received were in perfect condition and I was the perfect recipient

The following days were miraculous. I couldn't stop smiling and my husband couldn't stop crying. God is good and we'd truly been blessed with a Miracle. I received excellent care and encouragement from the entire staff at UPMC. I made a great recovery and was home in two weeks. That was over four years ago and I can still feel the exuberance of those first few days after receiving my new lungs.

That was June of 2006 and in December I wrote a letter of gratitude to my Donor Family. That was very hard to compose. It was sent through Center for Organ Recovery and Education (CORE). I heard from the donor's family in May of 2007. It was a wonderful letter from my donor's Mom. It broke my heart and I cried for two days.

My donor Michael Corea was born with a rare liver disease. He was sick most of his young life. At the age of 13 he received a liver transplant. He went on to thrive. He made it known from that time he wanted to be an organ donor. On June 5th, one week before his graduation from Ohio State University, Michael was involved in a tragic motorcycle accident, which ultimately claimed his life.

Thanks to Michaels's gracious generosity I am alive and able to witness to the love and generosity of him and his family. Our families met on November 8th, 2009. It was a wonderful afternoon. One that was very emotional yet truly healing for both of our families.

The past four years have been filled with many joyous occasions. Graduations, birthdays, anniversary and holidays plus enjoying the accomplishments of my children and grandchildren are things I would have missed, not having had a transplant. Most of all for being able to breathe without difficulty and having a second chance to live an active and fulfilling life, I am most grateful.

Recently on August 14, 2010 my husband Jim and I participated in a Memorial Run/Walk sponsored by Lifebanc of Cleveland, Ohio. It was held at Blossom Music Center, a beautiful park with a Legacy Garden. There along with Michael's family and friends we were able to pay tribute to him and so many other donors. We took part in a very emotional memorial service, followed by the run/walk. Michael's lungs enabled me to participate in this wonderful event along side the people who were closest to him. I am truly blessed. The fact that my donor was also a transplant recipient made this very rare and unique transplant experience. I am grateful to everyone who made this possible.

Isaiah 40:31 "Those whose hope is in the Lord will renew their strength, they will soar on wings like eagles, they will run and not grow weary, they will walk and not be faint." This is a Bible verse my Mom claimed for me when I was first diagnosed with Primary Pulmonary Hypertension in March 2000. It remains a favorite of mine.

Barbara Roupe, 69
Washington, Pennsylvania
Primary Pulmonary Hypertension
Double Lung Transplant, June 8, 2006
University of Pittsburgh Medical Center, Pittsburgh, Pennsylvania
Michael Allen Corea - Donor
Read Lynda Corea's Story, Mother of Michael, in this Edition of Taking Flight

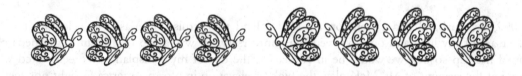

"How'd You Like a Lung?"

"How'd You Like a Lung?"
By Judy Russell

My pulmonologist first said the word "transplant" to me during an appointment in October 1998. Five months later, I had gone from working full time as a legal secretary to being confined to a wheelchair and on oxygen 24 hours a day (24/7) in the matter of about six weeks. As the American Lung Association says, "When you can't breathe, nothing else matters." During my illness and wait, I discovered that things were a lot easier if I found humor in what I was going through.

After being released from the hospital in 1999, I attended a presentation by Mark Kistler (a children's artist) with my son, complete with wheelchair and oxygen tank. Mark said that he never had someone come directly from the hospital to see him. As part of his program, he drew pictures on an overhead projector. He drew a picture of a scuba diver with oxygen tanks, called it "Scuba Judy" and gave it to me. I've been Scuba Judy ever since.

On August 15, I was attending the transplant picnic in Madison, Wisconsin, when one of the transplant coordinators slapped me on the back and said, "Judy Russell, how'd you like a lung?" I received the Gift of a left lung early on August 16, 1999, after only being listed for 52 days. The letter instructing me how to get a pager and to make arrangements for ambulance service arrived the day of my transplant. I could write a whole story just on the events of August 15.

In 2009, my husband and I went on an 11-day land tour/cruise of Alaska to celebrate the 10th anniversary of my lung and our 25th wedding anniversary. It was a trip of a lifetime. I specifically planned the trip so that we would be in Alaska on the day of my transplant. We celebrated while looking at the summit of Mt. McKinley, the highest elevation in North America (a sight not seen by many because it's usually hidden in clouds).

I had a pretty rough time during a recent hospital stay and had some sleepless nights when I returned home. I searched the Internet for my favorite jazz pianist, Keiko Matsui. My son and I had attended a Dave Koz concert where he had announced the performers who would be along on his 2010 Jazz Cruise to Alaska. Ms. Matsui was one of them, along with some great jazz sax artists. Since my son plays jazz tenor sax, I told my husband that I would have loved to take him on that cruise. I said that I would like to see Keiko Matsui perform once in my lifetime. I almost had a heart attack when I checked out her tour schedule on her site and found out that she was going to be playing at the Racine Zoo Animal Crackers Jazz Series on July 7, approximately 35 miles from my house! The next night, I looked her up on Wikipedia and found under charitable causes the following: "Proceeds from Matsui's 2001 mini-CD *A Gift of Life* went to the National Marrow Donor Program and the Marrow Foundation in support of their program Asians for Miracle Marrow Matches, which promotes the registration of people of ethnic minorities as marrow donors in hopes of improving the chance of finding matching donors for people of similar descent in need." I sent Ms. Matsui an e-mail telling her how excited I was that she was going to be performing in Wisconsin and explaining that I had listened to her music as part of my biofeedback therapy to relax while awaiting my transplant. I mentioned that for all these years I had no idea that she had any connection to transplantation. I also told her that Wisconsin has the first organization in the nation to have all four areas of transplantation under one roof: organ, tissue, bone marrow and blood. I asked if it would be possible to meet her so that she could sign the CD I had listened to while I was sick and *A Gift of Life* CD, which an on-line friend had found and purchased for me. I bought our tickets the first day they went on sale and asked the marketing rep at the zoo if she could possibly help arrange a meeting with Ms. Matsui in case she didn't read her e-mails while on the road. The afternoon of the concert, I was told that Ms. Matsui had agreed to meet me. We met and the director of the program took our picture and she signed my two CDs. My son still can't believe that I managed to get my own personal meet and greet with Keiko Matsui! I felt that somebody was watching over me and thought I needed something good to happen.

Since I have been unable to return to work, I have tried to give back by crocheting comfort shawls for donor families with Threads of Compassion, a division of the Wisconsin Donor Network. I am currently waiting to be trained to be a volunteer for the Wisconsin Donor Network to promote organ donation.

A big event in my life was attending the 2010 US Transplant Games in Madison, Wisconsin this summer. I walked 1.1 miles in the 5K Race for Organ, Eye & Tissue Donation. I attended a Lung Gathering, the only organ-specific meeting at the Games, and met lung recipients from around the country. The highlight of the Games for me was attending the Donor Recognition Ceremony with Threads of Compassion. After the ceremony, my group presented over 650 comfort shawls to the donor families. That night, my sister, son and I attended a coffee house gathering and sat behind a table of women wearing their shawls. One of the women got up and told her story about her son, who had been a donor. After she spoke, she came over to our table and talked to my son, who was working on a very unique shawl. All of a sudden, my son said to me, "Mom, isn't that your shawl?" Sure enough, it was. I attach a special tag on my shawls that says, "Stitched with love by a grateful lung recipient." We talked about Threads of Compassion and she is interested in helping make shawls with our group. We exchanged addresses and I hope that we will meet again at a Threads meeting.

Through my donor family's generous gift, I was able to see one son graduate from high school, a second son get married and another son graduate from high school and get accepted to the University of Wisconsin. I am so thankful for all the many wonderful things I have experienced as a result of their gift. I hope one day to meet my donor family to thank them personally for making my last 11 years possible. Lastly I would like to thank the people who made my new life possible: Dr. Paul Guzzetta, Dr. Richard Cornwell, Dr. Robert Love (my transplant surgeon), Dr. Kenneth Presberg, Dr. Thomas Cantieri, Jill M. Simaras, B.S., R.N., my family support system, many friends and most of all, my donor family.

I am considering writing a book, if not for publication, at least for my family. So many people have told me that I should tell others about my exciting post-transplant experiences. I am living proof that there is life beyond the five year projected survival rate!

Judy Russell, 56
Waukesha, Wisconsin
Chronic Obstructive Pulmonary Disease
Single Lung Transplant, August 16, 1999
University of Wisconsin Hospital and Clinics, Madison, Wisconsin

From Oxygen Tank Back to the Ski Slopes:
My Journey Through a Double-Lung Transplant
By Armand Sadlier

My journey through lung transplantation started about 10 years ago. I'm now 53-years-old. I was very active and noticed a gradual loss of function. I finally went to a very reputable hospital in my area, and was followed there and loosely diagnosed with some sort of pulmonary fibrosis disorder, and had slowly declining lung function. I was never put on medication, which was good in retrospect, as prednisone would not have helped my condition. Then, in 2007, I got a case of double pneumonia that took me from still being able to walk miles (albeit, shorter of breath than others might have been), to needing to be on oxygen in the space of a weekend. Something I had seen coming, but still frightening to be at that juncture.

I asked if I would be a candidate for lung transplant. I was told, I would be, but that being said, they didn't see that as being 'any time soon'. I was transplanted just 10 months later. That's soon, in my book. Mind you, no on had ever uttered the word 'transplant' to me in three to four years of being followed. I was quite relieved to know at least there were options. The point of this is not to cast aspersions on that hospital, only to say that even the best doctors sometimes can misjudge the course of interstitial lung disease, and the fact that ANYONE with this type of disorder should be told of the possibilities that exist. Lung transplant is certainly a risk, but dying was a certainty. Easy choice, in my mind.

I knew that Duke University Hospital, Durham, North Carolina had some of the best three year survival numbers of any center performing over 50 lung transplants a year. Fortunately they were covered under my health insurance policy. I knew it could mean being away from my family for months, but it meant having the best chance for long-term survival; it was a small price to pay.

First and foremost, getting involved in a pulmonary rehab program is about the best thing you can do prior to this surgery. (In some lung illnesses, exercise may be prohibitive – ask your lung transplant team.) You can't underestimate the contribution of being in the best shape possible; to face what is ultimately quite an ordeal. Then, after transplant, you must make exercise a routine part of your life. You owe it to your donor.

Several things you may want to ask about when being evaluated at the center you ultimately choose are fairly new procedures designed to improve long term outcomes. One such would be the use of Nissen Fundoplication to prevent acid reflux from damaging the new lungs. Also, the discovery that the cancer drug Rituxan can help remove unwanted antibodies that may attack the new lungs.

I moved to Durham and within a month, I was in the best shape I had been in since even before I had gotten pneumonia. By the end of the wait, I needed 33 liters of oxygen per minute, just to walk around the track and keep my oxygen (O2) saturation (SATS) about 88%. I was in the right place at just the right time. Just five and half weeks later, on October 27th, I got "the call". Suffice to say that the next month or so was not an easy time. But thanks to the outstanding surgeons and quality of the nursing, it was as painless as possible. I was lucky to only need 36 hours in the intensive care unit (ICU), and was out of the hospital in nine days! They get you up and walking in a day or two, if there are no complications. Again, being in good shape helped greatly with all of this. Another thing to pay attention to in your decision making process, the more time they've seen the complications with your lung illness, that can occur, the better.

I was walking around the Sarah P. Duke Gardens, just 12 days after having my lungs replaced. Walking up steps, not coughing; I have been given a new lease on life. Not everyone's experience will be this way, and the side effects of the medications are something everyone may need to deal with. But compared to the alternative, there is no comparison.

I left Durham after a total of seven weeks, and having completed my 23 rehab sessions. A week later, I went on a ten-mile bicycle ride with my 13-year-old son. Luckily, the wind in my face quickly dried the tears I shed as I thought about my donor, and the phenomenal gift that all donors give. Just four months afterwards, I skied in Vermont with my family.

Like my donor's family, I took a tragic situation and made the best of it that I could. A little over three months after surgery, I got a letter from my donor's Mother. Turns out her name is Gail, the same as my only sister, who was there with me when I got the call. The lungs were from her 18-year-old son, Jody. As I read the letter and she described him, it was the most profoundly moving experience I've ever had. To know that my good fortune was borne out of the depths of the sadness she was experiencing, was about as conflicted as one can feel. We have corresponded several times, and maybe one day I can thank her in person. Several times a day, when I take a deep, clear breath, I think of Jody and the life he never got to finish. I hope I can do him proud.

In the two years since my transplant, I have approached life with a renewed vigor. I have been very lucky to have minimal complications, but I also do constant research into improving my chances of long-term survival, such as the recent discovery that Vitamin D deficiency may play a role in rejection, especially early on. I have gotten involved with the newly formed Lung Transplant Foundation in Durham, started as a means to fund the research of Dr. Scott Palmer to improving long-term outcomes for lung recipients. Despite many advances, it still remains the most difficult organ to keep viable. We raised almost $60,000 in our first benefit, 'Lungapalooza', and I am trying to use my music business connections to create a yearly benefit.

Armand Sadlier, 53
Highland, Maryland
Pulmonary Fibrosis
Double Lung Transplant, October 27, 2008
Duke University Hospital, Durham, North Carolina

Life Begins Anew
By Richard and Karyn Schad

May 17, 2009 – Life Begins Anew
Dear Life-Giver,

How do I say thank-you, to you, that my wife is alive today because of your gift of her life-saving lungs? How I do really say thank-you; that my wife is alive to live?

I want you to know that my wife, Karyn, cried when she was told the operation today was "a-go", that she would receive your lungs. Karyn cried because she knew that somewhere a family lost a loved person in their life. My heart goes out to you and to your family, and my heart will always be there. I am overwhelmed with feelings, a curious mix of joy and sorrow. Second-hand pain is the hardest to bear, and my heart is filled with barbed-wire sadness.

Karyn had a short window to live. The clock was winding down too quick, nearing midnight, and the tolling of her breath escaping much too fast. It seems like yesterday that I met Karyn at a dance in December 1965, and then all-too-soon, she could no longer dance, had limited mobility, was on oxygen 24 hours a day (24/7), and could not catch her breath.

Thinking back to the June afternoon in 1999, when Karyn was diagnosed, and the doctor saying, "Do you know what LAM is?" Karyn responding with only that look she owns, "If I say no, can I have something else?" That weekend was one of the worst of our life; being told my wife's life has an expiration date, "There is no cure. You only have ten years to live. You will die."

Karyn has Lymphangioleiomyomatosis (LAM) – just saying it takes my breath away. LAM is a nasty progressive and frequently fatal lung disease. I am sure you never heard of it, it is very rare - I always knew my wife was one-of-a-kind, and with your lungs she remains one-of-a-kind. The disease prevents the lungs from providing oxygen to the rest of the body. Having LAM is like sucking air through a straw – did you ever try that? LAM is like picturing a color you have never seen.

Know this about Karyn; that LAM exploded in her body, but it never ever touched her heart, her soul, and that's where hope lives. "I tell myself, that no matter how each day goes, I win, the LAM wins, or it's a draw – I can get through it, for another day. I am after all a Lammie." I love the way she devours life, savoring every bit. The hope that Karyn has and shared with so many others cost her nothing, but to me it is priceless. Maybe if Karyn charged a fee for hope, I would have a better sense of its value – of course, I could not afford it, for the value of hope and breath is indeed priceless.

No more dances, no more showers, no more playing with our granddaughter Avah, no more walks with her dogs and me. LAM turns off the lights one by one.

Please remember that no matter where I am, or what I am doing. I've got a special place inside my heart that's all for you. Know that your giving of yourself is a kind of feedback loop, with no beginning and no end.

Thank you for the miracle of giving me back my wife – there is no greater gift.

In awe and admiration and love,

Richard
~~~~
May 17, 2010
Dear Life-Giver,

Thinking of you again today, and wondering what you see when you look down upon Karyn and I. We wish there were magic glasses; others could wear while walking, in the mall, or at a sporting event, glasses that would clearly show them your gift, and letting them know all who have been transplanted.

I reminisce to the days immediately after Karyn's transplant. A doctor came to me and took me back to Intensive Care Unit to visit with Karyn. I said, "Hi" and Karyn responded back with a puzzled, "Hi". All her answers were one word. I asked her, "What do you see when you look at me?" Karyn answered, "Butterflies." Karyn at this point did not realize I was her husband. I knew that due to the surgery and anesthesia, Karyn was having hallucinations. My wife did not know she had had a lung transplant and that she could breathe on room air. You gave her the "Gift of Life", and she did not know.

Finally, just before dawn, God answered the phone (as you know personally, God's phone is never busy), and a wave of peace settled over me, and I knew with whatever there was to deal with, we would work through it, I still felt hollow, shell-shocked, but I knew then, that I could get through this, no matter what. The roller coaster of LAM and lung transplant, you buy the ticket, you take the ride.

Each day brought a little bit more of my wife back to me. The main transplant anti-rejection drug caused this reaction, and with a change from Prograf to Cyclosporine, and the miracle of your lungs, and God, my wife came back to me. I knew my wife was back when she gave me my marching orders a week later, to stop by one of the markets and get a huge basket of fruit for the staff, with very specific instructions on what to buy. "Private husband Rich, reporting for duty." It never felt so good to be told what to do.

Having a double lung transplant and LAM is like being trapped on a roller coaster – a really good one with lots of twists and turns, and huge drops. The kind that makes your stomach turn over.

As much as the twists and turns of the ride affect you physically, the ups and downs play havoc with your emotions also - you look for hope where you find it. You yearn to return to Duke University Medical Center, Durham, North Carolina, to learn there is no rejection. You brace yourself for bad news, and when it comes, acute rejection, aspergillus, it still hits harder than you were prepared for. Karyn smiles and reassures all those around her, that the ride isn't too bad. Your ticket is truly a wild ride, and there's really no way to get off. A roller coaster, a ride that can make you feel frightened, scared, sick, excited, and so thrilled all together. I know we will one day walk off the ride, shaky legs perhaps, but still walking, with big smiles on the faces of those around us who have watched, cheered, and loved you. I see your big smile.

It hits me on the head and I realize how much those of us living without LAM, or a double lung transplant, take for granted our life on the ground.

Now when I see a butterfly, I think of Karyn and you, and I smile. Butterflies are always with me on the roller coaster. Butterflies, like Karyn, go where they please, and pleased where they go.

The book of life, which you have given my wife and me with many new changes, is a difficult read. But read we must, I try not worry about life too much. I have read the last page of the book and it turns out all right. Walking with our dogs, Emma and Jake, and our grand-daughter, Avah, I am struck by the simple truth that sometimes the most ordinary things are made extraordinary simply by doing them with the right person.

Remember that no matter where I am or what I am doing I have a special place inside me that's all for you. I remember it all, because I remember it all. Maybe all I should say is that reliable old line that goes on almost every postcard …

"Having a great time, wish you were here."

Richard

Scott Spencer, <u>Man in the Woods</u>

"Walking through the woods, it's step by step, one foot in front of the other. What could be more fundamental? It's like breathing – inhale through the nostrils, exhale through the mouth, the taste and tickle of your own mortality coursing over your lips like running water over stones. We are under a sea of air, to which we have adapted just as fish have adapted to their life underwater."

Much truth – I remember Karyn before her transplant, looking like a fish out of water, going "glub – glub", and trying to get enough air. Now she is like a fish out of water, but with the gift of lungs, she, too, has adapted.

Richard and Karyn Schad
Karyn, 61
Louisville, Colorado
Karyn, Lymphangioleiomyomatosis
Karyn, Double Lung Transplant, May 17, 2009
Duke University Hospital, Durham, North Carolina

When I am Taking Flight
By Joanne Schum

The creation of this 2nd Edition of Taking Flight has been a hard decision for me. My life has been full of the greatest times, and the saddest times these past nine years. Once I was able to realize the grief for both my sister and mother will last my lifetime, it also rekindled what my two favorite ladies wanted for me, "Be happy, life goes on, stop and smell the roses, enjoy your great health, we walk just beside you forever loving you, forever happy for you."

The story of my achievements over the past years would take pages and pages in this book. I have so many fond memories to remember, of my family and friends, of vacations around the United States of America. With joy and jubilation I attended four Transplant Games and part of the Lung Gatherings that I organize both at the Transplant Games and back home locally. My never ending offering to help with a fundraiser, raising awareness for organ donation, in hopes to help others, is a proud accomplishment that means a great deal to me. Happiness is part of my everyday life now.

My flight over the past 13 years has been one that has the appearance of forever soaring and filled with new adventures and flight patterns, jam-packed with excitement. So what have I planned for my upcoming years? My list is painted with a rosy picture of travel, education, exercise and good health.

The path I take may change, may vary, may take wide twisting turns, but that is the road that I enjoy and all within reach because of this wonderful, "Gift of Life". My, "extreme" goals; the list of dreams I will push myself to reach, but realize every day I am breathing and living in itself, is "an extreme goal", are to pursue further education – not so much for a career (though that would be a pleasant benefit) but rather to enjoy the return to further my college education in new fields of study. I have learned to appreciate the world of medicine, genetics, and discovering more therapies, treatments and medication to advance the field of eliminating organ rejection is fascinating to me. Now that I have new lungs, I can sit back, relax and truly envelop myself in studying hard, where long ago, I was just there to experience as much of life as possible, but not setting any real goals....lung transplantation has allowed me the gift of desire to learn and make real goals I can "earn wings" with.

When I was in college back in the 1980's, I received a degree in Food Administration. I soon learned that it was not a field that someone with Cystic Fibrosis should be looking at, both for my own health, but the health of others. In 2010, I have re-discovered enjoyment of cooking. Cooking healthy, affordable, and fun food is a return to my past college degree.

I sometimes dream of being the next, "Julie/Julia" and cooking my way through a Julia Child cookbook! "Joanne/Julia" does not sound bad at all!

The 1st book I published in 2002, "Taking Flight: Inspirational Stories of Lung Transplantation" can still be acquired through Trafford or Amazon.

Joanne Schum, 47
Webster, New York
Cystic Fibrosis
Double Lung Transplant, September 12, 1997
University of North Carolina Hospitals, Chapel Hill, North Carolina
Read Joanne's Lung Transplant Story in the 1st Edition of Taking Flight

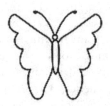

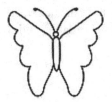

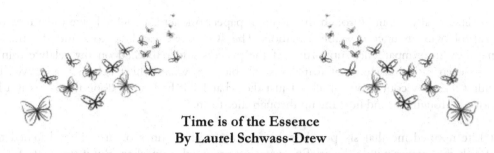

Time is of the Essence
By Laurel Schwass-Drew

On May 10, 2001, I lost my husband of nearly 19 years, James S. Drew, to a brain aneurysm. He was 43-years-old, 10 days away from turning 44, and in seemingly good health, having had only asthma since early childhood. I was working full-time, and concurrently attending graduate school for art.

We were quite busy with numerous work, home and family issues at that time, but we felt we had much to look forward to.

Jim and I met in the late 1970's as undergraduates at what was then the Philadelphia College of Art. Jim enjoyed painting, drawing and, more recently, making digital images. We had no children, but we shared a very happy life of creative pursuits such as screen printing and doing other printmaking media; as well as outdoor activities like camping, swimming, hiking and kayaking, among other things. Thus, the shock of losing Jim so unexpectedly was almost overwhelming to family, friends and everyone who knew him.

The aneurysm abruptly manifested itself as an annoying headache. At first Jim thought it was a sinus headache and proceeded to endure it for a week. At the end of that week, the headache suddenly got extremely severe, and Jim collapsed and had to be rushed to the hospital. Looking back, I recalled that Jim had been uncharacteristically tired and irritable at times, in the weeks preceding the rupture of the aneurysm; however, I attributed that to over-work and stress.

Jim's doctors tried very hard to save his life, but warned us at the beginning that there were no guarantees. The aneurysm was large, in a major blood vessel and couldn't be repaired easily. At first it looked like he might survive the ordeal, but serious complications set in, and after 10 days in the intensive care unit (ICU), the doctors told me that brain death was imminent and he was not going to be with us much longer. As soon as they said that, I told them that I wanted his organs to be donated. I felt, in every fiber of my being, that something positive had to be done to offset this nightmarish event. I considered the fact that Jim wouldn't need his organs anymore, and I knew I couldn't have lived with myself if I hadn't at least offered to do this, and possibly help others in the process. I knew Jim had the organ donor designation on his driver's license, but we had not talked about organ donation together: that is, until the previous year. Almost prophetically, just after his mother died, we had a brief conversation about our final wishes. We both agreed to donate our organs if one of us predeceased the other.

The topic of death is difficult to confront, but this was one of the easier discussions we had. It was this talk, and knowing the kind of person Jim was, and that he would heartily approve, that got me through the donation. The Gift of Life Donor Program, Philadelphia's organ recovery agency, treated us like royalty. Going through the required paperwork actually helped give me a measure of some control over an uncontrollable situation. The ICU nurses and doctors and the transplant coordinators were sympathetic, supportive of the process and remarked on my relative calm and courage ----even though a storm of fear, indescribable sorrow and sheer exhaustion brewed inside me. I didn't feel very courageous at all – I just did what I felt had to be done then – as if a larger force moved through me, and held me up through the storm.

Gift of Life notified me that six people subsequently received Jim's organs. They listened to my stunned daily discoveries within the grief process and provided counseling. But it started to feel like I had joined a whole new honorary family, made up of the Gift of Life staff, and of other organ donors, transplant recipients and their families. It is a powerful emotion, to know that there are others out there who have walked a similar path as oneself.

In time, I heard back from three of Jim's recipients. First there was Lorraine, one of his kidney recipients. I received a simple but sweet thank-you card from her a few months after Jim's donation. It was about all I could handle at the time, but I was glad to get it. A year after Jim's passing, a very important milestone for all concerned, I heard from the family of Richard, Jim's liver recipient. Richard was a father of five whose life had been saved on the day of Jim's donation. They sent me a beautiful and heartfelt message of gratitude. At that time I was happy to have survived a year without Jim, painful as it was at times –and, as this card reminded me, I was also grateful to hear that Richard was doing so well, a year after the donation.

In September of 2004, just before my wedding anniversary, I heard from Ann, Jim's left lung recipient. This communication could not have been timelier. I had just been thinking about Jim's recipients, and about whether I would hear from any more of them, then Ann's letter arrived. Her letter to me was very detailed about how sick she had been before the transplant (I believe she had severe emphysema), and how her life had so changed for the better after it. I was amazed and gratified, because I had heard that lung recipients had a more challenging time with receiving transplants, due to the more delicate nature of the lungs ---and because Jim was an asthma patient for most of his life. Yet here was Ann, apparently doing well three years after her transplant –and kind enough to share this with me. She described being able to once again do her shopping, cooking, cleaning, gardening, enjoying family and especially her grandchildren. All the small but crucial things in life that some of us sometimes take for granted. Ann asked me specifically to write back to her, which I did right away. I have not heard anything further from her, or any of the other recipients since then, but I am totally okay with that. Even though I would jump at the chance to hear from, or even meet any or all of Jim's organ recipients and their families, I know that much time has now passed for all of us, and perhaps it may not be appropriate. The most important and comforting thing for me continues to be the fact that Jim was able to help people, even through his untimely death.

To be honest, receiving these communications from Jim's recipients was a bittersweet, but uplifting experience. I felt, of course, grief at my loss once again; yet coupled with that was extreme gratitude and joy, affirmation that the right decision was made, to give someone else another chance at life through my husband's organ donation. *It has made Jim's death seem less senseless.*

After Jim's loss, I learned to never take anything for granted again.

These experiences shaped my decision, six years ago, to become a Gift of Life volunteer. I have never been a big "joiner" of groups, nor do I feel it's my mission to proselytize. The decision to be an organ donor is highly personal, and one must be ready, willing and able to make an informed decision about it for oneself. But I observe that the donor family perspective is quite under-represented (compared to the still-greater numbers of transplant recipients whom I see more regularly coming forward to share their stories), owing perhaps to the burden of grief and the connection to a tragedy; however, in recent years I have noted an increase in donor family volunteers at my local Organ Procurement Organization (OPO), which is wonderful! I think it is important to relate my experience with organ donation, to help others understand that this option exists, and that it is vital to those many people who are now waiting for organ transplants and life-enhancing tissue transplants. If sharing my story has educated someone in their decision to be an organ donor, has enlightened a bereaved person negotiating a path of grief, or has helped a donor family member find the courage to tell *their* donation story, my job has been done.

I am now a volunteer speaker and writer, telling Jim's story to various groups. I have started doing memory-box-making workshops with other donor families. Additionally, I co-chair a committee for Gift of Life's annual poster contest, giving local high school students a chance to design (and receive recognition for) a poster on this humanitarian health and social theme. Sharing my time and energy with Gift of Life and the transplant community has helped me to process Jim's death more fully, and provided a place for healing to occur. People still tell me that Jim's story moved them, and I am humbly gratified. I make sure to tell all the donation professionals and transplant recipients I meet, that hearing the words "Thank You" for Jim's donation is indeed enough; nothing else is required.

I also have attended several sessions with Gift of Life's Donor Family support group, Hearts of Gold, to learn about subjects related to the loss of a loved one and the facts about the organ donation process. I had an excellent school counselor, whose services I was able to utilize while I worked on finishing my degree.

I read several books on the subject of widowhood, the brain and brain death, trying to understand what had happened to Jim. (I'm sure the bookstore clerks thought I was nuts, when I walked up to the register with a pile of books on widowhood, shortly after Jim's death!) I was so hungry for this knowledge; I even recently attended two sessions of Drexel University's Mini-Medical School, to learn more about the body and brain. I am one of those people who specifically must read, watch and learn more about a traumatic or life-changing event, in order to make sense of it. All of these experiences helped me begin to come to terms with Jim's death and gain some perspective on my loss.

It is essential, in going through a grief process, to allow <u>time</u> for it to happen. In our society, grief is unfortunately rushed through, faster than the time it really takes to process a major loss. I have had to learn to make friends with my grief, to not push it away. Grief is inconvenient, but it insists on always having its way. You have to learn to let it come and pass through when it must. You learn to rely on yourself, but also when to ask others for help, which is not an easy thing. Jim's untimely loss, although easily the most emotionally painful process I have been through, has served to make me appreciate and try to use my own time on earth more fully. I have realized that much of what we concern ourselves with in life is really very petty. I try to look at the larger picture and I prioritize my actions. I try to not "sweat the small stuff". I try to take time to simply enjoy being alive, right here and right now. You never know what can happen. Never in my wildest imagining would I have thought it could happen, but experiencing widowhood at the time I did has proven to be a galvanizing and growth experience. With determination, and the support of family, friends and colleagues, I was able to finish grad school and get my degree. After the loss of a spouse, you learn how important that support is, if you didn't quite know it before. I don't think I would change anything about my experience, as difficult as it has been. I am so glad that Jim's organs went to help others.

I continue to be in the process of building a new life for myself, both artistic and personal. I have learned to be obstinate (yet kind to myself) in creating new rituals; celebrating holidays, anniversaries and birthdays in my own ways, even if sometimes they are smaller and quieter. Scary and empty feeling at first—but I had to make myself do it. Gardening became even more important---to learn to trust nature again and to create new landscapes, to honor Jim's love of flowers. I have learned to cultivate gratitude for all good things that come my way.

I know Jim can't be with me physically, and it has taken a long time for me to accept this situation. Many times I still have dreams about Jim, and even in these dreams I know things have vastly changed and he isn't supposed to be on earth with me anymore. Early on, that fact caused me a great deal of pain; now I know things happened the way they happened and time can't go backwards, no matter how much I might wish it.

I feel he is still with me in spirit; I strive every day to remember Jim and to make my life, even surviving without him, something he would still be proud of. However, at this point in my life, after nine years, I also realize the importance of moving forward.

This realization almost feels like a weight lifted off of me; again, I would have never thought that I could get to this miraculous point in my grief process.

Time is of the essence.

Laurel Schwass-Drew, Donor Wife of Husband, James S. Drew
Philadelphia, Pennsylvania
James Passed Away, May 10, 2001
Organs Donated: Heart, Lungs, Liver, and Kidneys;
Pancreas for Islet-Cell Research
James, "Forever 43"

God Helped Ease My Mind
By Pete Schwob

After receiving a transplant most people are able to do their normal activities. Some have a few medical problems associated with their transplant and some do not. I am fortunate that my life got back to normal very fast. I could not walk around the block, even with oxygen, a year and a half prior to my surgery. Three weeks after transplant I could.

Living a fairly normal life for 4 ½ years allowed me to train for the 2010 Transplant Games. I started playing racquetball and swimming again. I won a bronze medal swimming the 100-yard Individual Medley.

But the best aspect of receiving a transplant for me has been watching my girls graduate from high school and college, and celebrating my 25th wedding anniversary. The second best aspect is being able to give back to the transplant community by volunteering for TransLife, my local Organ & Tissue Donation Services.

I believe these items below are necessary to increase the chances of having a long lasting, successful transplant:

1. A positive attitude
2. A good support team
3. Exercise
4. A healthy diet
5. Staying away from situations that could put your health in jeopardy

I do all the above to a high degree and have had no major problems with my lungs. I did have two bouts of acute rejection that were easily fixed – neither affected my breathing or lifestyle and both were gone in about a week.

While we all may have our doubts leading up to transplant, I found great relief in God's word, which helped ease my mind and soul. Hopefully you can too so that after your transplant you can live a full life and do all the things on your list that you want to do! Maybe you want to go skiing, mountain climbing, or just walking in nature looking at the butterflies.

Pete Schwob, 51
Longwood, Florida
Idiopathic Pulmonary Hemosiderosis
Double Lung Transplant, November 14, 2005
Shands Hospital at The University of Florida, Gainesville, Florida

My Ultimate Gift
By Diana Shackleton

I was only nine weeks old when I was diagnosed with Cystic Fibrosis (CF). Later in life I was also diagnosed with Rheumatoid Arthritis and CF related diabetes. By the age of 22 my health began to quickly deteriorate. I had four hours out of the day designated just to taking breathing treatments. I was on oxygen at 10 liters, twenty four hours a day. My pulmonary function had dropped down to an FEV1 of 28%. I couldn't even walk to the bathroom without getting exhausted. I was slightly in denial about having a lung transplant, but it was the thoughts of what I could do after the surgery that helped me with the decision. It was November 6th, the day after my 23rd birthday, that I received "the phone call".

My family and my husband joined me at the hospital. My transplant surgery lasted around eight hours. It only took five hours after waking up to be taken off of the ventilator. I was in the hospital for four weeks. The day after I was released, I was Christmas shopping at Wal-Mart and had a new love for fried shrimp!

I've done very well since my transplant. It's hard sometimes to even remember being sick! It has never once seemed to me that these lungs came from somewhere else. They always felt like they were mine. I've accomplished so much since then.

I work at a pharmacy and volunteer for mental health. I've become very involved in Community Theater. Also on the board at the local theater and am now in charge of their youth program. It's been so much easier to do daily activities, any activity! I can actually do things with my husband now. We were so limited before.

I have two nieces now, who I never would have met, and they are two very bright lights in my life. The one thing that was always a struggle for me, were stairs. There is a place here where I live that has 300 steps. Every year on the anniversary of my transplant, I walk down them and back up, just because I can.

I had the opportunity to meet my donor's mother and sister three months after my surgery. My donor was 26 and she had a son. Her mother almost didn't donate her daughter's organs, but after hearing all different stories of the other recipients, she was very glad that she did. We found out that my donor's step father is related to my uncle's ex-wife.

But what she gave me was truly the ultimate gift, life. I try every day to live for her. Every year on my anniversary, not only do I climb the stairs, but I also visit my donor to thank her. I leave a rose on her grave for every year that she has given me. This year I will be leaving five roses!

I am very grateful to have a family who has supported me through everything. Not once have they ever treated me like someone who had a life threatening illness. I've also had great friends who have always taken interest in my CF and even gone to doctors' appointments with me and helped keep me out of trouble.

I met my husband before my transplant and he was there before and after my health began to fail, but he stayed with me. These are the people who have kept me going and there are not enough ways to thank them.

I definitely have a new respect for life, since I am now able to live and breathe. I look forward to the future and what it will bring for me. Hopefully I will be able to become a phlebotomist. I will continue to be involved in theater. Hopefully I will finally be able to go on a honeymoon, since I was on the transplant list on my wedding!

Life brings new possibilities and it's those possibilities that I look forward to the most.

Diana Shackleton, 27
Oscoda, Michigan
Cystic Fibrosis
Double Lung Transplant, November 7, 2005
University of Michigan Medical Center, Ann Arbor, Michigan

 The Simple Things
By Elaine Short

You don't know how important it is to be healthy
Until it is taken away from you.

The simplest things in life
Can be such a burden.
To take a shower
Can be such a chore.
To hang the wash
On the line
Or unpack the dishwasher
Every time.

To go shopping all alone
Would be a disaster without my phone.
Shadow follows me wherever I go.
He makes me breathe at an even flow.

The stares
And the giggles
Behind my back
Just want me to hide
Inside my shack.

Waiting, waiting
Until the very day
When the change of life
Will come my way.
Dreams and visions of a healthy me
Running free as can be.

(Elaine wrote the above poem before her lung transplant surgery.)

Strength & Courage
By Elaine Short

I am a 54-year-old woman from Sulphur Creek, Tasmania, Australia. I suffered with alpha-1 antitrypsin deficiency and received my double lung transplant in November 2006.

I was diagnosed with the disease in 1988 and slowly deteriorated over the years. In the year of 2003, I spent most of the year in and out of hospital with chronic infections, to the stage where 24-hour oxygen and confinement to a wheelchair were needed. At this stage I was recommended to apply for a lung transplant. After numerous tests at the Alfred Hospital in Melbourne, Australia, an appointment with the lung transplant team delivered the devastating news that I was not accepted for a transplant. The team explained that I was too sick for the operation and would probably not survive. Overwhelmed with tears I left the hospital with determination I would fight to improve my health for another review with the team.

I wanted to see my granddaughters grow into young women and get married and have children of their own. I wanted more time with my daughters and my husband to enjoy the days together until we were old. Part of me said I have had a wonderful life for 50 years, and the other part of me said I am not ready to die - I still have too many things to do and see. I was eventually listed for a lung transplant.

After waiting three long years, the call came. I traveled to the nearest airport and departed near midnight with my husband. The one-hour trip by plane was very quiet with almost silence. On arrival to the hospital I had many more test procedures before being wheeled down to the surgery theatre. This was the stage when the tears started to emerge. A very emotional time for my husband and myself, not knowing whether I would survive or not. I can still remember that room this day. The next thing I can remember was waking up in intensive care unit (ICU) with a tube down my throat and many lines and tubes elsewhere. In particular I wanted my false teeth; I can remember pointing to my mouth, indicating to the nurses. I spent a week in ICU before been transported to a day ward.

I knew the weeks ahead were going to be tough, but I was alive and very determined to achieve my dream. I experienced pain, but it was all worth it.

The transplant was the hardest thing I have ever done. It takes so much strength, courage and faith. My family and my friends were my strength. They were there to walk with me to regain strength; they were there to love me when I wasn't even aware they were there.

Life is so amazing now, I feel so well, I can do almost anything I choose. Each morning when I open my eyes, I am thankful for this gift of life.

I felt sorrow knowing that somewhere a family was grieving while I was rejoicing in receiving new lungs. I learned to be patient while waiting to receive the much-awaited call, eagerly looking forward to being strong enough to walk and breathe, at the same time without the assistance of oxygen.

Since my transplant I have enjoyed my hobbies of photography and traveling. With my hubby and camera in hand we have traveled this beautiful land of ours.

I am much more appreciative of life since my transplant. I welcome each day as a precious gift and a wonderful new beginning. No, life will never be the same for me...but without the lung transplant experience, I might not have experienced my **remarkable** spiritual journey.

LIFE IS BEAUTIFUL
LIFE IS SWEET
LIFE IS A JOURNEY
HERE TO STAY

Elaine Short, 54
Tasmania, Australia
Alpha-1 Antitrypsin Deficiency
Double Lung Transplant, October 26, 2006
Alfred Hospital, Melbourne, Australia

❧ **My Story Living with Alpha-1 and Lung Transplant** ❧
By Gary Singleton

My name is Gary Singleton. I am married and have two stepchildren. While I live a good life with decent health now, it has not always been that way. I was 31-years-old, single, a smoker, but in good health, or so I thought. Since my teen years I had worked on and off in the Christmas tree business. I then worked for GDS garbage disposal and pulled a hernia. The hernia was fixed as an outpatient procedure and I woke with pneumonia. The doctor told me if I continued to smoke, I would keep getting pneumonia, so I threw my cigarettes in a hospital trash can while I was leaving and never picked up another one. I kept getting short of breath and wheezing.

I married Connie in 1995. Anytime I walked up hill or any exertion; I was short of breath and wheezing. Connie thought it was asthma. Dr. Hill in Morganton, North Carolina said, "Gary, I do not know what is wrong but you have the lungs of an 80-year-old man." I went to see Dr. Bazemore, in Asheville, North Carolina. After some tests, he told me, "It looks like you may have a rare lung disease called Alpha-1 Antitrypsin Deficiency." The only cure was a very expensive Intravenous Therapy (IV) medication you receive weekly called, Prolastin. I began IV's to slow the progression of the disease but after eight years, it never slowed down. Then I was sent to Duke University Hospital in Durham, North Carolina in 1999 for a transplant evaluation.

As we needed to relocate, I required a place that would allow my dog, Little Bit, to come too, or I was not going. Luckily we found an apartment in the same building our daughter lived in.

After five dry runs, "the call" came on March 19, 2003. Upon awaking the next morning, I thought, "Well it's not hot, so where ever I am it's okay." Then I took my first deep breath and I cannot explain that feeling. No oxygen. I walked one and half miles that first day around the hospital corridors with pumps and IV poles and a chair holding lots of stuff, but man it felt good to breathe.

I stayed in the hospital only six days, moved back home to Morganton, North Carolina by mid May. That spring I built a deck for the house, went to a race, and went to see the Washington Redskins/Panthers game all without oxygen. My joy when I first went home was playing with my first granddaughter, Hannah. We moved to Sanford to be closer to Duke University Hospital, but also to enjoy my second born granddaughter. Kinsey. The last three years have been wonderful to be able to jump, run, and play and not be out of breath doing it.

Since transplant, I have had Cytomegalovirus (CMV), rejection, and diabetes all due to the transplant, but these are all treatable diseases and just small hurdles to overcome. Being able to breathe makes it worth it all and I feel I have a better quality of life.

Gary Singleton, 47
Sanford, North Carolina
Alpha-1 Antitrypsin Deficiency
Double Lung Transplant, March 19, 2003
Duke University Hospital, Durham, North Carolina

Because Life is a Precious Gift!
By Tiffany Smith

In 2000 I was diagnosed with Primary Pulmonary Hypertension. I had put on some weight and started to take back control of my "life" and was turned on to a diet pill (muscle builder, fat burner) can't release the name of it, but it contained Ephedra in it. Although it had started to work, I was down 40 pounds, I noticed during my workouts, I was getting fatigued and had this pain up the side of my neck. Long story short, I was admitted to the hospital for 2 ½ weeks where they ran dozens of tests and I was given the news of needing a double lung transplant. I waited on the list in California for over two and half years before I got my new breathers.

I had a tough time. I had an extended stay in the hospital due to some complications. They never thought I would make it; I showed them. I was considered their miracle patient. I think just getting a transplant was a miracle in itself, and found myself being lucky and truly blessed.

After about two years I moved to Arizona, and would go back to California every three months to see my team. In the 3rd year I spent time at University of Southern California University Hospital (USC), Los Angeles, California on oxygen and photopheresis for rejection. I did this procedure for almost four years. My team from USC opened up a new heart and lung program in Phoenix about three years ago, so again lucky me; they could follow me in Arizona instead of me making the long commute. In January 2010, I was blessed with another transplant!!! A quick recovery and I was released 10 days later.

I am here for some reason. Not only to give support to those in our group meetings we have once a month but to encourage those whom are waiting, that it is worth it, and to fight hard, live strong and laugh often, because life is a precious gift....

Tiffany Smith, 46
Avondale, Arizona
Primary Pulmonary Hypertension
Double Lung Transplant, June 3, 2002
University of Southern California University Hospital, Los Angeles, California
Re -Transplant, Double Lung Transplant, March 6, 2010
St. Josephs Hospital and Medical Center, Phoenix, Arizona

2nd Generation Hope
By Heather Snyder

My story started long before I even knew what lung disease was or what it felt like not to be able to breathe. In 1972 I was the second of three daughters born to Gary and Dottie Snyder. We had a close, fun loving and active family that spent a lot of time together.

Unfortunately, when I was three-years-old my father started feeling short of breath. Since his older sister, Clara was already diagnosed with Sarcoidosis; he quickly received a lung biopsy and was diagnosed with Interstitial Pneumonitis and prescribed high doses of prednisone. After no improvement, his pulmonologist referred him to the National Institutes of Health (NIH) in Bethesda, Maryland for further testing and treatment.

Although my father was finally diagnosed with a rare lung disease called Idiopathic Pulmonary Fibrosis (IPF), he was never told he was dying. It wasn't until he read sealed documents that he discovered the truth about his fate. To make this diagnosis even worse, the doctors told him that it was possible that this disease could be hereditary. He was truly devastated and scared, but faithfully commuted to NIH to participate in several drug studies to help find a cure. He felt that the only thing that could make his situation worse is if one of his daughters inherited this dreadful disease.

The winter of 1980 -1981 was hard and my father's lung capacity was failing fast after surviving pneumonia. His last hope was a lung transplant. He read an article about a 45-year-old mother of three in Stanford, California surviving her 24th day, after a heart-lung transplant. My father cut this article out of the paper, kept it in his wallet and showed it to his doctors and asked for a transplant. My mother even wrote to Stanford asking the hospital to consider my father as a candidate for transplantation.

One June 15, 1981 at the age of 41, my father lost his battle with IPF. The heart-lung transplant article still tucked away in his wallet, my mother finally received a response from Stanford indicating that my father was considered too ill for transplantation. (My family still has that article from the newspaper that Dad carried in his wallet, after all these years.)

While growing up without a father was very difficult, it made me a stronger person. I have always been independent and determined just like my father, but also always refused to believe that his lung disease was hereditary. However, after 10 years of the "asthma" and "anxiety" diagnosis, I demanded a chest x-ray because I was severally out of breath with exertion.

At age 37, a lung biopsy was performed. The diagnosis was – Familial Pulmonary Fibrosis (PF). My new best friends were a team of pulmonologists. All of them disappointed to hear that none of my previous doctors ever ordered a chest x-ray considering the severe clubbing of my fingernails that started in high school. Familial PF is not common and from what I was told, most doctors do not familiarize themselves with this disease because the odds of them ever having a patient, especially a patient in their 20's or 30's with it, are slim to none.

Now with the diagnosis in, what happens next? I was thinking that 28 years after my father's death, there should be some kind of drug therapy or some medical advances. Right? Well, the answer is "no" and "yes". The truth is that, there is still no cure or even a Food and Drug Administration (FDA) approved medication on the United States market that slows the progression of the lung scaring. Good news is that, yes, lung transplantation has become more successful over the last 28 years. So, with no other choice, lung transplantation is what I plan to do.

It has been a year and five months since my PF diagnosis and a lot has happened. I have met so many incredible people and even though I am sick, the world feels like a happier place. So many have pulled together and volunteered to help raise money for my transplant fund and awareness for this disease. This journey has been easier because of them. It is not possible to express my gratitude for the champions that have been part of my life recently. They have inspired me as much as they say I inspire them.

But now it is time for surgery. I am officially listed and waiting for the call from the hospital. Many of my doctors feel that I will receive new lungs before my 39th birthday, which is just around the corner. I am not sure if I feel terrified or excited, but every day I dream about a life that is not consumed with gasping for air and mucus filled coughs. To all that have persevered and passionately made lung transplantation what it is today, thank you. Without you, I would have no hope.

June 15, 2011 will be the 30th anniversary of my father's death. I am happy to say that by that date, I will have successfully made hundreds of people aware of Pulmonary Fibrosis and survived a double lung transplant….something that was my father's dream. I know his spirit watches over me and I know I have made him proud.

Update: Heather wrote this story pre-lung transplant. I am happy to report; Heather received her double lung transplant, February 8, 2011.

Heather Snyder, 38
Mechanicsburg, Pennsylvania
Familial Pulmonary Fibrosis
Double Lung Transplant, February 8, 2011
University of Pittsburgh Medical Center, Pittsburgh, Pennsylvania
Daughter of the late Gary Snyder
Idiopathic Pulmonary Fibrosis
Gary diagnosed in 1972, Research Study Participant, for a, Cure for Pulmonary Fibrosis

 To Wish Upon a Star
By Sammi Sparke

Well, I can't think of a better way to celebrate my eight-year transplant anniversary than looking back to my life before that lucky day on the 13th of August 2002 and the vastly different life I have now, thanks to it.

I was born in 1978 to Jackie and Brian, who soon learned I had been born with Cystic Fibrosis (CF). I was in and out of hospital from age three, some years good, necessitating two stays in hospital, some not so, meaning I was in and out all year.

From age three to twenty, aside from the regular health problems, there were three significant times mum and dad were told to take me home and make me comfortable because I was dying. On each of these occasions however I managed to amaze medical staff by getting better. Mum always says that I just wasn't taking, "No" for an answer.

I got well enough to make it through school and even made it to university but this is where my health deteriorated very seriously. Everyone lives it up when they first go to university and this included me. However this wasn't the primary reason for my health hitting rock bottom. The main problem was that I'd developed a growth in my lung called an Aspergilloma (often known as farmer's lung). I came back from university after my first year and they found the growth. Not only that but I developed pneumonia and was in hospital for weeks. I was too ill to go back to university in the autumn and in 1999 was told I was going to die if I didn't get a transplant.

This was a huge shock as I'd always bounced back before. I went into a massive depression, the idea of standing on death's doorstep was petrifying… but all the while I knew I wanted this transplant more than anything I've ever wanted. After speaking with the surgeons they told me that with the Aspergilloma there was chance they wouldn't be able to do the surgery. So they told me I could go on the list but the chance was that if the call came for me and they opened me up and saw it was too difficult to do the operation they wouldn't do it.

[288]

Blind faith got me through the next two and half years on the list. I transferred my studies to the Open University and so I could study while at home. One of the main things that kept my spirit up and kept me hopeful was my dream to travel the world. In the years I waited on the list I went from being seriously poorly, to being unable to breathe even with a Nippy ventilator, hours away from dying.

One of the last things I remember was the night before I got the call, saying to my mum that there was going to be a meteor shower and that she should go out and find a shooting star and wish upon it. She did and in the next 24 hours I was on the operating table undergoing a double lung transplant.

One of the first things I remember on coming round was my mum telling me I'd had the transplant, which I wanted to hear knowing they might have not been able to do it. The second and overriding sensation was that I didn't need to cough! I had no tickle, no anything. It felt like the most peaceful feeling.

Because I had been so poorly prior to my operation I had no muscle tone, body mass, basically no strength at all. This meant my stay in hospital and rehabilitation took months. From Christmas onwards, my body had acclimatised to what had happened and began to heal and progress quickly.

Little by little I could do things I had previously only dreamt of doing, not just during the time I was waiting for my call but things, due to the CF, that I hadn't been able to do for ten years. Walking, running, sports, having an appetite, graduating with a 2:1 in my History of Art degree, but most of all getting my long awaited independence back!!

The one thing that had really got me through was my need to travel and see the world and a year after my transplant, two friends and I jetted off to Barbados to celebrate my amazing year of being alive. The next three years I journeyed to Egypt, South America, Africa, South East Asia, Australia, New Zealand, Fiji and Singapore. These were the most amazing years of my life.

There are many places I am still desperate to see but all that is put on hold while I am doing a second degree, this time in Photography. Photography was something that I realized when travelling and that I wanted it to become more than just a hobby. I wanted it to be a significant part of my life and now it is.

If it weren't for my donor none of this would be possible. I think of her often and never more than on this day, because she had signed the donor register, she gave me my life back…. and what a life indeed!

Sammi Sparke, 32
St. Neots, Cambridgeshire, United Kingdom
Cystic Fibrosis
Double Lung Transplant, August 13, 2002
Papworth Hospital NHS Foundation Trust, Cambridge, United Kingdom

🦋 **Dying to Live** 🦋
By Ashley Spigelman

Waiting. Such surreal terminology; waiting for someone to die, so you can live. Waiting in an "invisible" line up to get called for a double lung transplant. It seems unfair, but this is the part of organ donation that gives someone like me, a second chance at my life.

I was born with a lung illness called Cystic Fibrosis. I lived a normal childhood like any other child would, however when I started entering my 20's my health started deteriorating. I endured a lot of hospital admissions, and taking more medication and wearing oxygen full time by the time transplant was needed. It wasn't until I was 24-years-old that the doctors suggested I be put on the transplant list. At first I had said, "No!" because I wasn't mentally prepared at that point and was in denial about needing one. But as my health started declining faster, I decided to have the doctors list me.

My status was put as 'rapidly deteriorating' and the doctors weren't even sure I was going to live long enough to receive the call. My lungs were drying up and I was literally drowning in my own mucous. I even went comatose for a week due to my lack of oxygen and ability to breathe. Finally after three long weeks of struggling and waiting on the list, I got the call for my lungs.

I was transferred from St. Michael's Hospital, Toronto, Canada, to where my lung transplant would take place; Toronto General Hospital (TGH). My double lung transplant surgery lasted eight hours, and went extremely well. My surgeon came to my family after and told them that it was perfect timing, and that I was lucky enough to have received the call.

My hospital admission at TGH lasted a month. I did have some complications, but that was taken care of. I was breathing well, my oxygen was 100%, the pain was under control but since I was in hospital eight months prior to transplant, I had lost all my muscle strength. The biggest thing for me to overcome was learning how to walk again and taking care of myself physically. After release from TGH, I was transferred to a rehab facility called St. Johns. I was there for only three weeks and within that time I was taught to walk, go up and down stairs and take care of myself. It was a great feeling and I was even more excited to get home and start to live my new life with my two new lungs.

Once home I was finally able to sleep in my own bed, was able to see my family all the time, started driving again (as I was unable to drive from being in the hospital so long as well as for three months after transplant), and just was so thankful I was back at home. It took a while for me to adapt to my new lungs and life – going from dying to living. It is all just such a miracle.

After five months, I went with my family on a trip to Ottawa, Canada and I walked everywhere. It was incredible; I was able to keep up with everyone and was able to do anything I wanted without getting out of breath. I even took a trip to Boston with my family for my one-year lung anniversary. The first year is said to have hardships, hurdles and possible rejection and I was lucky enough to not have to experience any of that.

Now, it is 18 months since my double lung transplant and I am doing amazingly well. I am back in school and graduating April 2011 with my second Marketing degree. I am spending tons of time with family (which without them I would have never even made it this far in life) and I am living every day, as if it was my last, enjoying every memory I make. I plan on traveling more and experience things I was never able to before. I couldn't be more thankful to my generous donor who was able to give me the second chance that I needed and deserved. My life is amazing, full of happiness, love and of course health. After all the struggling I have been put through, I can honestly say that it was worth it.

To be here, to be a part of the world, to be able to appreciate and enjoy every single breath I take, and everything I do. I have become the person I've longed to be and I couldn't have asked for anything more.

Ashley Spigelman, 26
Thornhill, Ontario, Canada
Cystic Fibrosis
Double Lung Transplant, May 27, 2009
Toronto General Hospital, Toronto, Canada

🦋 To Have a Second Chance at Life 🦋
By Dan Spurrier

My name is Danny Spurrier. I received a bi-lateral lung transplant on September 18, 2005 at Duke University Hospital, which is located in Durham, North Carolina.

The reason for my transplant was Emphysema caused by many years of smoking, and I think my work environment was also a contributor. I was officially diagnosed in 1999. I was actually only on the "active" waiting list for three days; however, I was attending rehab at Duke for several months prior to being made active on the list.

My surgery, I am told, lasted between 11 and 12 hours. I came out of surgery without supplemental oxygen, breathing on my own. This was quite an accomplishment. I was in intensive care unit (ICU) less than a day and walked to my next room without any problems. I had no complications during or after surgery other than the pain we all experience from such an ordeal. I left the hospital five days later.

Now I am able to do almost anything I want to do. I walk and lift weights several days per week. I am able to go fishing anytime I desire. I can actually do anything I want to at almost anytime. I am not currently working as I am on disability from my workplace, and plan to retire soon. I have been spiritually revived as a result of my experience and attend church regularly. I have married since my surgery, and been so for almost three years.

My plans for the future are just that: to actually have a future is great. I will continue to live life hopefully to the fullest.

I want to thank my donor family, doctors, my family, and Duke University for this second chance at living life. I have been in contact with my donor family on several occasions and we email each other on occasion. It is still very hard for them and me as well, to talk much after such a devastating occurrence for them.

Dan Spurrier, 63
Southmont, North Carolina
Emphysema
Double Lung Transplant, September 18, 2005
Duke University Hospital, Durham, North Carolina

 Greedy for Breath – Re-Transplanted, Re-Awakened
By Ana Stenzel

I looked into the mirror, unable to recognize the person I once was. A short walk from my bedroom to the bathroom left me panting, leaning over the sink to catch my breath. The light above the mirror shone on my face, pale and sunken with fatigue. Dark circles surrounded my eyes like runny mascara. In disbelief, I asked myself "What the hell just happened?"

The last six months were like a bad dream. It had been six years since my double lung transplant for cystic fibrosis (CF). I had absolutely no complications since the transplant, not even diabetes, and my health had not impeded my fitness, travels or career in any way. I was at the peak of health, training for a half marathon. My chest felt tight after running one day, which led to a lung biopsy. That led to the diagnosis of "Stage-2 Acute Rejection". *Rejection*- the dreaded, most feared word of all for transplant recipients. To me emotionally, it signified the end of my party and the beginning of the end.

"All lung transplants have an expiration date," my doctor told me. Truthfully, he too didn't understand why rejection started so suddenly years after transplant. *Did I overdo it? Did I catch a virus that woke up my immune system? Was my donor mad at me?* Despite numerous attempts to stop the rejection with new immunosuppressive medications, acute rejection spiraled into uncontrollable chronic rejection, which persisted in a rapid, relentless, downhill spiral.

I welcomed the cool breeze that entered through the bathroom window. Oxygen hissed from the tube under my nose. I sucked briskly trying to find relief. Only the painful sensation of hypoxia consumed me; the tingling fingers, the weak muscles, and throbbing headache. I stared at my shoulders pumping up and down for breath, moving the port-a-cath needle on my chest, where I was infusing antibiotics intravenously for an infection I caught by being so immunosuppressed. It was as if God was playing a bad trick on me, teasing me with good health for six years only to take it all away again. Chronic rejection was like free falling into the world of illness again, fast and furiously, with an unforgiving sense of suffocation worse than anything CF had ever dealt me. In a bewildering de-ja-vu I was back on oxygen, inhalation treatments and intravenous antibiotics (IV's), but this time, within seven months I could no longer walk and had to use a wheelchair. All the privileges of my healthy life - exercising, volunteer work, socializing, and even my job - were tossed aside, my life

[292]

imploding into a hole in which the mere goal centered on just trying to breathe. I had jumped from the ship of the living to the sea of the dying so quickly, amidst a raging immunological war within me against my beloved donor. I was on survival mode, so the emotional implications of this crash could not even surface. With a lung capacity of 16% and lungs that were slowly turning solid like a rock, I sucked air like breathing through a straw. *Haven't we been here before?*

My breathlessness threw me into a panic, and I began to breathe faster and heavier, my mind wandering, fearing I was going to faint. I tried to calm myself, closing my eyes, gripping the edges of the sink. *You've been here once before with CF; you can do this again. Hang in there. Breathe. Just breathe.* In tears, I collapsed over the closed toilet seat, my spirit and body broken, tears running down my face. I prayed to my donor's spirit, pleading for our unity, and apologizing for my body's rejection of his gift. The end was coming.

I faced dying with acceptance, as I had been given six years of near perfect health. I had seen many of my fellow lung transplant friends die of rejection and now it was my turn. If they could get through this, so could I. It was time to harness the lessons I learned from CF and face the end with peace and gratitude. It was finally time to surrender, to let go.

But my identical twin sister, Isabel, who received her lung transplant for CF two years earlier, was not ready for me to die. We had just begun to live our lives together, free of illness, when I got sick again. We were in the midst of publishing our memoir, *The Power of Two*, which was set for release in late 2007. I had to survive. Isabel begged me to fight, to not give up.

Later that week, the mood was somber at a clinic visit. All the treatment options for chronic rejection had been exhausted, to no avail. With stern and sincere eyes, my doctor leaned forward and asked, "How about a second transplant?" My eyes met his, widening in disbelief as a glimmer of hope enveloped my defeated spirit. For a moment, he was like God, holding my life in his hands. He could let me die or he could offer me another chance. But second lung transplants were rare and extremely risky. *Could I survive? Was it fair for me to get a second transplant when so many people died waiting for their first due to the shortage of organ donors?* My life had been fulfilling and privileged; how could I ask for more?

In a depressed state, I told my sister, "I've fulfilled all my goals. I don't know what else I have to live for." She broke down and pleaded, "What about me? Don't you want to live for me?" Isabel was training for an 18-mile relay race for organ donation; she was traveling and hiking, living the full, healthy life I had enjoyed for six years. Now, I wanted her by my side more than ever. "I feel guilty for enjoying my health," she said. "But your rejection is just so painful to watch. It reminds me I need to make the most of this." The inevitability of rejection just reminded us both how vulnerable we really were. I begged her to keep living.

After careful consideration, and a faith that God was handing me the option of a second transplant for a reason, I decided to be listed for a second transplant. I was greedy for breath; I was selfish for wanting to live more and breathe more. After a rigorous evaluation deemed the rest of my body healthy enough to withstand another transplant, I was re-listed for another double lung transplant.

With the new lung donor allocation system based on recipients' critical need, I was placed at the top of the waiting list.

Two months later, on July 13, 2007, I was called for my second transplant. I relived the nostalgic events of June 14, 2000 on that day - the phone call from the surgeon stating that lungs were available, the anxious rush to the hospital, the waiting room buzzing with supportive friends and family, the farewells before surgery. This time, however, familiarity and trust replaced the intensity of the moment. I had no fear; only faith in God's hands. He would decide if I lived or died. He would take care of those left behind.

At the hospital, I looked around the waiting room with its high ceilings, bright lights and sterile smell. Night had fallen and it was quiet in the halls. Calmness of spirit accompanied the stillness. My mother, siblings, brother-in-law and a half a dozen of my closest friends stood by me, their expressions a mix of relief that a donor was found and nervous anticipation. I had been the symbol of transplant success to them for so many years that when my rejection happened they mourned in disbelief with me, remembering what a vibrant athlete I was less than a year ago. These loving friends were the ones who had pushed my wheelchair, brought me food and given me a reason to live. They believed in me. Although I had fulfilled many goals post-transplant, I made new ones and realized how much I had to live for. I couldn't let my friends or my donor family down. With unspoken exchanges, love was shared. We feared the worst, but hoped for the best. With a 25% chance of death with second lung transplants, I bid each person farewell with greater conviction than with the first transplant. I was about to embark on the ultimate test of strength.

My twin and I embraced, "Whatever happens, we are always together," I said to her, pressing into her body as if to fuse our spirits one last time. My eyes welled up, fearing the unknown and the possibility of leaving her.

Fortunately, the second transplant went smoothly, a rare occurrence that I attribute only to Divine intervention. The familiarity was comforting, as I experienced the same sense of delirium in the intensive care unit, the same shortness of breath from the deflated new donor's lungs, the same scar, and the same challenge of re-learning how to eat, sit, stand, and walk again. Steadfastly, I told God I had too much to do to die.

I left the hospital in 16 days. Standing upright in front of the mirror of my bathroom a month later, I smiled. My lips were bright pink, my face colorful, and my chest breathing effortlessly. I was whole again. I silently thanked my new donor family for giving me the gift of life. I found peace with my guilt through talking to my first donor's family, who offered understanding and forgiveness about rejection of my first donor's lungs. On Oct. 18, 2007, I declared my transplant recovery over by stating, "Enough of this being sick shit. Time to get on with life." My nightmare was over and I had woken to glorious sunshine.

Despite a few bumps in the road, like finally developing diabetes, and a bought of acute rejection and Cytomegalovirus (CMV), I am cautiously stable and pray daily that chronic rejection will never return. I decided that if I were to die from transplant related complications, I would take cancer or some other issue over chronic rejection in a heartbeat. Suffocation is just not my thing. Some days I feel like I have aged ten years from my re-transplant and lost a few brain cells in the process. Yet, since my second lung transplant I have been able to resume traveling, hiking at high altitudes, and swimming again. When our memoir was published in late 2007, Isabel and I drove 10,000 miles across America on a book tour to 24 states, sharing the message of cystic fibrosis, organ donation and the twin bond, to over 35 conferences and book signings. A year later, our book was translated into Japanese, and we traveled there with a documentary film crew for a book tour to promote organ donation awareness in a country where organ donation is rare, highly controversial and painfully inadequate.

On the one-year anniversary of my second double lung transplant, I swam in the 2008 United States Transplant Games, winning three medals. I had to pinch myself as my life had normalized, grateful that the nightmare of chronic rejection was just a bad dream from which I awoke. In 2009, my boyfriend who had endured the drama of my re-transplant, proposed, and we were married on June 5, 2010. Together we have been able to enjoy traveling, companionship and good health together. My memoir will be the subject of a documentary film, *The Power of Two*, and it will be released in 2011. Now I have so much to live for. Not a day goes by without a sense of disbelief and gratitude that I am still alive, thanks to my two wonderful donor families. Each day I live is in honor of them.

With deep breaths.

Ana is co-author of her memoir, "The Power of Two: A Twin Triumph over Cystic Fibrosis." To learn about this book search online for "The Power Of Two Movie".

Ana Stenzel, 39
Redwood City, California
Cystic Fibrosis
Double Lung Transplant, June 14, 2000
Re-Transplant, Double Lung Transplant, July 13, 2007
Stanford University Medical Center, Stanford, California
Read Ana's Lung Transplant Story in the 1st Edition of Taking Flight
Read Isa Stenzel Byrnes Transplant Story in this Edition of Taking Flight

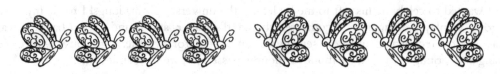

My Donor's Gift of Bagpiping
By Isabel Stenzel Byrnes

Six weeks before my transplant, I sat in a wheelchair with three tanks of oxygen strapped to the back, and I was pushed by my husband and his family around Disney World's Epcot, Orlando, Florida. I had spent a lifetime coughing and feeling short of breath due to cystic fibrosis (CF), but now my lungs were at their worst. I had just done a treatment and napped at the infirmary, and was ready for a few more hours of energy expenditure on this over-stimulating, exhausting 'vacation'.

As we approached the 'Canada' exhibit, my ears caught the majestic sound of a bagpipe. My Canadian-American father-in-law loved the pipes, and always talked about wanting a piper to play "Amazing Grace" at his funeral. We approached the large Caucasian man wearing a kilt playing the bagpipe. I watched in amazement as his large chest rose and fell with each steady, slow breath as he filled the bag. I noticed how the veins in his neck popped out with each blow. His fingers danced on the chanter while everything else remained completely poised. He looked refined, royal, and historical in his Scottish attire. I was in awe of his controlled breathing, his lungpower, and the spectacular cacophony that could be heard across the entire corner of Disney World.

When I got home after New Year's Day 2004, I surrendered to Stanford Hospital in Northern California. It was clear that my CF lung disease was progressing to its natural end. I was placed on the waiting list. My last shower brought the sensation of suffocation, despite 10 liters of oxygen. I gasped at the slighted movement. Soon I could not brush my teeth, then eat, then sleep. Breathing became torturous. After coding and experiencing a spiritual near-death experience, I was placed on a ventilator. At the time, lungs were allocated based on time on the list, not severity. My chances were slim. My family prayed for a miracle.

Thankfully, on February 6, 2004, a miraculous donor family said yes to donation just two days after I was intubated. I woke up two days later, pink, with slow, relaxed respiration. After 32 years, my CF was gone. But I struggled to get up from the toilet, to walk again, to climb stairs, to breathe deeply. Coming back to life took time. I later learned my donor was an 18-year-old Hispanic man named Xavier Cervantes. Following a car accident, he became brain dead. He was on a ventilator just like I was, at the same time. I could not understand why I was chosen to survive and he wasn't. Even now, I think of him every day.

Two months after my transplant, I attended the California Transplant Donor Network (CTDN) Donor Recognition Ceremony. I felt fragile, but volunteered to stand on stage in front of 1,200 donor family members, along with my twin sister Ana, also a lung recipient, and a group of other grateful, successful transplantees. Afterwards, I sat in the audience and watched a professional bagpipe band perform a beautiful 'Amazing Grace'. I got goose bumps. The entire auditorium seemed to vibrate with a sacred boom. Something stirred inside. I wanted to play that song for my donor. I wanted to celebrate his gift to me by letting the universe *hear* his lungs! I made my decision; I was going to play the bagpipes. I contacted the band's leader, and found a local bagpipe teacher. She was medical technician, and very sensitive to my needs for hygiene. I got busy with traveling, exercising and writing my book, so about 15 months passed before I began lessons.

For the first six months, I learned to play a practice chanter. This is like a plastic recorder. I would blow for a few seconds and stop, gasp for breath, and ask myself, "Why do I want to be short of breath again?" I'd sweat, my mouth would ache, but I'd rest and keep going. I sounded like a dying duck but I kept going. My finger muscles ached as I learned the nine notes, but I practiced consistently several times a week.

After six months, I borrowed a bagpipe from my teacher, and wiped it down thoroughly with alcohol. I quickly learned that bagpipes could make some pretty horrible squeaks and squeals! But I kept at it. It took concentration and focus, and fierce defiance against my "Prograf Brain".

Around my 3rd anniversary of my lung transplant, I joined the San Francisco Stewart Tartan Pipes and Drums. The Scottish-American band welcomed me, despite my Japanese-German heritage! After so much sickness, it is very refreshing and healing to be part of a 'normal' group of regular people. I needed this social connection, since I haven't worked regularly post-transplant. The fabulous leader has a great sense of humor, and honors that our participation should be fun. That's what we're still here for, right? To enjoy life and have fun.

The band members are all very compassionate to my special requirements in the band. Ironically, many of them have health challenges of their own. Every fall, I send out an email reminding members to stay away from me if they have a cold or flu. I wash my mouthpiece before use, and disassemble my pipe completely after each practice to thoroughly dry all parts to avoid mold growth. I never let anyone use my mouthpiece! I also say no to piping gigs at crowded, indoor concerts in the wintertime.

Thankfully, my healthy donor lungs have allowed me to learn with the same pace as the other beginners. I started with all drones plugged, and as I gained lungpower and muscle strength in my lips and abdomen, I opened one drone at a time. My first concert, believe it or not, was 'playing' one tune on the chanter only (no drones) while marching down Main Street at Disneyland! It took me about one year to play all three drones… and my FEV1 increased proportionally. My lung function has increased 25 % since I started to play the bagpipes! I have never seen my numbers go up when I had CF! I think the pipes keep my lungs healthy, and serve as a form of airway clearance. Sometimes, after I recover from a cold, I notice coughing up phlegm after I play for a while. When I feel tight, my lungs feel much more open after I practice. I also swim, jog, hike and bike regularly, and this level of fitness allows me to keep up with marching and playing the pipes at parades throughout the year.

Thankfully, since I played the violin as a child, I've been able to read music and memorize 22 tunes in three years. Our band does parades, weddings, funerals, and graduations all over the San Francisco Bay Area. We wear a red Stewart tartan kilt, a sporin, ostrich feather bonnet, spats, and plaid (a blanket-like cape that inspired the term, "whole nine yards"). The band looks spectacularly awesome, if I may say so myself.

Now, I practice the pipes inside my house while my husband winces and my basset hound howls alongside me! She won't move to another room; she likes to sing along! I also occasionally play at the beach, on a cliff or at a park. I usually draw an audience, which can be embarrassing when I am just practicing.

Playing pipes in nature is truly a spiritual experience. The volume of the pipes is like calling out to God, saying, *"I'm still here! Thank you for this lung power!"* I want to call out to my donor, and tell him he's still with me, that his spirit is very much alive through me. I want to show him what he has allowed me to do. This is *him* playing.

I've been privileged to play solo for the 2008 United States Transplant Games Donor Recognition Ceremony, the Cystic Fibrosis Foundation Great Strides, Stanford Hospital, and at organ donation and CF awareness events in Japan. My bagpiping dreams culminated when I played the Nation Anthem at the 2010 United States Transplant Games Opening Ceremony. I stood before 10,000 people, in full uniform, playing each note slowly as the audience swayed and sang along. My spirit was transported to a different place as all those touched by donation could hear the holy sound of my donor's lungs.

In all my years of serious lung disease, bagpiping is something I never, ever, ever imagined I'd be doing. This is the true miracle of lung transplantation. Transplantation truly is human resurrection, and the gift of music through bagpiping is indeed redemption after decades of illness. I am incredibly grateful to my medical team, my supporters, and my family for allowing me to call myself a bagpiper. I know I won't be able to pipe forever, so I cherish each moment, and allow the tears to flow when I think of losing my lungpower. Bagpiping started as a hobby and has become my passion, my emotional and physical therapy, my greatest joy and my highest tribute to my lung donor.

Isabel is co-author of her memoir, "The Power of Two: A Twin Triumph over Cystic Fibrosis." To learn about this book, and to view videos of piping go online and search for: "The Power of Two Movie"

Isabel Stenzel Byrnes, 39
Redwood City, California
Cystic Fibrosis
Double Lung Transplant, February 6, 2004
Stanford University Medical Center, Stanford, California
Read Ana Stenzel's Lung Transplant Story in the 1st Edition of Taking Flight
Read Ana Stenzel's Lung Transplant Story in this Edition of Taking Flight

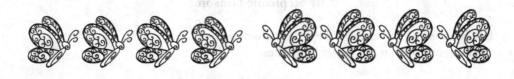

Dedication
By Stephanie Stinson

"To my Family, the Donor, and their Families, the Doctors, Nurses and staff at the University of Utah Medical Center, Transplant and Pulmonary Program; for their sacrifice, generosity, dedication, long hours, compassion, caring, and sometimes even a sense of greatly needed humor!"

~~~~

Donors, Doctors, and Me

The Donors have donated while their families grieve; the Candidates get the phone call they hope to receive.
It's the Doctors on the line; they think they have a match!
But come in very quickly, for this is the catch.
It's now or never, it's to do or die, it's a hope for your future it's the blue in the sky.
You're nervous, you're scared, but you're flying on high!
The Donors have donated while their families grieve they gave in the hope that those who receive would live on with their families, with the love that they share and make certain that the memory of how they got there, would never be forgotten, for the ones that they loved live on inside you looked upon from above.
The Doctors have "patients" of both kinds; they say you will need it because it takes time. I'm sure this will work for it's all on the line.
You'll have to stay positive for there will be bumps in the road; but those are expected, sometimes you'll feel like a toad!
But I'll always remember the gift I've been given – all the effort and times that I have been driven – to appointments, tests, clinics and more, it's been a busy schedule and there's more in store! I'll be a patient, patient you've all been so kind, thank you for listening to these things on my mind.

Very Gratefully Yours,
Stephanie Ann Stinson

Beginning of life 10/18/68, Second chance with life 5/18/09

~~~~

Life is But a Journey...
By Stephanie Stinson

Life is but a journey through the blue uncharted skies
And we but flutter through it like lovely butterflies.........

While we have made a change from our quite unpleasant past
Our future looks more promising the more flowers that we pass.

As we encounter others in our travels along the way
We talk and tell and wish them well and then are on our way.
    We enjoy each and every moment
    Of each and every day

    Because of a gift a stranger, gave to us one day

    We honor them in memory, as we think of them each day
As we spread our wings in wonder and flutter on our way.

    Life is but a journey through the blue uncharted skies
And we but flutter through it like lovely butterflies.........

~~~~

Connections – Unsure of Our Beginnings but Grateful to the End...

My name is Stephanie Stinson; I am 42-years-old. I became ill in 1995, but was not diagnosed until 2001. I became the recipient of a bi-lateral lung transplant in May of 2009. The surgery was performed at the University of Utah Medical Center, Salt Lake City, Utah.

I am a wife, to Craig, and mother to four wonderful boys – Houston, Tyler, Morgan and Ian, and have two beautiful granddaughters, Lilly and Jasmine. Prior to becoming ill, I enjoyed traveling, camping, fishing, and time spent with my family. During the time waiting for diagnosis and treatment I was unable to do anything. It was so horrible I can't put it into words. Being rushed into the Emergency Room, time spent in comas and the constant stress put on my family... I spent too many days in the hospital to count. I was on oxygen constantly.

At the time I was transplanted my life and time was very limited. If it had not been for the generosity of a stranger's last gift, I would not be here today. Since my transplant I am able to do most of the things that I enjoyed before. Please consider Organ Donation. There are so many in need and one person's gift can help save many.

"You might be only one person in this Whole World... but to one person you might be the Whole World." ~~Anonymous

Stephanie Stinson, 42
Kearns, Utah
Cryptogenic Constrictive Bronchiolitis
Double Lung Transplant, May 18, 2009
University of Utah Medical Center, Salt Lake City, Utah

Not Going to Live a Normal Life
By John Sullivan

In 1981, at the age of 35, I was diagnosed with Alpha-1 Antitrypsin Deficiency, which is a genetic disease where your own body attacks your lungs. The doctor told me that I wasn't going to die in two years, but that I would not live a normal life. At that time I had no idea what he was talking about. My children were eight and six, and all I could think about was that I had to live long enough to get them through college.

I continued to work and my lungs continued to deteriorate until in 1989 my doctor suggested that I might want to consider a lung transplant. First of all I had never heard of a lung transplant; secondly, I wondered how I could be sick enough to even consider one? In 1990 I was evaluated at the University of Pittsburgh Medical Center, Pittsburgh, Pennsylvania. At that time the doctors informed me they would give me a heart/double lung transplant, which is all they knew how to do. They would give me a double-lung/heart and then give my heart to someone else. I was very fortunate during the 14 months that I waited; surgeons had developed a procedure to transplant a double and single lung without transplanting the heart.

On April 30, 1991 I got the call and received a single, right lung transplant. I was in the hospital for about five weeks and then returned home with no oxygen and resumed my life. I did very well for about six months when I developed pancreatitis. I was air lifted from Detroit, Michigan to Pittsburgh to be treated. One of the medicines caused the pancreatitis so the adjusted my medicines to save my life. However, then my right lung rejected. I was huffing and puffing, but not back on oxygen.

I was fine until April of 1994, when I came down with a fungus. I spent three months in Cardio-Thoracic Intensive Care Unit (CTICU) trying to get off the vent. They told my wife four times I was not going to make it. I left the hospital on a vent and was placed back on the lung transplant list. I started to work at home from an office connected to my bedroom. It was very important for me to work because it took my mind off my illness and waiting for another transplant. I waited for 32 months; in October of 1996 I got the long awaited call. My wife Claudia and I flew to Pittsburgh. But it turned out to be a dry run.

Once again in January 1997, we got the call and Claudia and I again flew to Pittsburgh, and again, it was a dry run. After a few days the transplant team advised my wife and I that they were taking me off the transplant list because my kidneys were failing. They could not waste a lung on a patient with multiple organ failure. Dr. Bartley Griffith, the director of the heart/lung transplant team, told me if my creatinine dropped to 3.5 he would put me on the list. It did, and I was once again on the list.

On February 4, 1997 a suitable set of lungs became available in Augusta, Georgia. I received a double lung transplant, but the operation was too much for my kidneys and I lost them. I was on dialysis but that was okay because I could breathe again. In January 2000, I received a kidney transplant. Now my kidney is working well and they tell me that my lungs are better than 98% of the people in the world. We had come a long way after 20 years of battles.

As I mentioned my main goal was to get my children through college. Both of them have graduated, and my wife finished graduate school. In May of 2000 I also was able to walk my daughter down the aisle. That was very emotional for me because I never thought that I would be here for that special occasion. I lost my wife in 2006, and the doctors told me that without her I would not have made it this far. I just want to remind the patients that the whole process is much more difficult on the caregiver than it is on the patient. We know how we feel but the caregiver suffers everyday.

I have attended to three Transplant Games with Team Pittsburgh. I did not win a medal at the games playing golf, but that is not why I was going. Also, just because my lungs came from Augusta, Georgia, home of the Masters, it hasn't helped my golf game a bit. I know that I have already won the biggest challenge of my life. I went to the games to participate in something that would not have been possible without the support of my family, friends, medical staff and Dr. Bartley Griffith who believed in me. Even with all of my support I know that without the love and generosity of the donor's and their families I would not be telling my story today

Thanks to all of you, I NOW HAVE MY LIFE BACK!!

John Sullivan, 64
Pittsburgh, Pennsylvania
Alpha-1 Antitrypsin Deficiency
Single Lung Transplant, April 30, 1991
Re-Transplant, Double Lung Transplant, February 4, 1997
Kidney Transplant, January 2000
University of Pittsburgh Medical Center, Pittsburgh, Pennsylvania

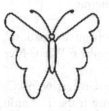

Reaching New Heights
By John Taylor

"Mark, I can't breathe." That's the first time I said aloud what had been going through my mind and body for a long time. But I didn't plan on it coming during my weekly golf outing with my buddy, Farmer Mark, and I never anticipated it would become a defining moment in my life.

Sure, I wasn't as fit as I'd been in my younger days. I was in my early 40's, watching more sports than I was playing. Work consumed those hours I might have spent working out. And while I could have walked to the store instead of piling in the car for a half-mile drive, who actually does that? The trouble had become more apparent during the last year. I gasped for air while walking short distances. I became expert at avoiding stairs and inclines. Even those closest to me didn't see how cleverly I hid my shortness of breath. But the secret was out that Sunday morning. In a sense I was relieved that it was time to face the fears and talk with the doctor.

Luckily, my dear friend and small town country doctor also happened to be a genius. After experimenting with some asthma medications and running a few inconclusive tests, he told me he wanted to rule out the "billion-to-one condition they talked about for five minutes in med school". A week later, I heard the term Alpha-1 Antitrypsin Deficiency for the first time. The pulmonologist described it as a form of genetic emphysema, manageable with medication.

In 2005, I experienced a noticeable change in my breathing. The tricks of avoidance weren't enough to get by anymore. I was tired unlike I had ever been. Just that quickly, the hurdle turned into an oxygen tank. I required over three liters just to sit and watch TV. Making it into the office for just a couple hours became a huge effort. Life had become a mortal struggle, and the tank by my side, and cannula in my nose were both my allies and my enemies.

When the pulmonologist said the words, "transplant evaluation", it was as if he was speaking a language I couldn't understand. Double lung transplant? What? Me? Where? When?

The trip from my home in Oklahoma, to the University of Colorado Hospital/Health Science Center, Denver, Colorado, did nothing to ease my fears. The airline sent my oxygen on the wrong flight, guaranteeing I would be late for the first of two days of evaluation. When I reached the thin air of Denver, I was certain that I was going to die. Even increasing the amount of supplemental oxygen left me wheezing. But with the help of the staff I made it through. I remember little of that whirlwind. All I know is that I left Denver living in a shocking new reality: the next time I saw their faces; it would be to receive new lungs.

So I waited. While most potential recipients have at least some prep time as they move closer to the top of the transplant list, I had a unique problem. At 6 feet, 7 inches tall (6'7"), I required a donor of similar size, and they don't come along everyday. I was placed on alert from the moment that I left Denver to be ready when the call came. Bags were packed for a three month stay, plans made to care for the animals, arrangements to leave my work at a moments notice without losing my job, even to have a car brought to me in Denver.

After being listed, I jumped each time the phone rang. The call came one June morning. My sleepy brain tried to process what the doctor was telling me. An inmate in a federal prison in California had died in an assault. He was my physical match. Due to the circumstances of his death, there could be no assurance that he had not been exposed to a sexually transmitted disease or infection during his incarceration or the attack. The lungs could be mine, if I wanted to take the chance. I spent the longest twenty minutes of my life making an irreversible decision. My health had been holding steady, and the thought of going through the surgery, only to be undermined by a lurking infection seemed too cruel an outcome to chance. So, hearing the words as if they were coming from someone else, so I said, "No".

A beautiful September day the next call came. But this time, the decision was not mine to make. The lungs wouldn't fit my chest cavity. It seemed that maybe my height, of which I have always been so proud, was going to be my downfall. But after two chances in just a few months, I thought my time was coming. Third time's a charm. Good things come in threes. Right? It was over a year until the next call came, in November 2007. This was it. I was whisked away to Colorado by air ambulance, rushed to the hospital, taken to pre-op. The preparation began…then stopped. An infection was discovered in the donor lungs. There would be no transplant. I was going home, in my mind, to die.

When the phone rang the morning of January 2, 2008, the caller identification (ID) reading, "transplant center", I wasn't excited. I figured it was my coordinator calling with best wishes for the New Year. Instead, I was on a flight to Denver in little more than an hour. Check-in at the hospital was a blur, and I recall little of the tests and paperwork. A nurse told me it was time, so I called my mother and siblings. The last call I made came from the gurney as they wheeled me to pre-op. So much happening so quickly.

I was surprised at how many people were in the operating room. Looking up at them, trying to stay focused enough to answer their questions. Making sure none of them had been up late, celebrating or drowning their sorrows after their team's big bowl game. Counting backwards.

The voices came and went as I tried to regain consciousness. I couldn't concentrate on them enough to know what was being said, and the paralytic drugs used post-surgery made it impossible to move. I tried to will my eyes open, to move a finger, to let them know I was okay. The tube in my throat felt the size of a trashcan. But slowly, it dawned on me that I was alive.

The next day I was out of bed, in a chair, eating the most delicious cheeseburger any hospital has ever served. The change in my condition was immediate. Three days later I was moved from intensive care unit to the transplant ward, practically free of supplemental oxygen. Five days later I was discharged to my temporary home near the hospital. Aside from a scary episode of dehydration caused by diuretics, and a minor infection, I was racing along the road to recovery. Within a couple weeks, I walked on a treadmill, crying with each step. To move, without gasping, without supplemental oxygen, without looking for the chair I would need when the breathlessness came, was a moment I thought I would never see again.

I left Denver less than three months after surgery, reclaiming the active life I thought was left behind. My daily exercise routine progressed from walks around the block to weightlifting and swimming. Thankfully, even the laundry list of anti-rejection medications that I take daily have not adversely affected my life in any way.

Less than a year after my surgery, I moved to Phoenix and married the love of my life. In September 2009, I swam the mile leg in a team triathlon event, and I hope to participate in the Transplant Games in the near future. My lungs have given me the ability to see my niece married, the birth of a great-nephew, and the faces of my loved ones once again.

I've even been blessed to have a wonderful relationship with the family of my hero, my donor, and to work with his mother to increase awareness of organ and tissue donation and transplant. That I can do anything to help ease the pain of losing their beloved son and brother, to honor this young man who selflessly saved my life, is the greatest chapter of an incredible story.

John Taylor, 52
Phoenix, Arizona
Alpha-1 Antitrypsin Deficiency
Double Lung Transplant, January 2, 2008
University of Colorado Hospital/Health Science Center, Denver, Colorado

Random Thoughts of A Caregiver
By Robert Tencza

While talking with some of my co-workers about my wife's pre and post-transplant experiences, some have commented that it must also be hard on me to go through this with her. Thinking about that for a while, I have honestly answered that it was NOT. I will readily admit that it was often times frustrating, sometimes tiring, and at other times depressing but never "hard". I say this since I have always tried to keep matters in the proper perspective. My wife has lived with her respiratory problems since childhood, and has adapted herself to deal with whatever comes along. Housekeeping does not come easy to someone who becomes exhausted easily; I did my best on the weekends to try and do as many house chores that I could. When I felt a little pooped out, I'd say something like, "Just give me a minute to catch my breath and I'll be all right". What Sylvia wouldn't have given to be able to say that, and get some of her strength back. Sorry, but that was only a dream.

Then there were the times when getting ready for bed and she would say, "Sorry honey, not tonight, I'm tired". That I realize was not being turned down but knowing that she is physically exhausted and that's just from trying to make it through another day. I got over feeling tired, but I know that she couldn't always do that with a little nap. She didn't know for her first 52 years that all of her problems were actually related to Cystic Fibrosis (CF).

At first she was told it was asthma, later on it's bronchitis, then it's chronic bronchitis, and then it's this or that and finally someone says it's Sarcoidosis. Well then, that explains everything, right? Nope! It wasn't until a very observant pulmonary specialist hears a sniffle and asks if she had sinus problems and if she was ever tested for CF. Yes to the problems, but no to the testing and then it all made sense, and maybe she could get a lung transplant. Life is hard not knowing what is wrong. There is nothing at all that I do that is hard compared to that. I only wished that there was more that I could've done for her.

Frustration and worry are just part of the package: Do we have enough liquid oxygen in the portable Helios for a few hours out of the house? Do we have enough spare E-tanks for just-in-case? Can I pull off the road fast enough to switch tanks before her headache starts. How about the frustration of getting those "dry run" calls only to hear a little while later to not even bother to leave the house due to the fact the donor would not be the right match for Sylvia. Worse yet? Get as far as the pre-operating holding room, and have a, "No Go" at the last minute. You say to yourself that it must be for the best but you question how many times that you've gotten "the call" and wonder how many more before you almost give up hope. As her caregiver and loving support, I was there with a shoulder for her to cry on or the arm to offer my strength, always holding back a tear knowing how disappointed she must be feeling. Somehow we found a way to keep a positive attitude believing that her time will come, that maybe the organs were not good or that they were not the best ones for her.

Her seventh and last call came at the beginning of January 2006, and somehow everyone that we spoke to knew that this was the one. Were they all just being supportive or did they have an insight that we weren't aware of? Maybe I should ask for the winning Lotto numbers. They were right, this was the one and by the grace of God, she survived the ten hours of surgery and in a matter of a little more than three weeks, she was sent home to enjoy her new lungs and a new life.

I am elated to say that so far she is coming along very well, good and healthy lungs showing up clear on the x-ray. What a miraculous way to start the New Year! Looking back at all of the little things that we have gone through, seeing her for the first time without the use of oxygen tubing, more than made it worth while. We tend to appreciate more things that don't come easy, and that we have to fight for.

It is obvious that I do believe in miracles but not necessarily the kinds that we've heard about in the past. You must have a belief in some Divine Creator to get through this and to witness things that you cannot explain. My personal belief is that He works His miracles in all of the little things that we either don't see or just take for granted. Never mind the parting of the Red Sea, I am amazed at how all of the heavy rush hour traffic suddenly parts so that I can maneuver over to the faster left High Occupancy Vehicle (HOV) lanes on the highway when we are running late for our appointment. Have you ever looked up and said a little thank you, as you are the last one to make a turn before your light turns red? If you can look at little things like this as mini-miracles, your travels can become a little more calming. After that, the miracles start getting better. God calls home another soul, and fortunately, the family honored their wish to donate the organs." You transplant surgeon and his team is having one of their best days, organs arrive on time and look healthy and the surgery is a success. Isn't modern medicine one of His greatest miracles? I have never asked God to cure my wife but I have prayed for the strength and patience to make it to our goal of transplant. I have also thanked Him many times for the wonderful doctors and nurses who have helped us along the way.

Last but not least, I have thanked Him for our donor and prayed for consolation for the donor's family.

Robert Tencza, Husband of, Sylvia Tencza
Sylvia Tencza, 59
North Lauderdale, Florida
Sylvia, Cystic Fibrosis
Sylvia, Double Lung Transplant, January 3, 2006
Jackson Memorial Hospital, University of Miami School of Medicine, Miami, Florida
Read Sylvia Tencza's Lung Transplant Story in this Edition of Taking Flight

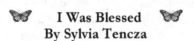

I Was Blessed
By Sylvia Tencza

It was June 14, 2004, when I learned the true nature of my failing lungs. Numerous pulmonary doctors, had diagnosed me over the course of nearly 50 years, but not one had the correct diagnosis. I had been treated over the years, for pneumonia, sarcoidosis, pseudomonas, allergies, asthma, and a host of other diseases. I was at one of my regular check ups, after having been listed with United Network for Organ Sharing (UNOS), being examined by the Jackson Memorial Hospital University of Miami School of Medicine's head pulmonologist, who was on the panel of transplant surgery.

I sniffed, as people with a runny nose, do. The doctor stopped her note taking, looked up and asked, "Have you been tested for CF?" "What is CF?" I answered. Two weeks later, the tests came back positive for cystic fibrosis (CF). I was moved up the list on UNOS.

I was so relieved to have a true diagnosis. All my life I had remained a human puzzle, a person without answers for the deep coughing, constantly apologizing for doing it. I recalled that in fifth grade, the class sweetheart turned around, and in front of everyone, announced, "Geesh! You sound like a volcano!" Of course, as a kid, I was mortified.

It seems that after being involved in a motorcycle accident in 1996, my lungs took a downhill dive. It became more difficult to breathe. Less than nine years later, I was on oxygen, and in a wheelchair.

The wait for new lungs was surreal. One moment, it was a blessing to be listed. The next moment I could not comprehend it. I grew weary of being on oxygen, and in a wheelchair, I was tired of fighting, and felt hopeless. My dear husband and caregiver rarely caught me crying, as I did so many times. I turned to my faith in God. After awhile, a calm peace came over me, and I just bore the wait as part of my life, a day at a time.

My husband decided that he would not let me just sit and wait. He drove me to places I liked to go, took me out for dinners. I spent my daytime hours with the computer, the television, and my cats and hobbies. I accepted the wait, for-- whatever Our Maker had in store for me.

The transplant staff said that on the first call, one must have a ready answer. We were not expecting the call when it came. My husband handed the phone to me, I had no idea why, "Are you ready to come for your transplant?" my coordinator asked. "Yes!" I immediately answered without hesitation. A few minutes later, she called back, to cancel the transplant. "You're a difficult match; these lungs won't work for you." I only cried for a few minutes, remembering hope, and my faith once again. I had a total of six dry runs over 23 months. I had learned to accept disappointment without tears, and keep a positive disposition that the next time might be my call to prolonged life.

On call number seven, January 2, 2006, my husband and I were cracking jokes and laughing as I lay on the hospital bed, awaiting the word that it was a "go". I had long ago made my peace with the Lord, and I was determined that my husband would remember me as being happy. I remember being placed into position on the special operating room bed, I remember nurses and doctors talking to me, everyone was smiling. I was asking questions about the equipment.

I knew my husband was near, I recall my coordinator telling me I was doing well. I knew I was out of surgery. I don't remember much else, until I fully awoke from the anesthesia a couple of days later, but I do not remember any pain, nor the surgery itself. I spent a total of 21 days in recovery after my transplant.

I never looked back. I am active, limited only by a weak knee, from the accident years before. I have an excellent quality of life, and although I am not a daredevil, I know I can do almost any physical thing I challenge myself to do.

As a wife, I live a normal life, with regular demands. No longer do I need for my husband to assist me when I take my shower, as I did pre-transplant for fear of weakness or falling. I now do cooking and housework without exhaustion, and do the laundry without effort. I have again enjoyed the challenge of walking the malls, swimming, keeping up with my active adult children, lifting heavier objects without effort, as most people can, and do, everyday. I can now enjoy playing with my cats, walking outdoors, and participating with friends in activities, such as outdoor games, and dancing, local volunteer work, and working out at the gym. I can climb flights of stairs without being winded. I am a member of two online transplant support groups, and I am a transplant mentor under the Transplant Foundation at Jackson Memorial Hospital. I am proud of my "ordinary" accomplishments, which would not have been possible without the transplant.

I am also proud of my personal being. Being close to death, and finding peace can certainly mellow a person, and I find my personal priorities are rearranged. No longer do I hold myself to deadlines, nor do I procrastinate to enjoy an activity. I am more carefree and forgiving than I used to be before transplant. I am a much more understanding and patient person, and I am blessed with numerous friends. The wonderful euphoria I *felt* after transplant has worn off for the most part, but not the *memory* of it, or the revelations it brought me personally. I am sometimes overwhelmed to tears at my good fortune; and all this due to the blessing of a miracle, I am living!

I will forever be grateful to my donor's mother and sister, when, at the worst moment in their lives, they generously choose to donate their loved ones lungs, saving my life, on call number seven.

I would like to dedicate this story to Gina, who gave me her lungs, to Si Pham, MD who was my transplant surgeon, and to Debra Fertel, MD, who diagnosed and cared for me, among others.

Sylvia Tencza, 59
North Lauderdale, Florida
Cystic Fibrosis
Double Lung Transplant, January 3, 2006
Jackson Memorial Hospital, University of Miami School of Medicine, Miami, Florida
Read Robert Tenzca's Story in this Edition of Taking Flight

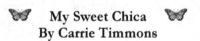

My Sweet Chica
By Carrie Timmons

Elinda walked into my life when she was only four-years-old. Never did I imagine that my life was completely about to change. At 16, I had never even heard the word 'Cystic Fibrosis (CF)' but soon found out every aspect to the illness. I married her uncle, and now Elinda is my niece and is a huge part of my personal family. She is a part of me. Here is her story.

When Elinda was born, she seemed healthy but soon her health started to decline. After another trip to the emergency room with 'pneumonia', her grandmother Carmen (and guardian) was accused of giving her peanuts (actually was mucus), which was lodged, in her chest. Carmen then rushed her to University Medical Center Health System Hospital, Lubbock, Texas, where Dr. Riff took one look at her and ran a CF test. This is where her journey began at four months old.

Elinda began the normal CF protocol of treatments with a few minor set backs along the way until she was about 10. At this time she began to have problems with her liver. Her liver was banded twice in a year to prevent the organ from shutting down. After missing most of her 7th grade year in school, Elinda was on the transplant list for a new liver. Her new life began February 9, 2004. This was Elinda and Carmen's first plane ride ever! A family that I was acquainted with, the Cooper's, who barely knew Elinda's story, flew her to Texas Children's Hospital, Houston, Texas. The Cooper's saved Elinda's life and will have a special place in Heaven because of the kindness they have given us. When Elinda was about to be wheeled in to surgery, she told the docs that if someone else needed that liver more than she did, that she wanted them to have it. I believe she made the surgeon cry with that request. The transplant took 10 hours and she recovered beautifully! Within 48 hours she was sitting up in a chair playing Nintendo. At 12-years-old she had a new lease on life.

Life was going pretty well for Elinda post liver transplant until 2007. This is when her lungs began to fight to stay healthy. She fought B-Cepacia and Methicillin-Resistant Staphylococcus Aureus (MRSA). Her junior year in high school is a distant memory since she only attended the first month of school before having to be put on oxygen and home schooled for fear of infection. Eventually Carmen and Elinda had to relocate to Houston to be closer to Dr. Marc Schechter (pulmonologist) and the transplant team. Elinda was officially listed for a double-lung transplant in April 2008. By this time, her oxygen saturation was dangerously low; she had no energy, and barely had the will to even live. One night Elinda got out of the bath, sat by her grandmother and told her she had a conversation with God. Elinda told God that it was all in His hands and that she was leaving the decision up to Him. Four hours later...she received "the call". Her third chance at life was given to her on July 31, 2008. I firmly believe that all God was waiting for was for her to be 100% ready and willing.

Elinda's recovery was absolutely remarkable. She was out of the hospital in only six days!!! The surgery itself lasted about 13 hours, on a vent for only 24 hours and off oxygen and breathing 100% pure air at three days post transplant!!! The only major set back was a minor rejection of her liver. The doctors acted fast, put her on steroids and chemo. In January she returned back to school for her last semester as a senior. Elinda attended her senior prom, had senior pictures taken and graduated from high school. There was not a dry eye in the auditorium. Elinda's next step? College!

Elinda thought long and hard on what she wanted to study. She decided to attend South Plains College in Levelland to become a surgical technician. Elinda is now in her second year of college. This is something the family and I prayed and prayed for. There have been times in Elinda's life that were a complete struggle and we prayed for her to see another day.

This remarkable young lady is the light of my life. Through most of her trials and tribulations Elinda has kept a positive attitude. I only pray that I stay as strong as her when I am having a bad day. Elinda definitely makes you think when you gripe about a stubbed toe.

As petite as Elinda already is, in September 2010, she developed pneumonia. Although we never imagined this would occur, on October 21, 2010 Elinda fought her last battle. Elinda took her last breath in her grandmother's arms at home, right where she would have wanted to. So strong and powerful, yet so small and sweet. Our Pastor, Michael Holmes led the beautiful memorial service.

Her headstone will be placed in spring of 2011. It will depict as much beauty as Elinda herself and will stand out among the land since she stood out in life. Elinda can now breathe easy.

Carrie Timmons, Aunt of, Elinda Margaret Timmons
Levelland, Texas
Elinda, Cystic Fibrosis
Elinda, Liver Transplant, February 9, 2004
Elinda, Double Lung Transplant, July 31, 2008
Texas Children's Hospital, Houston, Texas
Elinda sadly passed away on October 21, 2010
"Forever 19"

 God Performed a Miracle
By Linda Tollakson

Linda Tollakson, a resident of rural Dawson, Minnesota, admitted to being a life-time smoker who quit in 2003 but was diagnosed with a lung disease; Mycobacterium Avium Complex (MAC) in 2006. Tollakson explained that MAC is in the tuberculosis family but is not spread from person to person. She reflected that her late father and her four siblings all had lung problems.

"In 2009 my husband, Roger and I drove to Minneapolis for an appointment at the University of Minnesota Medical Center Fairview." Before her appointment, her husband had a hard time waking her. An ambulance took her to the emergency room at the university hospital. "My carbon dioxide (CO2) levels in my body were at 160; the normal is 40. Therefore, my body was being taken over by the CO2 levels, and was starving me of oxygen."

Linda was placed at the top of the waiting list, for a double lung transplant in the tri-state area of Minnesota, South Dakota, North Dakota and western Wisconsin. Miraculously, she received lungs fourteen days later.

"I had antibodies in my blood, so a cross-match had to be done – a blood test for patient antibodies against the donor's antigens. A positive cross match shows the donor and recipient do not match. A negative cross-match means there is no reaction between donor and recipient and that the transplant may continue," Tollakson explained. Her incision goes from under one arm across the chest to under the other arm. They also opened the sternum. She was taken off the ventilator and oxygen two days later, and was breathing on her own. After sixteen days, the doctors were amazed that she could be discharged from the hospital.

Here caregivers were her daughters, Melissa and Angela, sister, Bonnie, and husband, Roger. In just six short weeks, Linda got the okay to go home.

She now pretty much has full strength back in her arms and hands, but still has a ways to go with her legs. She is still shaky, but this has gotten a lot better. Tollakson is grateful that she can cook, do laundry, and light housekeeping. She attempts to attend the support group meeting for lung transplants at the university hospital once a month.

"Since seeing first-hand the importance of organ donation, our family has decided to be donors, and have this put on our driver's licenses. Think about being a donor. Since 1986, the university has done 381 single lung transplants and 216 double lung transplants. I was number 214."

Tollakson concluded, "Yes, February 17, 2009 was a good day for me and my family. I was in the right place at the right time, and God was watching out for me, and this was all meant to be. We know that this was a great day for me, but we also know that a life was lost, and family and friends were grieving. With all the many, many people praying for me, I believe in the power of prayer, and I was truly blessed, God performed a miracle."

Since the interview, Linda Tollakson received a letter from the donor's mother and was told that the donor was a 28-year-old male from Indiana.

Linda Tollakson, 59
Dawson, Minnesota
Chronic Obstructive Pulmonary Disease,
Mycobacterium Avium Complex
Double Lung Transplant, February 17, 2009
University of Minnesota Medical Center Fairview, Minneapolis, Minnesota

       ## I'm Still Alive, Healthy & Happy
By Dana Trude

I am Dana Trude, 49. I had a heart and double lung transplant on December 12, 2006. As I was unaware of the first few critical days and still cannot remember some stuff, I have taken excerpts from my Care Pages, which immediate family only had access to and you can read the very beginnings. I do not remember seeing to many people the first day or two or even three.

Care Page Excerpts: Entries that my husband, Sam wrote.
"Good Morning everyone... this is our third day here and Dana is progressing awesomely! Her breathing tube was taken out early this morning and she is now sitting up. We will be posting another update later today."

"Good Evening everyone! Here we are again in the waiting room but this time we are awaiting a phone call that the move to the step-down unit was successful! So... by this you must realize how well Dana is progressing. Her voice is starting to come back now so she is now able to whisper, and she is wide-awake and looks absolutely great! So we will be back online tomorrow for further updates after we have had time to visit her."

"A good Sunday Morning everyone! I am writing this from home as I took the boys home with me last night, realizing they need to get back to some normalcy, back to school etc."

"On Friday she had such a great day, very alert and bright although she still has a lot of pain but all she has to do is push a button, and she likes that too. Her heart surgeon saw her Friday afternoon and called her, "Their Poster Child" as he was just thrilled with her progress."

Care Page Excerpts: Postings I made on December 14, 2006.
"I made it home in record time according to the nurses. In and out in eleven days.

I had a bronchoscopy on December 27 and a clinic visit on the 28th; NO REJECTION AND NO INFECTION." "I feel GREAT!"

Care Page Excerpts: Postings I made in the most recent years.
"I returned to work on November 11, 2008." "Everything is going GREAT! I hardly have any down days anymore. I help my husband do lawn maintenance in the summer; which I find is great exercise. I love to walk; in fact I am participating in a 10K on the same exact day of my operation December 12, now four years ago. I went through a terrible lose, my mother. She passed away November 24, 2009 of lung cancer; she was my main support, best friend, and confidant. I miss her dearly. But health wise everything is good. My pulmonary function test continues to slowly slide, so in terms of life expectancy, I have no idea. BUT, I am a fighter and will fight for every day and every moment on this earth. My husband Sam is an extremely hard worker, and works an endless amount of hours to keep our family fed and sheltered. He was no able to come with me for the 10K walk in Hawaii however, as he had a ladder slip out from underneath him and he fell 10 feet thus resulting in a fractured spine (Lumbar 1). I have an upcoming event May 15, 2011, which is a ½ walk marathon. Still healthy and strong."

Dana Trude, 49
Kitchener, Ontario, Canada
Pulmonary Hypertension
Heart/Double Lung Transplant, December 12, 2006
Toronto General Hospital, Toronto, Canada

    Not a Breath Too Soon
By Melissa Tweedy

Growing up is hard to do,
I've known this since age of two.
Lasting more than twenty days,
They thought it was just a phase.
Crying, sobbing, screaming all night,
My family put up an outrageous fight.
What will happen who's to know,
Will I see the Lord's radiant glow?
30 years full of strife,
Cystic Fibrosis rules my life.
It gets me up, it gets me down,
I strive on without a frown.

Breathing for me is hard to do.
But if you find me I'm standing true.
One of these days I'll breathe free,
I can't wait for you to see.
Standing there on the other side,
With my wings I'll just glide.
Gone from my lungs, gone forever
Will I look back? Probably never.

~~~~

Not a Breath Too Soon
By Melissa Tweedy

Crying, fussing, screaming all night. My family put in a tremendous fight. It was 1982, two years since I was born, and yet no one got rest during the day or night.

My grandparents had chosen to raise me due to the fact I was sick and yet no one could tell them what was actually wrong. Then an angel came to my grandmothers' front door raising money for "The Great Strides Walk" a fundraiser for the Cystic Fibrosis Foundation (CF). This woman who came to our door that day changed my life and the lives of my family forever.

I was hospitalized so many times over and over, but I still was able to complete college and get my degree in four years. I decided that I would keep dealing with my CF, but I also wanted to get out on my own. I took a job in the Kansas City area and enjoyed my "Freedom". I started getting sicker and hospital visits were getting closer and closer. I decided to move back to my hometown of Wichita, Kansas. It wasn't long before I got the word from my doctor; the news I knew was coming; that I needed to think about a double lung transplantation.

I went to the University of Colorado Hospital in Aurora, Colorado, in the Denver area. I was evaluated and immediately put on the "active" list. Now all I had to do was wait for "the call." Days, weeks, and months went by and I was getting sicker and sicker. On May 20, 2008 I got "the call".

It took me awhile to recover. I had to relearn to breathe again. It was weird taking a breath and not coughing. I had to get used to the fresh air I was breathing in and out. After one month in the hospital, I made a full recovery and left walking and without an oxygen tank on my back. It was then I decided my life was worth living. I was walking, talking and eating. Some of the things I never experienced before. I exercised more, I gained weight and I was a "Survivor" of Cystic Fibrosis.

The first thing I did with my new "life"; we went to the mountains in Colorado, and I slowly but excitedly, climbed Boulder Mountain. I had never seen anything so gorgeous in my life. The waterfalls, the wild animals, and the love of my family who were so happy to see me accomplish this feat, were part of the joyous experience.

Finally I returned to Wichita, Kansas; and got my life back in order. My reunion with my dog Stoli was first, and then I looked for a job, hung out with friends and family that I hadn't seen. I still like to do the things I did before I got sick; like swimming, bowling, and movies. My new interest of course is my lung donor.

I decided to finish up my Master's Degree in Forensic Psychology, in which during this time, I am working with juveniles that have been placed in psychiatric facilities, and juveniles that have a diagnosis that parents cannot understand or work with them at home. I plan to become a psychiatrist in a prison on death row eventually. I know that will take time but I know I will get there.

Now two years post transplant living in Wichita, I celebrated my 30th birthday in March of 2010. I am breathing better than ever before. I have another year to celebrate, because of my anonymous donor, "Rest in Peace". I could not want anything better than what the Lord has given me.

Melissa Tweedy, 30
Wichita, Kansas
Cystic Fibrosis
Double Lung Transplant, May 20, 2008
University of Colorado Hospital, Aurora, Colorado

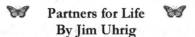

Partners for Life
By Jim Uhrig

My name is Jim Uhrig. I have a very full, robust family life – five very supportive children and married to my second wife for 34 years - and continue working in the same industry into my fifth decade.

Three years ago, ordinary things in my life literally started to take my breath away. I found that mundane tasks, like tying my shoes, caused difficulty breathing. I could not catch my breath. In 2008, I felt like I had the flu. After a visit to the pulmonologist, a review of chest X-rays and Computerized Axial Tomography (CAT) scan led to a diagnosis of pulmonary fibrosis (PF). PF was unknown to me, so on my way home that day I made two calls. The first call was to my wife, Donna, who searched the Internet and found hundreds of pages to print, giving some insight into the disease and treatment options.

The second call was to my friend of 40 years, John Sullivan ("Sully"), who had a double-lung transplant in 1997. (See his amazing story in this edition of Taking Flight). Sully connected me with the Dorothy and Richard Simmons Center for Interstitial Lung Disease at the University of Pittsburgh Medical Center, Pittsburgh, Pennsylvania (UPMC). I met my "new partners," the professionals dedicated to the research and treatment of this disease. I felt an immediate high level of confidence. They helped me understand the unknown clinical course of my disease, gave me confidence in treatment options, and the hope that none of my four sons nor two grandsons from my bloodline had the same fate. The doctors I've asked don't feel there is a genetic link, but from talking to other patients, I've observed that there could be a tendency. Even if this tendency doesn't exist, I want to help with treatment of future PF patients.

I was evaluated for my transplant in March 2009. Within a month, I was blessed with a donor, albeit a high risk one. But it was a donor that my doctors believed was a good match for me. So I had my double-lung transplant in April 2009. That's when fate and luck shined on me. My excellent surgeon, Dr. Jay Bhama, removed my old lungs that he later described as "bricks." He estimated that they might have held out another six to eight weeks. Was this timing lucky? Maybe, but I'm definitely blessed. After a few setbacks, I came home from the hospital two months later. But I came home without oxygen and was back to work full-time that fall. I also returned to work part time in our family's custom picture frame business.

The fate of a generous donor gave me new lungs, which came just in time, but my confidence in the medical staff, their competence and strong support of my wife, family, Sully, and many old "partners" or friends and business associates gave me the encouragement, and courage to take flight again. While I have always been competitive, it sure helps to have supporters rooting you on to keep trying to do your best. My family, especially Donna, and Sully were the best support anyone could ever wish for. But there were so many others who came back into my life to cheer me on with their encouragement of messages, words and visits. The networking was incredible and culminated in a fundraiser in the fall of 2009 with a golf course full of supporters and diners that helped me raise money for the medication I needed until I returned to work.

I participated in the 2010 Transplant Games, and already I am planning for the next games in 2012. This year I was a golfer, and while golf will remain some of my focus, I also want to be a sprinter at the 2012 Games. Participating in the Games is exhilarating, but having the chance to continue life is a wish any chronically ill person dreams about.

Stay positive, get the best medical and emotional support and hope for the luck that the opportunity of a transplant can give. Work on your physical therapy to rebuild or maintain your strength. Do this under the watchful eye of a trained physical therapy specialist with knowledge of the oxygen needs of a patient with PF. The stronger you can make yourself, the better you will come through the surgery. Once you are diagnosed, keep learning and listening to those who provide support. Their experience and ideas for your well being will help you deal with the reality of your plight and recognize the options that can lead to your return to a productive life, or perhaps to a cure for those similarly afflicted.

I have seen that my return to good health is inspirational to others, some who also have the misfortune of developing PF. The disease is a game-changer, but can be an incredible experience that puts life, family, activities and life's work in perspective.

There is no time for pity or sorrow ... only time to listen to your doctors and your supporters; and to get yourself in shape for the challenge of transplant.

Jim Uhrig, 65
Venetia, Pennsylvania
Pulmonary Fibrosis
Double Lung Transplant, April 21, 2009
University of Pittsburgh Medical Center, Pittsburgh, Pennsylvania

A Second Time Around
By Valerie Vandervort/Boyer

I was diagnosed with Cystic Fibrosis (CF), a genetic and digestive system illness and failure to thrive at the age of six weeks. From then on I lead a pretty normal life except for being admitted to the hospital around two times a year for "tune ups", where I was given intravenous (IV) antibiotics, breathing treatments, chest x-rays and lots of blood work performed. I went to public school, took dancing and tumbling for 13 years, I played softball one summer, and was a cheerleader. I graduated 8th in my class from high school in 1990. In 1989 I met the "love of my life", Rick, and we have been together ever since.

I was listed for transplant in October of 1999. Waited almost two years to the day for a double lung transplant. I was transplanted, October 4, 2001 at Barnes-Jewish Hospital, St. Louis, Missouri. I was on a ventilator for 17 hours, and was out of intensive care unit (ICU) in 48 hours. I was released on the 8th day after transplant. Wonderfully, I was released to go back home, to Oklahoma, on December 21st just in time for Christmas and then my 30th birthday!

Since my transplant, now nine years ago I can breathe without oxygen, talk complete and LONG sentences, sing, eat till I am full, take showers instead of just baths, go shopping, clean house and do laundry. The energy I have now has allowed me to change much of my life; feeling good and not being tired all the time allows me to put these "gift of life lungs" to good use. I swim, climb stairs, jump on my trampoline, run, lift weights, and most of all I can dance again.

For these past nine years I have had so much joy in my life. I have been able to watch both of my sisters graduate high school, been a maid of honor in one of my sister's wedding. I have two nieces and two nephews now. I have been able to watch Rick advance in his umpiring career, and fulfill some of his "bucket list goals". I have traveled to places that have been on my "bucket list". Hiked up and down a mountain, seen beautiful waterfalls. I have participated in the United States Transplant Games in 2002, 2004, 2006, 2008, and 2010. I have won three medals in swimming events, one silver and two bronzes, out of the five years. This past year, 2010, my donor's parents were able to attend the games and cheer me on and support me. I have run several 5K runs, and I will soon climb 36 flights of stairs for a Cystic Fibrosis fundraiser. I also am a mentor to CF patients who will be in need of a transplant. I love promoting organ donor awareness and transplantation. Making the public more aware of the need for organ donation is very important to others and myself; who have received, or need a transplant. Recently I had an article in the New York Times about my donor and me and her family published.

In February of 2011 I am going to attempt my very first indoor triathlon. I like to challenge myself and set new goals periodically.

Life post transplant just has a new meaning and I view life so much more differently. I take each day as it comes, and I take time to stop and smell the roses along the way. Letting each day bring new meaning, and blessings to me. I know God has so much more for my life than I will ever realize or I wouldn't have been given this gift of life "A Second Time Around."

I thank God for all my blessings, and my donor, and her family. Thank you Rick for showing me what life is like spending it with the, "love of your life". Thank you family and friends for all your support as well. For I know I am truly BLESSED!

Valerie Vandervort/Boyer, 39
Claremore, Oklahoma
Cystic Fibrosis
Double Lung Transplant, October 4, 2001
Barnes-Jewish Hospital, St. Louis, Missouri
Read Valerie's Lung Transplant Story in the 1st Edition of Taking Flight

 My One and Only Friend
By Eileen VanValkenburg

Joanne and I met at our first job; working at the local library. We quickly became great friends. We also attended out local community college together. There wasn't much to do, back in the 1980's. We tried to make the Rochester nightlife as exciting as possible. We used to joke that we were each other's 'one and only friend'. I don't know what I would have done without her, really. When other friends went off to college or to other ends of the world, Joanne stayed in town with me. Joanne was instrumental at my meeting my husband. She reminds me of that often!

She didn't tell me about her cystic fibrosis (CF) until after my son was born in 1992. My family and I thought she had a 'nervous cough' or had an eating disorder because she was so thin. However, I had eaten out with her many times over the years and that girl could put away a meal bigger than herself, so I knew deep down she did not have an eating disorder. And when we went to bars, Joanne was anything but nervous or soft spoken! She taught me how to get rid of an annoying guy with one, simple, dismissive word or a wave of her hand. I don't know why she didn't tell me sooner about her CF. Maybe she thought I was a shallow person and I would have not wanted to be with her. However, I believe, I would have been too shallow to ever give up my 'one and only friend'.

There were years, later in our lives, when we barely saw each other. Joanne discovered e-mail first and urged me to start using it. We started to connect again. When she went off for her transplant, I was very nervous for her. But, I really had no idea all that was entailed with it. I wish I could have been there for her. But, with two small children, it was difficult for me.

Luckily, she had her wonderful family and her man, Mitch, there for her - every step of the way. Joanne has been through so much, but she was always a fighter. She came out the other side swinging. The past 13 years have proven that. She is going strong. In the past, she sometimes had trouble talking because of shortness of breath – no one can shut her up now with those new lungs of her!

Now, I tease Joanne, because on Facebook, she has over 3,400 friends. I ask her if I am no longer her 'one and only friend'. She assures me that I am. But, I know that all those other people are good, supportive friends and Joanne inspires many. With her two books, she has moved and motivated so many people. She has taught us all not to complain, to enjoy our lives, to appreciate what we have - along with each and every day, to not take our organs to heaven with us and to 'breathe deeply'.

We are all very grateful to her donor's family, because our lives would be nothing, a very boring place indeed, without our beloved, our 'one and only friend' - Joanne.

Eileen VanValkenburg, Friend of Joanne Schum
Joanne Schum, 47
Churchville, New York
Joanne, Cystic Fibrosis
Joanne, Double Lung Transplant, September 12, 1997
University of North Carolina Hospitals, Chapel Hill, North Carolina
Shannon VanValkenburg, Artist for the Front Cover for this Edition of Taking Flight
Eileen VanValkenburg is Shannon's Mother
Read Joanne's Lung Transplant Story in the 1st Edition of Taking Flight
Read Joanne's Lung Transplant Story in this Edition of Taking Flight

🦋 Wings of Hope 🦋
By Imelda G. Vasquez

I was born in Mexicali, Mexico. At seven months old I was diagnosed with a congenital heart defect called a Ventricular Septal Defect (VSD). By the time I turned a year old, the enlargement of my heart and pressures that the VSD caused in my lungs, developed into Eisenmenger Syndrome. Eisenmenger's is a combination of having a VSD and Pulmonary Hypertension. They were not able to surgically close the opening of VSD, before it caused pulmonary hypertension due to my small size. I was three pounds, and too small to survive the surgery. I was so small I could fit in my dad's size eight shoebox. My parents were told to go home and pray and hope for the best. My chances of survival were slim to none. My disease was considered terminal and my only chance of surviving was a heart/double lung transplant. But that was a path that would come later in life.

My parents sought medical care for me in Guadalajara, Mexico. They decided to come to the United States when I was five-years-old. I led a relatively normal life most of the time. As a teenager I was very limited in my activity. My parents never spoiled me or treated me any different than my younger siblings. Given my prognosis, it must have been difficult not to treat me like a delicate porcelain doll. I am eternally grateful to them for not giving me a complex about my condition.

I was referred to University of California at Los Angeles Medical Center (UCLA) Los Angeles, California. That was the best recommendation any doctor had ever given me. I was evaluated by pulmonologist, Dr. Saggar. He put me on Tracleer and Sildenafil. He also warned me that I could not wait "too" long, so I should start thinking about the idea of getting listed. I did great on the medications with periodic increases to the doses for about three years. Dr. Ardehali told me that I would be his first heart and double lung transplant patient as normally he only did either hearts or lungs by themselves. Also, UCLA had not done a heart/double lung transplant in five years. I was scared but I didn't care. I didn't have time to find another doctor or another center that may or may not accept me. The wait was short compared to others who waited much longer and many who are still waiting…. but still I kept thinking they'd forgotten about me. At times I was afraid that I might not even make it to transplant. I felt worse and worse every day. I'd call the center once in a while just to make sure they hadn't forgotten.

I finally received my transplant on June 1, 2007. The nurses and doctors that were assigned to my care at UCLA were wonderful. They always made sure I was well taken care of. I spent two months recovering at the hospital and a 3rd month on home health. Once I regained my strength I started to actually live.

I am now going on 37-years-old and loving life. I live in Riverside, California with my boyfriend and two puppy kids. I can walk again without the use of a wheelchair, talk without becoming breathless, play with my puppy-kids, cook, dance and return to my love of drawing! I can now enjoy my life and spend good quality time with my family and friends.

If you are not an organ donor please consider signing up. You're not going to need them where you're going!

I have many thanks to give, mainly to my mom and dad for giving me life, never giving up on me and putting up with so much over the years. To my donor and her family I am eternally thankful for this second chance you have selflessly given me. To my best friend Francisca Ambriz, who has always been a true friend, through the good, the bad and the ugly. I am forever grateful to my excellent pulmonary doctor, Dr. Rajan Saggar and his staff, and my surgeon Dr. Abbas Ardehali for everything they did for me. Also big thanks to the entire nursing staff at UCLA. And last but not least, my wonderful and loving boyfriend Al Lopez who for months suffered many long and sleepless nights at my bedside and long drives to and from UCLA. He gave me so much love, care and support through it all. I'd be lost without him. I love you baby!

Imelda Vasquez, 36
Riverside, California
Ventricular Septal Defect, Eisenmenger Syndrome, Pulmonary Hypertension
Heart/Double Lung Transplant, June 1, 2007
University of California at Los Angeles Medical Center, Los Angeles, California

True Strength
By Amy Vickers

My name is Amy Singleton Vickers. I have Cystic Fibrosis and my transplant journey began on June 3, 2004. It was a very overwhelming decision to make, as I didn't know of anyone who had had a double lung transplant. I soon found out a friend received his "Gift of Life" and from then on my decision was made. I can do this!

I received my miracle on September 7, 2004 and had an amazing recovery. I was out of the hospital in just 11 days! From start to finish, my first transplant seemed to go so smoothly, having to wait just three months to receive my life-saving call. The actual surgery was eight hours in length, after which the doctors told my family that the lungs had come just in time, as I may not have even made it until Christmas time of that same year. This is when I realized that miracles really do happen, and that God was definitely on my side.

My recovery went very well, and within just three short months I was on my way back to my home in New Brunswick, to begin the new life I had been given. For the first time in my life, my breathing was no longer a struggle. I could walk my dogs, go shopping for hours, travel, and enjoy time with my friends and family. My mom joked that I must have gotten my new lungs from a traveling man, as I was constantly on the go! Unfortunately, my new life was about to change.

After bouts of pneumonia, my respirologist in Toronto discovered that I had Bronchiolitis Obliterans, which meant one thing: Chronic Rejection. This came as a complete shock as I had just lived the best four years of my life. After the shock wore off, I decided I had to go through this again, as my love for life outweighed my fear.

My husband, two dogs, and I relocated back to Toronto, but little did I know this second journey would be nothing like the first, right from day one. This time, as weeks of waiting turned into months, and the months turned into years, I realized that my strength, patience, and faith would all be put to the test over and over again.

On January 28, 2010 I received my second "Gift of Life". I had a lot of bumps this time around, that I had to overcome. With the help of the amazing doctors and nurses at Toronto General Hospital I felt very safe. We have met so many wonderful and courageous people that we had our very own transplant family. I had so much support and prayers from our own families and friends that it was very inspiring, and from this I was able to draw my strength and courage to fight.

Although this journey hasn't been an easy one, it has been one that has transformed me into the fighter I am today. I realize more and more everyday that anyone can give up; it's the easiest thing in the world to do. But to hold it together when everyone else would understand if you fell apart, that's true strength!

NEVER GIVE UP!

Amy Vickers, 33
Barnettville, New Brunswick, Canada
Cystic Fibrosis
Double Lung Transplant, September 7, 2004
Re-Transplant, Double Lung Transplant, January 28, 2010
Toronto General Hospital, Toronto, Canada

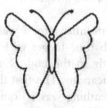

Breathlessly
By Alice Vogt

My name is Alice Vogt, I'm 26-years-old and I received my bi-lateral lung transplant on the 22nd of January 2008, at Milpark Hospital in Johannesburg, South Africa (JHB). The reason for my transplant was Cystic Fibrosis (CF). It's a genetic disease, and I was diagnosed at age two after my grandmother heard a radio program about the disease and insisted I be tested because the symptoms matched mine at the time. I had a pretty normal childhood despite doctors being negative about the prognosis. It was only after my 21st birthday that my lungs deteriorated rapidly, and I realized that something drastic was needed. I had always belonged to a CF mailing group called Cystic-L where they often discussed transplant, but before then I didn't pay much attention to it, thinking it was something I would only need in the VERY distant future. However when I reached the point where I had to start sleeping with oxygen I seriously started researching it and paying more attention. I found out they actually did lung transplants in South Africa, and through my local doctor, managed to organize an appointment in Johannesburg for me. At that stage I was on oxygen 24 hours a day (24/7), and spent hours every day nebulizing and doing chest physiotherapy. I didn't have time or energy for much else.

I was immediately admitted for my work-up, and listed a few months later after all the administration was sorted out. They say you get listed for transplant when you have a 50% chance of surviving another two years... At that point I seriously doubted if I'd last another two years. I was living in Port Elizabeth (PE) at the time, a city 11 hours drive away from Johannesburg where the only transplant centre in the country is. My dad had in the meantime accepted a job in Johannesburg, with my transplant and recovery in mind, so I had the option of waiting there, 8km from the hospital. I decided against it though, because all my friends were in PE, and Johannesburg has an altitude of about 1700m, which made it so much harder to breathe than at sea level. I just hoped and prayed for the best. The worse part of the wait was the questions running through my mind... "Will I get lungs in time?" "What if they call me at a time when there are no flights to JHB?" What if they call me and I have a bad infection?"

Eight months after I was listed I received the call that changed my life forever. With more than enough time to get to Johannesburg on the first flight the next morning, everything worked out perfectly in the end. Surgery was seven hours long and I was in hospital for 14 days with no complications. The first thing I noticed when I woke up in intensive care unit (ICU) was the fact that my breathing was so quiet for the first time since I can remember... no wheezing and crackling noises! I had a really smooth recovery with no issues, for which I am very grateful!

Life after transplant is COMPLETELY different. Physically I can do almost anything. My lung function is 100%, I attend gym regularly, I enjoy swimming and hiking for fun. I work full-time for the first time in my life, and don't have to worry about missing work due to being sick all the time.

Medically the only thing I need to do is take my anti rejection tablets (Prograf, Cellcept and Prednisone) and a few others twice a day. Which is absolute heaven compared to the HOURS I spent on treatments with little difference in how I felt. I've been EXTREMELY lucky and have only spent three days in hospital post transplant for some minor infection. I have also had no rejection up to date.

One of the highlights post transplant is without a doubt meeting the love of my life, Chris. I met him eight months post transplant, and we got married on the 7th of August 2010. If it weren't for my donor I would have missed out on this amazing event and definitely one of the highlights of my life.

Other highlights were participating in the 2009 World Transplant Games in Australia last year and I won a gold medal for squash. I also participated in the 3km race walk and 800m track event. Other high points have been starting my career, buying a house together with Chris, and becoming independent financially, especially with regard to my medical expenses. It's also amazing just feeling "normal" everyday, even though there's always the fear of chronic rejection at the back of your mind and an awareness of having to take my meds and avoid sick people etc. The worse part post transplant for me has been losing transplant friends… either because they died on the waiting list or because of some complication afterwards. You don't always understand why things happen the way they do, good or bad.

I appreciate every breath and try to never take it for granted. I get irritated when people complain about minor things when they don't know what it's like to fight for your life every day, or they don't appreciate their good health. Even though I work in the financial industry, my passion is promoting organ donation and doing talks wherever needed, from high schools to medical students. If I could, I would do it full-time! As you can imagine I'm very excited about South Africa hosting the 2013 World Transplant Games!

I would like to thank my parents, family and my sister Chrislie for always supporting and cheering me up when things were really bad; my doctor in Port Elizabeth, Dr. Paul Gebers, my doctor since transplant in Joburg (Johannesburg), Dr. Paul Williams. My friends who stood by me when I couldn't do much, and my new husband Chris, I love you very much! And last but not least…. My donor family… without you I would not be living this life I was meant to live.

If you would like to read my blog, Google – Alice Vogt.

Alice Vogt, 26
Johannesburg, Republic of South Africa
Cystic Fibrosis
Double Lung Transplant, January 22, 2008
Milpark Hospital, Johannesburg, South Africa

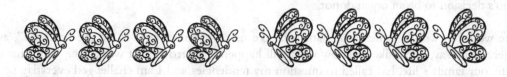

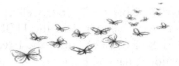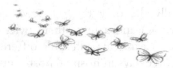

"Forever 16"
By Jessica Packhem Waters, Paula Martorelli,
And Timothy Packhem

Energetic, comedic, passionate and kind; loyal, honest, gentle and humble; these words simply touch the surface on an array of qualities Timothy Packhem embodied.

Tim, or Timbo, was my younger brother and great friend. Nine years divided us, though the development of our relationship continues to heal my heart to this day. We had such great times together through the years and I smile just thinking about him. Our kinship was unique for a brother and sister because beyond having our mother, he sometimes had me trying to act like another mother. He was developing into a fine young man, and I wonder everyday what he would be like today. We shared dreams and ideas together and I can only hope my life emblems the good in his short life.

My family members will each tell you a different story of my brother, exposing the diverse and interesting person that he was. Yet the common threads through all these stories are how amazed we all are at his unwavering loyalty to friends and family and his gentle heart. We have learned from his life, and are better people for having experienced Timbo!

In March of 2007 my family was faced with an unthinkable tragedy. My then 16-year-old brother was involved in an accident that took his life. My world fell apart, for my family and myself. We were also faced with a decision to donate his organs. For my family, it wasn't even a question. Tim was preparing to obtain his drivers license and just weeks before his accident had a conversation with my mother that made this decision for us. He expressed his wishes to be an organ donor. He made it clear that this was his intent. To this day, the power of that conversation helped us through such a difficult time.

Our paths have led us to grieve and communicate with one another in different ways. We, as a family, are different and have changed. Holidays come and go and new traditions are made, though we never forget the power of Timbo in our lives. With tragedy hope can come, the hope of new beginnings, the hope of meeting an organ recipient, the hope of spreading the word about organ donation.

We have become dear friends with Timbo's lung recipient, Robert. He embodies the kind, gentle soul that Timbo personified. Robert *is* our new beginning and has helped my family see the result of Timbo's decision to be an organ donor.

In life we often wonder where our path will take us. For me, I tend to be the "planner", as my mother would say, and I like to know what will happen tomorrow, next week, etc. This change to my life, our family's life, has called to question my tendencies and I am challenged everyday by that.

What I do know is that the life my family shared with Timbo will forever impact our lives going forward. Rather than be knocked down by the tragedy, I hope my family continues to be uplifted by the opportunities that have come our way since his passing. We are in a unique position to advocate for organ donation and represent donor families. We were blessed with the opportunity to go to the United States Transplant Games in 2008 in Pittsburgh, Pennsylvania. We met many, many amazing people. It was comforting to be with others who knew what we were battling and to experience such a unique event. We'll never forget that trip to Pittsburgh, especially since it ended in our meeting Robert. While this chance meeting is a story in itself, it has really helped my family heal and learn about this wonderful man. Robert has impacted our lives and is a part of our family now. I was blessed to have him apart of my wedding this past August. How awesome is that?!

On behalf of myself, my mother, Paula Martorelli and father, Timothy Packhem we thank you for the opportunity to share the life of an amazing young man. We also want to thank the National Kidney Foundation and New England Organ Bank for continually thinking about us and supporting us. Words do no justice to your kindness.

Jessica Waters, Sister to Donor: Timothy Packhem
Paula Martorelli, Mother of Timothy
Timothy Packhem, Father of Timothy
Timothy Packhem – "Forever 16"
Charlestown, Massachusetts
Timothy Passed Away: March 13, 2007
Timothy Packhem's Double Lung Recipient – Robert Juneau
Read Robert Juneau's Lung Transplant Story in this Edition of Taking Flight
Story Written by Mary Juneau, Robert's wife

My Brother –My Guardian Angel
By Stephanie J. White

Every day for thirty-two years, my brother, Edward W. Wlodarski, struggled to manage his cystic fibrosis and, as an adult, to remain independent and fulfill his financial obligations. At 32-years-old, he applied for and was accepted for a double lung transplant. However, his financial stresses grew with the expected transplant costs so together we began an aggressive fundraising campaign.

Growing up, Eddie and I were as typical as siblings come; we argued, wrestled, irritated each other and, had a stronger bond than either one of us would ever admit to.

Eddie could be angry, arrogant and mean spirited at times, but he was also strong, proud and gentle hearted as well. He most respected those who also did not treat or look at him differently - and being his sibling it was easy for me.

Eddie did not do anything in life that would be recognized by the casual observer as "memorable", "fantastic", or "historical", and he didn't go to college, or have a retirement plan, and he didn't save lives. BUT he was a great and amazing person. He would be the first person to help a friend in need, even if helping would make it difficult to breathe. No matter what the weather was like, he would always enjoy working on cars.

We were almost always together. As a young child he shoveled snow-filled driveways to earn his own money. I was never much help and often we were invited in for warm cookies and hot chocolate. But he always persevered. While he battled the cold, he'd send me inside to keep warm. My sole purpose of being with him was so I could be sure he was safe, although I would never tell him that. Eddie also took on a paper route...so I joined him. He was thinner than I was, less meat on his bones and with cystic fibrosis to boot; he was pulling me in the wagon as I cried because I was so cold! Yes, he was amazing.

In grade school I took on the responsibility of being a crossing guard -and he'd stand right there against the metal fence patiently waiting so we could walk home together. I also signed up for trumpet one year and then complained about how heavy it was and he'd carry it home (later I decided to switch to the flute!). Eddie always watched over me and one day I "had his back" so to speak. A neighborhood boy had said something mean about Eddie, so I defended him. Now picture this petite little girl wailing on a larger older boy - we all laugh about it now but his mother wasn't too happy and told my mother to "keep your daughter away from my son".

In October 1994, Eddie married his wife, LeAnn.

During all these life events Eddie struggled - financially and emotionally. He also was a hard worker and believed in taking care of himself and not asking for handouts. To get his life-saving oxygen, through state social services, he had to come up with a spend-down (co-pay) that he couldn't afford. His wife earned, what social services, considered "sufficient" income to live on (mind you, she worked in a fast-food restaurant – minimum wage - there was rent, food, bills, medical care, health care, hospital stays, general care, transportation, etc). This co-pay put an even further strain on his

[327]

finances and grudgingly he turned to family for help. It reached a point where it was just getting too difficult to keep coming up with these rising fees, even collectively as a family.

I remember looking everywhere I could for help. Not much came up on the Internet searches (at the time), the state program couldn't help because of his wife's "income" and I even went to national well-known organizations only to be turned away because the assistance we needed didn't exist, and they did not know where to direct us.

"What do I do?" I felt powerless. You know the old saying, "you can't fight city hall"? That's how I felt. It was so obvious of his needs and yet the state system that was put into place to help exactly these individuals was turning their backs on him. I told him LeAnn should leave her job and he should stop paying the co-pay. My rationale at the time was he needed this medical care and how could he be refused life saving oxygen just because he couldn't pay - and couldn't work to pay the costs? It was the worst solution I've ever had to come up with. Eddie's fight was my fight as well, and it just made me more furious that we even had to consider this as an "option" just so he could live from day to day.

Needless to say, we never reached that point. Eddie became ill and was hospitalized. To this day, I believe the stressors he endured in trying to figure out how to live day to day drove his last hospital stay. Sadly, just weeks before our annual family Thanksgiving in 1998, Eddie passed away peacefully - on his own terms. LeAnn, my parents, me, our whole family – all struggled greatly with Eddie's passing.

I have many happy memories of my brother and I will always remember him fondly. I will also remember the emptiness I felt the day he passed away. As much as I didn't want him to suffer anymore I also didn't want to lose him either.

In the months following Eddie's funeral I was just heartbroken and full of sadness - the best way I could describe it was that I felt alone. I struggled with picking up the pieces, carrying on and wondering how I could provide to others with CF the very assistance my brother so desperately needed - to give hope - to improve quality of life. Time passed, I thought a lot about Eddie, visited his gravesite often and then I met my husband, Robert. I told him all about Eddie, his struggles and the fundraising we did. His response was so clear and yet it had never entered my mind, he said, "You should start a charity that provides this assistance." In less than two years after Eddie's passing, and with the support of my loving husband, my resolution to help others like Eddie was memorialized in the establishment of the Lungs for Life Foundation.

I may not visit the cemetery as often as I used to and that is because I have come to know in my heart, my guardian angel is always there looking over me...

Stephanie J. White, Sister of, Edward W. Wlodarski
Rochester, New York
Edward W. Wlodarski, Cystic Fibrosis
Died Pre-Lung Transplant – 1998
"Forever 32"

Break on Through
By Eric Wright

Born in 1969 with Cystic Fibrosis (CF), at a time when very little was known about the disease, the prognosis was bleak. I grew up as a "normal" child, and aside from medication and treatments, was relatively healthy. As I grew, the balance needed to stay on track and keep up with the demands of the disease was a tricky thing to accomplish.

The stresses imposed on me as I matured forged an extremely mentally tough attitude and iron will. I read books about mental toughness and enlisted the help of a psychiatrist to help me cope. Even though your body is breaking down physically, your mind becomes stronger.

I had a demanding career as a Director of Human Resources. Five years ago, the disease won and I took a disability retirement and began to focus on what it would take to stay alive. I had a wife I love very much, along with my family and friends that I care for tremendously. I was not ready to leave them.

Despite my physical challenges, I was gifted athletically in the sport of racquetball. I rose through the ranks of racquetball skill level to champion status.

We choose University of Pittsburgh Medical Center (UPMC) in Pittsburgh, Pennsylvania for transplant evaluation and I was accepted August 2006. The waiting period for the call was very stressful. We reside in Rochester, New York. The trip was 4 ½ hours away. We enrolled with Angel Flight to fly me to the transplant center when the call came in.

On November 5, 2006, the call came in. We arrived in Pittsburgh, with several family members traveling from Syracuse, Rochester, Buffalo and North Carolina to support us. The brief moment before they came to get me, I slipped off my wedding ring and handed it to my wife, "I'm coming back for that" I said as we kissed each other. My family lined up on both sides of the hallway they high fived me and cheered as they wheeled me into surgery.

Right after surgery I had several problems. The care I received was exceptional. I came home to Rochester two days before Christmas. That year was the best Christmas ever. I had received a, "Gift of Life".

My recovery had several ups and downs. Finally I broke free and began working out and playing racquetball again. My life is now back to what I dreamed it could be. I credit my personal trainer for preparing me well to survive the difficulties I experienced immediately after surgery. I am convinced that if I was not in top physical shape things may have been dramatically different.

I am amazed how simple the act of breathing is taken for granted. Also, how important health is to everybody. I have become involved with the local Cystic Fibrosis chapter in Rochester. I will participate in the 2010 Transplant Olympics as well. I owe a great debt of gratitude and thanks to my donor family. For more information about my experience, I authored "Strive and Defy CF for Life" (coming soon).

Eric R. Wright, 41
Rochester, New York
Cystic Fibrosis
Double Lung Transplant, November 5, 2006
University of Pittsburgh Medical Center, Pittsburgh, Pennsylvania

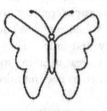

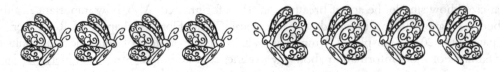

Life Has Wings
By Terra Yert

An anonymous writer on MySpace stated: "Life has wings...or rather life should have wings. When an interstitial lung disease damages the lungs from scarring because boils that grow on and around the air sacs, and no antibiotic or other medication can give the relief they once did, the quality of life is stalled. The length of your life is shortened, and when you are told, "You don't have long to live. You want those wings back to fly. Lung transplantation is the option to get those wings once again and live your life dreams."

For those who are fortunate enough to witness the actual lung transplantation surgery, they describe it as a moving experience that is emotional and awe inspiring. When the old lungs are removed appearing much like raw liver and the new lungs are taken from the cooler they have been transported in, the light, pink, white, new lungs, are in such contrast to the old. But the more breathtaking experience is to see the new lungs take life. When they are connected it is described as similar to, "Beautiful butterfly wings opening for the very first time." They expand and you can see the beauty in life, in "good lungs"... a comparison that has great meaning to those with an interstitial lung disease who received the gift of new lungs, and a chance to live their dreams.

On April 3rd 1999 I became a beautiful butterfly! I was nine-months-old when I was diagnosed with a rare, hereditary lung disease. My Father and aunt both had it. The name of the disease is Idiopathic Desquamative Interstitial Pneumonitis (DIP). This disease forms boils or big sores on the alveoli or air sacs. After the sores heal, it leaves scar tissue around and inside the alveoli, which prevents the lungs and body from getting the oxygen it needs.

I was on oxygen and medications all through my toddler years. My mom would hook me up to a 100-foot oxygen hose and I would crawl or walk around like it was no big thing. If the oxygen ever fell off or kinked up I would say "uh oh", and either try to put it back on myself or cry for my parents too put it back. At two-years-old I was finally able to get off the oxygen, and at five I was able to get off the medication. With the help of vitamins and the right care, I was able to start school and live a pretty normal life. There were times when I couldn't keep up with kids my age during recess or physical education, but I would just stop and rest and then go right back to what I was doing.

My disease seemed dormant most of my childhood, but when puberty set in I took a turn for the worse. It was the summer before I started 6th grade when I was hospitalized for the first time since infancy. Over the next two years I would be in and out of the hospital with several bouts of congestive heart failure. Congestive heart failure means that the heart is working inefficiently or pumping to weakly. When this happens, fluid builds up in the lungs, and among other organs creating a feeling of breathlessness.

Soon after, my pulmonologist started talking to my family and me about lung transplantation and maybe even a heart. When my parents heard this they were very shocked. Although I seemed to be doing okay to my parents, I really felt like I was slipping slowly into the dark and wondering what the outcome of this awful disease was. I was no longer able to attend school regularly and missing out on the social aspect of school, really upset me.

After a lot of praying and talking, my doctors, parents and I came to the conclusion that my only chance for survival was a double lung transplant. My Mother started looking up information on the Internet, reading books; anything she could do to find information on lung transplantation. After months of research, and getting opinions from other doctors, we decided to give St. Louis Children's Hospital at Washington University Medical Center in St. Louis, Missouri a call. St. Louis Children's Hospital had done the most lung transplants in pediatric patients. They had the best survival rates and not to mention the best doctors any patient could ask for! In 1998 my parents and I took a trip to St. Louis to see if I was a candidate for a double lung transplant. One of the tests, the heart catheterization, was to determine if I would need a heart as well. The results came back that I was a candidate for the double lung transplant, but I would not need the heart.

Within a year I started going downhill very fast. I was hospitalized three times in four months with more congestive heart failure and random infections. My illness was now so bad! I had to be on oxygen 24 hours a day (24/7). I was on 15 liters of oxygen by a nasal cannula and a non-rebreather mask. 15 liters is a whole lot of oxygen but that still wasn't enough. The transplant team also wanted me to relocate to St. Louis as well. I was very upset when we had to move. I wanted a lung transplant, but at the same time, I didn't want a transplant done. I was so scared but I wanted to be able to breathe, and walk around without getting tired. I had felt like I was suffocating all my life and have never know, what it feels like to breathe normally. The thought of getting to breathe made me so happy and I couldn't wait! My mom and I moved to St. Louis.

My Grandma, two cousins, aunt, dad, and sister had all come down to celebrate Easter with my mom and me. We all went to bed like a normal family, but on April 3rd 1999 my prayers had finally been answered. I finally got the call that would change my life forever! I was so scared and didn't know what to do. Finally I asked my mom to come pray with me, and she did. We sat on my bed held hands and prayed. I felt such a huge weight lifted off my shoulders. It was almost like God whispered in my ear and told me that everything was going to be okay.

We arrived at the hospital and as I waited for my surgery, nurses came in and drew blood, blood, and more blood. I don't remember how many tubes there were exactly. Before I went through the double doors, my family had to stop there and say their good-byes and I love you's. This was the hardest thing that I have ever had to do! Not knowing if I would ever wake up or get to see my family again was heartbreaking. I carried my stuffed bunny in my hand gripping tightly as I was wheeled in to the operating room. The last thing I remember was when a mask went over my face and doctors and nurses in funny outfits telling me that everything was going to be okay! I was now in "la la land" while my family waited anxiously for reports on how my progress was. Around an hour later my family saw a doctor rushing in carrying an ice chest with my last name on it. This was the gift that would finally give me a second chance to live! I was hooked up to a heart/lung machine that would circulate blood through my body while my lungs were being replaced.

As each lung was removed and switched my family was informed and anxiously awaiting the moment that they would get to see me again. I requested that my mom take pictures of my old lungs. I wanted to see the scars of this awful disease and know that I was now set free from something I thought could never happen. The lungs were brought out in a stainless steel bowl. They were about the size of small chicken breasts with little black spots confirming that they were diseased.

The doctors warned my family of the many tubes that would be in place when I was wheeled out, but never in a million years did they guess they would see their loved one in this kind of shape. They all realized though that it was all for the better and that soon I would be able to breathe with no hoses whatsoever. I was on a ventilator for about three days. The doctors were very surprised. I woke up not needing any oxygen and the feeling of being able to breathe is still unexplainable to this day. My immune system was very suppressed, because of anti-rejection medications. This caused me to catch Respiratory Syncytial Virus (RSV) and I was treated for the virus with a medication called Ribavirin and within a couple of weeks I was a healthy spontaneous 13-year-old girl.

As I mentioned at the beginning my Father and aunt both had this awful disease that I was born with. My aunt passed away in 1986 after the birth of her second child. The doctors didn't know exactly what the disease was when she had it so they never gave her a diagnosis. My Father was diagnosed with his disease 10 days after my transplant. That was a big shocker to all of us as he had been sick for a while but no one ever put two and two together. My Father was put on the list for a double lung transplant but unfortunately passed away less than a year from his diagnosis, on February 27th of 2000. My family made the decision to give the gift of life just as we had received. We were able to donate his eyes, and about six months after his death we received a letter that someone could now see because of our unselfish decision. When we received that letter I felt such a sense of relief. Knowing that we were able to give was the most gratifying experience. I know that's what my dad would have wanted. He was such an unselfish man!

I don't know a lot about my donor except that he was a 10-year-old boy that got hit by a car. I have written my donor family recently and hope to get a response in the near future.

I am now 25, and I have been able to see and do things my family and I never thought possible. I was able to graduate high school in 2004, and attended the Pharmacy Technician Certification Program in the fall of that year. I also learned how to drive a car, go on that 'first date', and many other things a child should get to experience. I am now able to sing, which is something I have loved to do since I was little but couldn't. I have sung the National Anthem at a Texas Rangers baseball game. I have been to Branson, Missouri and sung in a gospel contest, sung at Johnny High's where Leann Rimes got started and many, many countless other places. I have always loved speaking to people about transplant and organ donation. If I can reassure someone to donate or someone that needs a transplant, then I am 100% there.

As of July 22nd 2010 there are 108,117 people waiting for an organ transplant. 12,578 of those are in Texas alone. 17 people will die today because of the lack of donated organs. One person can save or enhance over 50 lives if they decide to be an organ donor.

Family discussion is a very important aspect with the organ donation process. Most organ donors die suddenly from a head injury or bleeding into the brain or a brain stem injury. It can be very difficult discussing organ donation when a loved one has suffered a brain death. Time is of the essence; organs must be transplanted quickly in order to save the lives of others. Discussing organ donation with family ahead of time can be beneficial to relieve one of the burdens, and knowing that something positive has come from a tragic event. In some states, there is now in place an Organ Donor Registry, that one can get their name onto, whereby the family cannot change the person's mind about organ donation. Some states the old system is still in place whereby the parents, spouse, or partner is the ultimate decision maker for donating loved ones organs. The decision will be much easier to make if family members know the wishes of their loved ones for whom they now have to speak for.

Terra Yert, 25
Denison, Texas
Idiopathic Desquamative Interstitial Pneumonitis
Double Lung Transplant, April 3, 1999
St. Louis Children's Hospital at Washington University Medical Center, St. Louis, Missouri

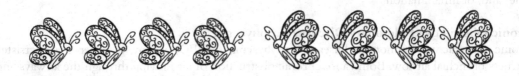

Appendix – Lung Illnesses

ABCA3 Transmitter Gene Mutation
ABCA3 Transmitter Gene Mutaiton is a member of the ATP-binding family of proteins that moderate the translocation of a wide variety of material or substance on which an enzyme acts, including lipids, across cellular membranes.

Alpha-1 Antitrypsin Deficiency
Alpha-1 Antitrypsin Deficiency (Alpha-1) is an inherited disorder that can cause lung disease and liver disease in adults and children. Alpha-1 antitrypsin (AAT) is a protein that protects the lungs. The liver usually makes the protein, and releases it into the bloodstream. Not having enough AAT puts you at risk of emphysema. If you smoke, you increase your risk.

Bronchiectasis
Bronchiectasis is a permanent dilatation (widening) of the bronchi (the large airways which begin at the bottom of the trachea and branch into the lungs).

Bronchiolitis Obliterans
Bronchiolitis Obliterans is a rare and life-threatening form of non-reversible obstructive lung disease in which the bronchioles (small airway branches) are compressed and narrowed by fibrosis (scar tissue) and/or inflammation.

Chronic Obstructive Pulmonary Disease/Emphysema
Chronic Obstructive Pulmonary Disease/Emphysema (COPD) is any disorder that persistently obstructs bronchial airflow. Both cause chronic obstruction of air flowing through the airways and in and out of the lungs. The obstruction is generally permanent and progresses over time. Emphysema is a lung condition featuring an abnormal accumulation of air in the lung's many tiny air sacs, a tissue called alveoli. As air continues to collect in these sacs, they become enlarged, and may break, or become damaged and form scar tissue. Emphysema is strongly associated with smoking cigarettes, a practice that causes lung irritation. It can also be associated with or worsened by repeated infection of the lungs, such as is seen in chronic bronchitis.

Cystic Fibrosis
Cystic Fibrosis (CF) is a genetic disease prevalent especially in Caucasian populations. It produces large quantities of thick mucous that clog the lungs and digestive ducts in the pancreas. The end result is progressive chronic obstructive lungs illness, and provides a breeding ground for bacteria. The pancreatic ducts are also clogged with mucous so most people with CF lack the enzymes necessary to digest fats, proteins and carbohydrates.

Eisenmenger's Syndrome

Eisenmenger's Syndrome is the combination of a congenital defect in the septum between the ventricles of the heart with early complications that include left to right blood flow through the defect, increased blood pressure in the pulmonary arteries, and hypertrophy of the right ventricle.

Familial Pulmonary Fibrosis

Familial Pulmonary Fibrosis is when multiple members of a family have a diagnosis of pulmonary fibrosis including idiopathic pulmonary fibrosis (IPF).

Idiopathic Desquamative Interstitial Pneumonitis

Idiopathic Desquamative Interstitial Pneumonitis is a lung disease includes disorders characterized by scarring and/or inflammation of the lungs.

Idiopathic Pulmonary Arterial Hypertension

Idiopathic Pulmonary Arterial Hypertension is a disorder primarily of small pulmonary arteries, which results in a progressive rise in pulmonary vascular resistance and right ventricular failure.

Idiopathic Pulmonary Fibrosis

Idiopathic Pulmonary Fibrosis (IPF) is a progressive form of lung disease characterized by scarring, or fibrosis of the lungs. Over time the fibrosis can build up to the point where the lungs are unable to provide oxygen to the tissues of the body. The term "idiopathic" is only used when the cause of pulmonary fibrosis is unknown.

Idiopathic Pulmonary Hemosiderosis

Idiopathic Pulmonary Hemosiderosis is a rare, generally fatal disease of unknown cause, typically affecting small children; characterized by infiltration of pulmonary alveoli with hemosiderin (iron-storage complex) containing macrophages progressing to diffuse pulmonary fibrosis.

Lymphangioleiomyomatosis

Lymphangioleiomyomatosis (LAM) is a very rare, progressive disorder of the lungs and lymphatic system. It affects women almost exclusively. Is generally diagnosed in women of childbearing age. LAM is characterized by an unusual type of smooth muscle cell, LAM cells, which proliferate uncontrollably. LAM cells invade the tissues of the lungs, including the airways, and blood and lymph vessels. The accumulation of LAM cells form cell clusters and cysts, which destroy healthy tissue. Over time, the LAM cells create holes in the lungs, preventing the lungs from providing oxygen to the rest of the body and progressively impairing lung function.

Primary Pulmonary Hypertension

Primary Pulmonary Hypertension (PPH) is a rare disease characterized by elevated pulmonary artery pressure with no apparent cause. The term idiopathic pulmonary arterial hypertension is now preferred.

Primary Ciliary Dyskinesia
Primary Ciliary Dyskinesia is a condition in which poorly functioning cilia (hair like projections from cells) in the respiratory tract contribute to retention of secretions and recurrent infection. The condition is inherited as an autosomal recessive trait and is due to mutation in one of several different genes located on chromosomes 5, 9 and 19. About half of patients have Kartagener's syndrome (bronchiectasis, sinusitis, and situs inversus in which the normal asymmetry of the body is partially or totally reversed).

Pulmonary Fibrosis
Pulmonary Fibrosis (PF) is characterized by progressive scarring – known as fibrosis – and deterioration of the lungs and the ability to breathe slowly declines. Sometimes PF can be linked to a particular cause, such as certain environmental exposures, chemotherapy or radiation therapy, residual infection, or autoimmune diseases such as scleroderma or rheumatoid arthritis. When no known cause can be determined, it is called idiopathic pulmonary fibrosis.

Pulmonary Hypertension
Pulmonary Hypertension (PH) is abnormally high blood pressure in the arteries of the lungs. It makes the right side of the heart need to work harder than normal.

Pulmo Veno – Occlusive Disease
Pulmo Veno – Occlusive Disease (PVOD) is an extremely rare form of high blood pressure in the lung area. In most cases, the cause of pulmonary veno-occlusive disease is unknown. The condition may be related to a viral infection or may occur as a complication of diseases like lupus, or a complication of leukemia, lymphoma, chemotherapy, or bone marrow transplantation. The disorder is most common among children and young adults.

Sarcoidosis
Sarcoidosis is a disease in which swelling (inflammation) occurs in the lymph nodes, lungs, liver, eyes, skin, or other tissues. The cause of the disease is unknown. Clumps of abnormal tissue (granulomas) form in certain organs of the body. Granulomas are clusters of immune cells. The disease can affect almost any organ of the body, but it most commonly affects the lungs.

Scleroderma
Scleroderma is a widespread connective tissue disease that involves changes in the skin, blood vessels, muscles, and internal organs. The cause of scleroderma is unknown. A buildup of a substance called collagen in the skin and other organs occurs in people. The disease usually affects people 30 to 50 years old. Women get scleroderma more often than men do. Risk factors include work exposure to silica dust and polyvinyl chloride.

References

1. Bharat A, Kuo E, Steward N, Aloush A, Hachem R, Trulock EP, et al. Immunological link between primary graft dysfunction (PGD) and bronchiolitis obliterans syndrome (BOS) Ann Thorac Surg 2008;86(1):189-95.

2. Avlonitis VS, Fisher AJ, Kirby JA, Dark JH. Pulmonary transplantation: the role of brain death in donor lung injury. Transplantation 2003;75(12):1928-33

3. Cypel M, Yeung J, de Perrot M, Karolak W, Chen F, Sato M, et al. Ex vivo lung perfusion in clinical lung transplantation - the "HELP" trial (Abstract). J Heart Lung Transplant 2010; 29 (2S):S88.

4. Cypel M, Liu M, Yeung J, Hirayama S, Anraku M, Sato M, et al. Functional repair of human donor lungs by IL-10 gene therapy. Sci Transl Med 2009;1(4):4ra9

5. Cypel M, Yeung JC, Hirayama S, Rubacha M, Fischer S, Anraku M, et al. Technique for prolonged normothermic ex vivo lung perfusion. J Heart Lung Transplant 2008; 27(12):1319-25.

6. Dong BM, Abano JB, Egan TM. Nitric oxide ventilation of rat lungs from non-heart-beating donors improves post-transplant function. Am J Transplant 2009; 9(12):2707-15.

7. Dong B, Egan T. Post-mortem and ex-vivo carbon monoxide (CO) ventilation reduces ischemia-reperfusion injury (IRI) in rat lungs transplanted from non-heart-beating donors (NHBDs) (Abstract). J Heart Lung Transplant 2010; 29 (2S):S95.

8. Egan TM, Haithcock JA, Nicotra WA, Koukoulis G, Inokawa H, Sevala M, et al. Ex-vivo evaluation of human lungs for transplant suitability. Ann Thorac Surg 2006; 81(4):1205-13.

9. Egan TM, Lambert Jr CJ, Reddick RL, Ulicny Jr KS, Keagy BA, Wilcox BR. A strategy to increase the donor pool: the use of cadaver lungs for transplantation. Ann Thorac Surg 1991;52:1113-1121

10. Egan T, Murray S, Bustami R, Shearon T, McCullough K, Edwards L, et al. Development of the new lung allocation system in the United States (The 2005 SRTR Report on the State of Transplantation). Am J Transplant 2006;6 (5 Pt 2):1212-27

11. Ingemansson R, Eyjolfsson A, Mared L, Pierre L, Algotsson L, Ekmehag B, et al. Clinical transplantation of initially rejected donor lungs after reconditioning ex vivo. Ann Thorac Surg 2009; 87(1):255-60.

12. Kim IK, Bedi DS, Denecke C, Ge X, Tullius SG. Impact of innate and adaptive immunity on rejection and tolerance. Transplantation 2008; 86(7):889-94.

13. Land WG. The role of postischemic reperfusion injury and other nonantigen-dependent inflammatory pathways in transplantation. Transplantation 2005; 79(5):505-14.

14. Land W, Schneeberger H, Schleibner S, Illner WD, Abendroth D, Rutili G, et al. The beneficial effect of human recombinant superoxide dismutase on acute and chronic rejection events in recipients of cadaveric renal transplants. Transplantation 1994; 57(2):211-7.

15. Matzinger P. Tolerance, danger, and the extended family. Annu Rev Immunol 1994; 12:991-1045.

16. Roberts CS, D'Armini AM, Egan TM. Canine double-lung transplantation with cadaver donors. J Thorac Cardiovasc Surg 1996; 112:577-583.

17. Steen S, Ingemansson R, Eriksson L, Pierre L, Algotsson L, Wierup P, et al. First human transplantation of a nonacceptable donor lung after reconditioning ex vivo. Ann Thorac Surg 2007; 83(6):2191-2195.

18. Steen S, Sjoberg T, Pierre L, Liao Q, Eriksson L, Algotsson L. Transplantation of lungs from a non-heart beating donor. Lancet 2001;357(9259):825-829

19. Ulicny Jr KS, Egan TM, Lambert Jr CJ, Reddick RL, Wilcox BR. Cadaver lung donors: effect of preharvest ventilation on graft function. Ann Thorac Surg 1993;55:1185-1191

20. Zanotti G, Casiraghi M, Abano JB, Tatreau JR, Sevala M, Berlin H, et al. Novel critical role of toll-like receptor 4 in lung ischemia-reperfusion injury and edema. Am J Physiol - Lung Cell Mol Physiol 2009; 297(1):L52-63.